ANTHROPOMETRIC ASSESSMENT OF NUTRITIONAL STATUS

Anthropometric Assessment of Nutritional Status

EDITOR
JOHN H. HIMES
Division of Human Development
and Nutrition
School of Public Health
University of Minnesota
Minneapolis, Minnesota

WILEY-LISS
A JOHN WILEY & SONS, INC., PUBLICATION
New York • Chichester • Brisbane • Toronto • Singapore

Address all Inquiries to the Publisher
Wiley-Liss, Inc., 41 East 11th Street, New York, NY 10003

Printed in United States of America

While the authors, editors, and publisher believe that drug selection and dosage and the specifications and usage of equipment and devices, as set forth in this book, are in accord with current recommendations and practice at the time of publication, they accept no legal responsibility for any errors or omissions, and make no warranty, express or implied, with respect to material contained herein. In view of ongoing research, equipment modifications, changes in governmental regulations and the constant flow of information relating to drug therapy, drug reactions and the use of equipment and devices, the reader is urged to review and evaluate the information provided in the package insert or instructions for each drug, piece of equipment or device for, among other things, any changes in the instructions or indications of dosage or usage and for added warnings and precautions.

Recognizing the importance of preserving what has been written, it is a policy of John Wiley & Sons, Inc. to have books of enduring value published in the United States printed on acid-free paper, and we exert our best efforts to that end.

Library of Congress Cataloging-in-Publication Data

Anthropometric assessment of nutritional status / editor, John H. Himes.
p. cm.
Includes bibliographical references.
Includes index.
ISBN 0-471-56876-7
1. Nutrition—Evaluation. 2. Anthropometry. I. Himes, J. H. (John H.)
[DNLM: 1. Anthropometry. 2. Nutritional Status. QU 145 A628].
QP143.5.A58A54 1991
613.2—dc20
DNLM/DLC
for Library of Congress 90-12813
CIP

Contents

Contributors

Linda S. Adair *[233]*
Carolina Population Center,
University of North Carolina,
Chapel Hill, NC 27514-3997

Stephen M. Bailey *[51]*
Department of Anthropology,
Tufts University, Medford, MA 02155

Eilene Z. Bisgrove *[233]*
Carolina Population Center,
University of North Carolina,
Chapel Hill, NC 27514-3997

Bruce R. Bistrian *[365]*
New England Deaconess Hospital,
Boston, MA 02215

Claude Bouchard *[213]*
Physical Activity Sciences
Laboratory, Laval University,
Ste-Foy, Quebec G1K 7P4,
Canada

George A. Bray *[383]*
Department of Medicine,
University of Southern California,
Los Angeles, CA 90033

Laura E. Caulfield *[259]*
Division of Human Development and
Nutrition, School of Public Health,
University of Minnesota,
Minneapolis, MN 55455

Noel Cameron *[347]*
Department of Anatomy,
University of the Witwatersrand
Medical School, Johannesburg 2193,
South Africa

Wm. Cameron Chumlea *[399]*
Department of Pediatrics,
Division of Human Biology,
Wright State University School of
Medicine, Dayton, OH 45435

T. J. Cole *[83]*
MRC Dunn Nutrition Unit,
Cambridge CB4 1XJ, England

Johanna T. Dwyer *[5]*
Frances Stern Nutrition Center,
New England Medical Center,
Boston, MA 02111

Stanley M. Garn *[123]*
Center for Human Growth and
Development, University of Michigan,
Ann Arbor, MI 48109-0406

Michael Gracey *[39]*
Health Department of Western
Australia, East Perth 6004, Australia

David S. Gray *[383]*
Department of Medicine, University of
Southern California School of
Medicine, Los Angeles, CA 90033

The number in brackets is the opening page number of the contributor's chapter.

John H. Himes *[1,141]*
Division of Human Development and Nutrition, School of Public Health, University of Minnesota, Minneapolis, MN 55455

Clifford Johnson *[319]*
National Center for Health Statistics, Hyattsville, MD 20782

Francis E. Johnston *[337]*
Department of Anthropology, University of Pennsylvania, Philadelphia, PA 19104-6398

W. Keller *[113]*
Route de Transchepied, 1261 La Rippe, Switzerland

Robert J. Kuczmarski *[319]*
Division of Health Examination Statistics, National Center for Health Statistics, Hyattsville, MD 20782

Michael C. Latham *[287]*
Division of Nutritional Sciences, Cornell University, Ithaca, NY 14853

T. G. Lohman *[173]*
Department of Exercise and Sport Sciences, University of Arizona, Tucson, AZ 85721

Robert M. Malina *[151]*
Department of Kinesiology and Health Education, University of Texas at Austin, Austin, TX 78712

Alan D. Martin *[185]*
Sport and Exercise Sciences Research Institute, University of Manitoba, Winnipeg, Manitoba R3T 2N2, Canada

Donald S. McLaren *[273]*
Department of Preventive Ophthalmology, Institute of Ophthalmology, London EC1V 9EJ, United Kingdom

Molly McMahon *[365]*
Division of Endocrinology, Metabolism and Internal Medicine, Mayo Medical School, Rochester, MN 55905

N. G. Norgan *[197]*
Department of Human Sciences, University of Technology, Loughborough, Leicester LE11 3TU, United Kingdom

Zhen Ouyang *[337]*
School of Public Health, Harbin Medical University, Harbin, People's Republic of China

Roberto J. Rona *[301]*
Department of Community Medicine, The United Medical and Dental Schools of Guy's and St. Thomas's Hospitals, St. Thomas's Campus, London SE1 7EH, England

Preface

Anthropometric assessment of nutritional status is often relegated to a single chapter or to an appendix in general nutrition textbooks and books on nutritional assessment. The principle aim of the present effort was to bring together in one volume contributions from a wide range of expertise and experience to consider state-of-the-art theoretical and practical issues regarding the applications and meanings of nutritional anthropometry. The contributions are aimed largely at professionals who plan and interpret research and practice protocols, including anthropometric assessment of nutritional status. Also, there is much of value for students in nutrition, anthropology, medicine, and public health.

Darleen Kenyon assisted with the editorial aspects of the volume and Catherine Carson provided the index. Preparation of the volume was supported in part by grant HD-24684 from the National Institutes of Health, Bethesda, Maryland.

John H. Himes

Anthropometric Assessment
of Nutritional Status, pages 1–3

1
Introduction

JOHN H. HIMES
Division of Human Development and Nutrition, School of Public Health, University of Minnesota, Minneapolis, Minnesota 55455

Assessment of nutritional status usually includes at least the most basic descriptions of body size. Whether self-monitored between one's toes on bathroom scales, or repeated aloud in laboratory protocols, measurements of body mass ubiquitously carry connotations of nutritional adequacy and surfeit. The nutritional connotations, of course, are not universal, and the exact meaning of a measure as simple as body weight generates as much discussion among professionals as among those at the spa.

The basic rationale for including anthropometry in the assessment of nutritional status is that antropometric dimensions provide morphological manifestations of nutrition. In children, these manifestations are primarily somatic growth; in adults, they comprise primarily maintenance of status. Of course, nutritionally mediated changes in adult morphology may be considerable. Nevertheless, the nutritional requirements for fuel and substrate associated with normal somatic growth and functioning provide a fundamental distinction between children and adults in the rationales for anthropometric assessment of nutritional status. In turn, there are related implications for methodologies, analyses, and interpretations of the anthropometric data.

It is clear that in severely malnourished children growth is retarded, and that extraordinary catch-up may follow nutritional rehabilitation. In less severe cases, qualitatively similar growth responses certainly occur, but there is less than complete agreement on their quantitative nature or value (Beaton and Ghassemi, 1982). Further, it is not clear what the exact mechanisms for these growth responses are (Golden, 1988). In terms of energy, growth is of relatively low priority compared with requirements for basal maintenance and even activity. Consequently, growth is sensitive to relative nutritional deficit and replenishment.

Because linear growth is completed in adults, morphological manifestations of changing nutrition are primarily composed of alterations in soft tissues. While attention often focuses on adipose tissue, there may be appreciable changes nutritionally mediated in the lean compartment as well (Forbes,

1987). Activity, disease, senescence, and health-related behaviors may complicate direct nutritional attribution of many adult morphological and compositional changes.

Anthropometry is said to be important for nutritional assessment because it has high validity, especially at the extremes of nutrition. With adequate training, anthropometric dimensions can be measured with high reliability, and there are standardized protocols and reference data available. Because it is noninvasive, anthropometry is acceptable to subjects. Most anthropometric equipment is relatively inexpensive and transportable for field efforts and surveys.

While these common summary statements concerning anthropmetry are true, they are superficial and incomplete. There are many issues concerning approaches to, and analyses and interpretations of, anthropometry in the assessment of nutritional status that are more difficult to discern, and upon which there may be considerable discussion. It is upon these latter issues that the contributions of the current volume focus.

The intent of this collection was not to provide a "how-to" book on nutritional anthropometry. Recent volumes provide excellent standard techniques for measuring (Cameron, 1984; Lohman et al., 1988). In this vein, the aim was to provide a "so-what?" and a "how-come?" book, with thoughtful discussions from those experienced in the methods and the issues.

Section II includes chapters addressing theoretical and background issues basic to the measurement of nutritional status and this application of anthropometry. Contributions in Section III consider commonly used anthropometric dimensions and their applications and interpretations, while those in Section IV consider the assessment of specific body components anthropometrically. Finally, Section V is composed of discussions of specific applications of anthropometric assessment of nutritional status, and issues arising in the analysis and interpretation of nutritional anthropometry.

The present volume is a comprehensive treatment of the anthropometric assessment of nutritional status, but it is not exhaustive. Some of the gaps in coverage are due to difficulty in obtaining contributions from authors in a timely fashion, while others simply reflect the emphases and preferences of authors, or editorial constraints. For example, the absence of a chapter on arm circumference is not meant to diminish its importance as a useful measure of nutritional status and relative limb composition (Velzeboer et al., 1983).

It is hoped that this volume will stimulate additional thought and discussion concerning the anthropometric assessment of nutritional status, and that others may in the future enlarge upon and refine our current thinking regarding this important topic.

ACKNOWLEDGMENTS

Preparation was supported in part by grant HD-24684 from the National Institutes of Health, Bethesda, Maryland.

REFERENCES

Beaton GH, Ghassemi H (1982): Supplementary feeding programs for young children in developing countries. Am J Clin Nutr 35:864–916.

Cameron N (1984): "The Measurement of Human Growth." London: Croom Helm.

Forbes GB (1987): "Human Body Composition: Growth, Aging, Nutrition, and Activity." New York: Springer-Verlag.

Golden MHN (1988): The role of individual nutrient deficiencies in growth retardation of children as exemplified by zinc and protein. In Waterlow JC (ed): "Linear Growth Retardation in Less Developed Countries." New York: Raven Press, pp 143–163.

Lohman TG, Roche AF, Martorell R (eds.) (1988): "Anthropometric Standardization Reference Manual." Champaign, Ill: Human Kinetics.

Velzeboer MI, Selwin BJ, Sargent F, Pollitt E, Delgado H (1983): Evaluation of arm circumference as a public health index of protein-energy malnutrition in early childhood J Trop Pediatr 29:135–144.

Anthropometric Assessment
of Nutritional Status, pages 5–28

2
Concept of Nutritional Status and Its Measurement

JOHANNA T. DWYER

Schools of Medicine and Nutrition, and USDA Human Nutrition Research Center on Aging, Tufts University; Frances Stern Nutrition Center, New England Medical Center, Boston, Massachusetts 02111

INTRODUCTION

Scope

This chapter defines nutritional status and describes its importance. The usual sequence of events involved in changes in nutritional status is described. The components of nutritional status and their measurement are reviewed, including dietary intake, anthropometry, history, physical and biochemical measures, and other issues. Several issues of practical importance, including the differences between dietary status and nutritional status, and the associations between anthopometric measures and other indices and nutritional status, are discussed.

Definition

Nutritional status is the condition of the body resulting from the intake, absorption, and utilization of food as well as from factors of pathological significance.

Nutritional status assessment usually includes anthropometric, dietary, and biochemical measurements, clinical history, and physical and other data (WHO, 1973).

Rationale for Multiple Indicators of Nutritional Status

The need for so many different types of indices arises from five realities related to the heterogeneity of malnutrition itself and to methodological limitations in measuring malnutrition.

First, many forms of malnutrition exist. At one extreme are problems associated with inadequate quantity or quality of intake, such as starvation, which in its severest form is known as marasmus; protein-calorie malnutrition, or kwashiorkor; and specific deficiencies of vitamins or minerals which are known clinically by a variety of names. At the other extreme are those caused by excesses in energy giving rise to obesity; imbalances or excesses of energy-yielding nutrients, vitamins, minerals, or other dietary constituents, which may lead to metabolic aberrations and increase risk of ill health; and toxicities due to excesses of alcohol or other substances in food which have adverse pharmacological effects.

Second, there is no single indicator for all forms of malnutrition, nor are specific types of indicators best in all circumstances. The best indicator of the presence of each specific form of malnutrition varies, in some cases consisting of a biochemical measurement, in others some different measure, depending upon the validity, reliability, and specificity of the indicator in question. Very few indicators are definitive and unambiguous in themselves. For example, a low hemoglobin and hematocrit may signal iron-deficiency anemia, blood loss, or the presence of chronic infection (Dallman, 1986). Several indicators are usually necessary to make a definitive diagnosis.

Third, the severity of the malnutrition may vary. Malnutrition in its most extreme form may be evident clinically with drastic effects on body size, appearance, and physiological function. Earlier, less severe forms of malnutrition may signal their presence only by decreased tissue stores or dietary intakes, which indicate increased risk of subsequent malnutrition. Since many forms of malnutrition are preventable, it is desirable to detect them as early as possible, before they have disrupted function. The several components of nutritional status assessment, each of which taps information about nutriture at different levels of pathology, often permit early diagnosis before malnutrition reaches the clinically apparent level.

Fourth, the causes of malnutrition vary. Primary malnutrition, due to insufficient quality or quantity of diet alone, is sometimes present. However, much malnutrition is secondary to disease, or social or psychological problems, and occurs even in the face of adequate and appropriate food in the environment (Cassell, 1976; Solomon, 1988). In most situations the nature and causes of the ill health are not easily assessed because none of the indicators of malnutrition are specific enough or precise enough to be indicative of a specific disease. Thus a process of differential diagnosis is involved which combines many different types of information to confirm or refute hypotheses about cause (Wadsworth, 1984).

Fifth, individual variability in human nutrient needs, genetic endowment, responses to disease, and diet-related behaviors is considerable. We never know an individual's precise nutrient needs. By using methods which provide measures of different states of nutrition and health status, it is possible to increase the certainty with which statements about the presence or absence of malnutrition in specific individuals or populations can be made.

Target of Interest

Table 1 provides some general guidelines to consider in planning nutritional status assessment. The target of the nutritional status assessment may be a single individual or a community. The objective may be to assess nutritional status in general or to detect the presence or absence of some specific

TABLE 1. General Guidelines for Assessment of Nutritional Status

Define the Problem
- Why is the assessment being done?
  - Describe purposes for which data will be used
  - Determine the precision necessary
  - Make sure the validity and reliability of assessment tools are adequate for the purpose

Design the Assessment
- Who is to be assessed?
  - Identify the target population as definitively as possible
  - Make sure sample represents target population or behaviors closely
  - Use probability samples if possible
  - Base sample size or number of observations on precision needed
- What is to be assessed?
  - Characterize the attribute or event as completely as possible
  - Build in method for independently corroborating results, especially if biases are present

Analyze Results and Draw Conclusions
- Make sure food or nutrient data bases are adequate for objective
- Make adjustments and corrections to account for inherent biases
- Use appropriate statistical techniques
- Interpret the biological as well as the statistical significance of results
- Compare data to appropriate reference standards

deficiency or diet-related risk factor for disease in a specific area or segment of the population. The specific tools for assessing nutritional status vary accordingly. Practical considerations, such as availability, cost, willingness of subjects or patients to submit to procedures, and time involved to do the assessment and to obtain the results of the test, are also relevant considerations in choosing assessment methods. It is usually recommended that three components of nutritional status assessment are mandatory to obtain reasonable estimates of nutritional status, and more are often required (Alfin-Slater and Mirenda, 1980).

Importance

Nutritional status assessment is important because it provides the nutritional diagnosis upon which rational interventions can be based.

Public health and community applications. On a community level, measurement of the extent of nutrition problems through the measurement of nutritional status is necessary for several reasons (Jelliffe and Gurney, 1973). These include, first, establishment of a baseline level against which planned interventions, unplanned changes, or secular trends can be assessed. Second, it helps in suggesting how best to use limited resources. Third, nutritional status monitoring can provide an early warning of potential nutritional problems. Finally, documentation of the problem often helps in stimulating political will to deal with it (Jelliffe and Gurney, 1973).

It has long been recognized that it is important to monitor and assess the nutritional status of the community, and that food consumption alone is insufficiently precise in providing a detailed picture of the nutritional status of the population. Ecological and indirect surveys of nutrition were first used, but more direct assessment of nutritional status in human communities is now the goal. Instead of surveys of food consumption, full-fledged nutritonal status surveys of communities, which include anthropometry, clinical signs, and biochemical and tissue tests, have become more common over the past half century (Jelliffe, 1966).

Periodic nutritional surveys of a population-based sample of Americans are conducted today in this country by the U.S. Department of Health and Human Services in its Health and Nutrition Examination Survey. These data bases permit the assessment of the nutritional status of the population and of risk factors associated with many chronic degenerative diseases (Yetley and Johnson, 1987). In addition to general reports, specific in-depth studies have been issued on a number of nutrients, including vitamin A (Pilch and Senti, 1984), iron (Pilch and Senti, 1984b), zinc (Pilch and Senti, 1984a), and folic acid (Senti and Pilch, 1984), among others. Diet-related risk factors which have been investigated include associations between diet and dental health (Burt et al., 1982), diet and other characteristics and blood lead levels (Annest, 1983; Mahaffey and Annest, 1986), diet and blood pressure (Gruchow et al., 1985; Harlan et al., 1984; Harlan et al., 1983), and diet and coronary artery disease (Harlan et al., 1983), among others (Sempos et al., 1986; Roberts et al., 1978). Other surveys of high-risk groups are also carried out by the federal government and other groups from time to time. (U.S. Department of Health and Human Services and U.S. Department of Agriculture, 1986). Methodologies continue to improve, with new facets of the epidemiology and faces of malnutrition in the population being explored.

Clinical applications. The assessment of the nutritional status of the individual is important if nutritional care planning is to be done on a rational basis. Emphasis has also long been directed toward especially vulnerable individuals within the population, who, by virtue of their health status, high nutrient needs, or extreme environmental or personal constraints, are deemed to be especially at risk for malnutrition.

Until the 1970s acutely ill, long-term medical, and surgical patients often received only the most cursory of nutritional assessments, often not even including monitoring of weight during hospitalization. If feeding by mouth or nasogastric tube was impossible, malnutrition was all but inevitable.

During the late 1970s and early 1980s new enteral and parenteral means of supporting acutely ill patients were developed. These new techniques, cost considerations, and the advent of expensive medical and surgical procedures to keep patients alive who even a decade ago would have died led to a rebirth of interest in nutritional status assessment for vulnerable groups consisting of the very ill. The costs of care for such individuals are so high that any means for determining which patients are most likely to benefit from interventions in terms of improved prognosis is worth consideration, and it was thought that rigorous nutritional status assessment would permit this. New biochemical indices of protein nutriture and immune function were thought to be especially promising (Myrvik, 1988; Heymsfield and Williams, 1988). The formal nutritional status assessments recommended for possible candidates for special enteral or parenteral feedings included indirect calorimetry to establish energy needs (Jequier et al., 1987); delayed hypersensitivity skin testing; biochemical tests including total lymphocyte counts, hemoglobins, hematocrits, serum albumin, transferrin, prealbumin, retinol-binding protein, nitrogen balances, and creatinine; and other biochemical measures which were thought to be useful for assessing bodily visceral and somatic protein compartments. In addition, an elaborate battery of anthropometric, clinical, and dietary measurements were also suggested (Buzby and Mullen, 1988).

Prognostic indices based on these nutritional status assessments were developed by several groups which were linked with later morbidity and survival (Mullen et al., 1979a; Mullen et al., 1979b; Seltzer et al., 1980; Buzby et al., 1980; Kaminski et al., 1977; Harvey et al., 1978; Simms et al., 1982; Hobbiss et al., 1984). It was initially thought that the correction of abnormal biochemical and other measurements could be brought about by nutritional means. However, enthusiasm was dampened when it soon became clear that many of these indices were often altered by the disease process itself rather than by malnutrition alone, and that abnormal values did not necessarily signal malnutrition (Ward et al., 1982; Hobbiss et al., 1984). A period of disillusionment set in when it was recognized that in acutely and chronically ill patients many of these measurements were invalid. Also, nutritional interventions did not result in the normalization of values or dramatic improvements in prognosis which had initially been hoped for. Finally, many of the biochemical measurements included in the indices were expensive and unavailable in many hospitals.

By the early 1980s the validity, utility, and cost of the elaborate nutritional status assessment batteries began to be questioned by many clinicians and a period of reassessment ensued (Greig et al., 1982). The metabolic basis for anorexia and cachexia was reemphasized (Lawson et al., 1982). While the need for nutritional support for many patients was evident, it was no longer regarded as a panacea, and therefore the elaborate assessment of nutritional status was no longer viewed as essential. The cost-effectiveness of routine nutritional support, especially for extremely ill patients, was increasingly questioned (Twomey and Patching, 1985; Roberts et al., 1982; Detsky et al., in press). Reimbursement for nutritional assessment and other nutritional support services became increasingly tenuous as cost containment measures were applied more rigorously with the advent of diagnostic related groups (Howard et al., 1986; Lifshitz, 1987). Concerns about the validity of nutritional assessment indices in severely ill patients, lack of demonstrable differences between full nutritional status assessment batteries as opposed to more global clinical assessments, uncertainty about the utility of formal assessments in improving outcomes, and growing concerns about the costs of care all led to an emphasis on more abbreviated forms of clinical and functional nutritional status assessment.

In recent years the focus has turned from prediction of favorable prognoses and the benefits of intervention to prediction of mortality. For extremely ill patients admitted to intensive care units, the APACHE II scoring system may predict patients who are likely to die even if total parenteral nutrition is provided. APACHE II scores are used to classify the severity of disorders of patients admitted to intensive care units. The score is a weighted index, depending upon 12 physiological variables, age of patient, presence of defined chronic disease, and need for emergency surgery (Knaus et al., 1985). In one recent study it predicted accurately which patients died despite the provision of total parenteral nutrition (Chang et al., 1986). This raises ethical as well as practical concerns (Zerfas, 1985).

The present view of the utility of prognostic indices is more skeptical than it was a decade ago. While it is probable that clinicians' performance can be enhanced by the use of a probabilistic approach based on hard data, "probability is only one factor to be taken into account in making a clinical decision. Statistics should be used as a drunken man uses the lamppost—for support rather than for illumination" (Editorial, Lancet, 1986). Such an emphasis is apparent in the current approach to nutritional assessment in hospitalized patients, which emphasizes functional or global clinical assessments (Shils, 1988).

USUAL SEQUENCE OF EVENTS IN DEVELOPMENT OF MALNUTRITION

Background

Because there is no single determinant of nutritional status, many characteristics which tap different levels of effects must be assessed. Nutrient requirements and nutritional status are influenced by diet, characteristics of the host, and environmental factors (Solomon, 1988). The component measurements from which nutritional status is inferred depend on each of these. Diet is measured directly or by report. Anthropometric measurements, history and physical examination for clinical signs or symptoms, biochemical measurements, and the like help the observer to assess the host's characteristics. Careful questioning can also reveal many environmental factors which influence dietary intakes and hence nutritional status. Such environmental factors include climatic conditions (ambient temperature, humidity, altitude); the living environment; the biozootic environment (including microbiological pathogens, parasites, and protozoa); and socioeconomic conditions (Solomon, 1988).

Development of Malnutrition

The basic model for the development of an alteration in nutritional status is well established. The pathophysiology of malnutrition is a process which consists of several phases, and the components of nutritional status assessment measure various points on the continuum between health and ill health with respect to malnutrition (Widdowson, 1988).

Changes in function, clinical signs of malnutrition, and changes in anthropometric measurements represent the end of a pathological process which earlier affects organ systems, tissues, and individual cells (Waterlow, 1986; Devlin and Horton, 1988). Alterations in biochemical measurements may reflect this earlier phase. If the cause of the altered nutritional status is due to diet, dietary alterations should be apparent for days, weeks, or months before metabolism is altered and changes in biochemical indices are evident. For example, decreased intakes of bioavailable iron are often evident months before iron deficiency is evident from hematological indices (Dallman, 1986). If the cause of the malnutrition is secondary to a disease, signs, symptoms, or biochemical indices indicating its presence are often present long before the malnutrition ensues. For example, biochemical signs of atrophic gastritis often precede development of iron or vitamin B_{12} deficiency by several months. While dietary data are therefore theoretically the most sensitive measures of all to dietary deficiency and disease-related alterations in nutritional status, they alone are of little value. Dietary data are less precise and reliable than some biochemical and anthropometric indices, are more subject dependent, and vary more in validity and reliability from one individual to the next. Thus findings of deficits or excesses in dietary intake may be due to diet per se or, in the wrong hands, to methodological error or poor sampling.

Nutritional status assessment is a diagnosis. Just as is the case in identifying other medical problems, the assessment of nutritional status represents a synthesis of all available information, not only dietary information. Conversely, nutritional status–related findings lack meaning and are difficult to interpret in the absence of dietary information (Devlin and Horton, 1988).

Dietary Status Versus Nutritional Status

Dietary status is a much more narrow assessment than is nutritional status. Dietary status measures only what an individual eats. Nutritional status measures what actually is metabolized. Thus dietary and nutritional status are different, and while appropriate dietary status is necessary for nutritional status to be good, dietary status can be satisfactory even when malnutrition is present. For example, an individual suffering from lactase deficiency might be consuming an excellent diet and still be undernourished because of the presence of large amounts of lactose which stimulate diarrhea and malabsorption of many nutrients.

The usual reason for using dietary status instead of nutritional status is that it is less expensive than a full-fledged nutritional status assessment. The food consumption surveys conducted by the U.S. Department of Agriculture are examples of dietary status surveys (Swan, 1983).

Dietary status can often be used to identify individuals who are at high risk of suffering from adverse nutritional status (Kennedy, 1988). For example, food records of children with chronic diseases such as Crohn's disease or nephrotic syndrome often reveal that these children are consuming far fewer calories than they need to grow, especially during illness spells, and only rarely is rehabilitation in hospital or at home complete enough to allow total catch-up growth to occur.

Dietary status also often clarifies and strengthens the presumptive diagnosis from biochemical, anthropometric, and other observations (Kennedy, 1988). For example, it was only when it became clear that vegan-vegetarian children of macrobiotics ate no animal foods at all that it became obvious that vitamin D was likely to be involved in the etiology of the growth retardation which we observed (Dwyer et al., 1979; Dwyer et al., 1982).

Functional Nutritional Status Assessment

The term *functionally based* or *global nutritional assessment* is often mentioned but rarely defined. The phrase usually refers to an emphasis on indices or tests which are clearly associated with the patient's health status, such as weight change, presence or absence of clinical signs and symptoms of deficiency, and ability to carry out activities of daily living.

The emphasis on functionally based assessment is evident in national nutritional status surveys of the elderly, which include items assessing activities of daily living, for example, in addition to more usual anthropometric, biochemical, dietary, and clinical indices.

On the clinical level, functional indices are also receiving attention. Most nutrition support services today rely on clinical nutritional status assessment which includes a full clinical history on the patient, with emphasis on all diseases and conditions from which the patient may be suffering; present and reported past measurements such as weight, weight change, gastrointestinal symptomatology (nausea, vomiting, diarrhea, loss of appetite); clinical signs of nutritional depletion; and clinical estimates of loss of subcutaneous fat, muscle wasting, and edema.

The focus of functional nutritional status assessment is on selected biochemical tests rather than on an elaborate battery of tests for all patients, and on very gross estimates of intakes rather than on more complete dietary intakes and dietary histories. Diet-related items include whether or not the patient has been eating at all, if a therapeutic diet is used, if patients report they are eating normally, if patients are restricting their intakes, and the like. Finally functional capacity, including fatigue in performing normal duties, activities of daily living, and the like is assessed.

The rationale for such a functional approach is that rather than establishing absolute cutoff points and values, using standardized test batteries, clinically oriented functional assessments are more cost-effective and more useful. Moreover, many clinicians continue to be disappointed by the lack of correlation between tests and prognosis.

It is not surprising that a consistent relationship between nutritional assessment parameters and prognosis is sometimes lacking. Prognosis depends not only on nutritional status but also on the nature and degree of illness or injury, prior nutritional status, type of treatment, and presence or absence of complications such as sepsis, as well as the insensitivity of nutritional status assessment parameters (Jeejeebhoy et al., 1982).

Today many excellent resources are available for making abbreviated nutritional status assessments in clinical situations among especially vulnerable patients such as high-risk neonates and infants (Brooke, 1987; Cox 1987); children (Hohenbrink, 1987; Trowbridge, 1988), adults suffering from various diseases (Grieg et al., 1982; Lang and Shulte, 1987), and the elderly (Munro et al., 1987; Chernoff, 1987; Russell and Sayhoun, 1988; Bowman and Rosenberg, 1982).

However, a caveat must be stated about relying too heavily on subjective estimates of nutritional status. While the criteria of clinical utility and cost-effectiveness are entirely appropriate considerations for choosing nutritional status assessment methods, they alone are insufficient. It is important to recognize that at present very few well-standardized "functional" tests of nutritional status exist. The goal of functional assessment should not simply be the recognition of clinically evident malnutrition. Rather, the goal should be to develop tests which provide early warning signs of alterations in biological functions of interest. Much research and development is necessary before such indicators will become a reality. In addition, appropriate standards for various populations, especially vulnerable populations such as pregnant women, infants and growing children, the sick and the elderly, need to be developed. And they must be linked to measures of quality of life.

COMPONENTS OF NUTRITIONAL STATUS AND THEIR MEASUREMENT

Dietary Intake

Rationale. Many dietary factors affect nutritional status. They include the physical and chemical form in which the nutrient is present in the diet, which in turn may be influenced by food processing and preparation as they affect nutritive value and destruction or transformation of nutrients. Other factors are the presence or absence of dietary fiber and other dietary components which may act as toxic agents or inhibitors, such as additives, carcinogens, and habitual intakes of energy, protein, ethanol, vitamins, and minerals (Solomon, 1988).

Usual focus: Habitual dietary intake. The focus in collecting dietary intake data is upon "effective dietary intake," that is, upon a representative sample of intakes over a sufficiently long period of time for its effects on nutritional status to be measurable and clinically meaningful (Jelliffe and Gurney, 1973). This is usually habitual dietary intake. If changes in intake have occurred, it is also helpful to obtain information on intake before the illness or whatever other event led to alterations. The effects of disease are often such that the patient cannot, will not, or should not eat, or he may be eating differently from what he did previously. The physiological effects may be primary, as is the case in anorexia nervosa (Dwyer, 1985), or secondary, as in some hypercatabolic states or malabsorption syndromes which lead to starvation at the tissue level although adequate food is consumed by mouth (Solomon, 1988).

Methods for assessing dietary intake. The methods for collecting information on dietary intake vary in their validity, reliability, precision, and whether groups or individuals are the focus of interest (Bingham, 1987; Block, 1982; Pao et al., 1990). Two major categories of dietary assessment methods exist: retrospective and prospective, based upon the time at which data are collected (Dwyer, 1988). These methods can be further classified on the basis of the time period of interest: the immediate past, reflecting a few days, or the "habitual" diet, reflecting a somewhat longer time. Habitual dietary intake is usually of greatest interest.

Retrospective data are collected days, weeks, months, or years after consumption has taken place. Retrospective methods include 24 hour recalls, which sample the immediate past, as well as food-frequency questionnaires, semiquantitative food-frequency questionnaires, and Burke-type dietary histories, which attempt to reflect the longer term. All retrospective methods are subject to considerable errors due to recall.

Prospective methods include food diaries, weighed intakes, telephone interviews, photographic records, electronic food records, records for monitoring specific foods, duplicate portion analysis, constant observation by a trained observer, and special records of other sorts. One of the major problems here is that respondent burden is great and there is a tendency on the part of subjects to shape answers so that intakes appear to be acceptable to the observer. The strengths and weaknesses of each of these methods are well reviewed in several recent publications (Dwyer, 1988; Bingham, 1987; Block, 1982; Alfin-Slater and Mirenda, 1980; Smickilas-Wright and Guthrie, 1984).

Dietary assessment methods which sample only immediate intake run the risk of failing to reflect habitual diet. They are unable to distinguish between intraindividual variability in intakes from day to day and interindividual variability due to true differences in habitual diet between individuals, making it difficult to link dietary intakes with other characteristics, such as anthropometric measurements, which often reflect a somewhat longer time. Rough estimates of the number of days necessary to collect dietary data to distinguish between interindividual and intraindividual variability are available, but precise estimates require pretests on the population or individual upon whom this method is to be used (Marr and Heady, 1986). The more stable the diet, the smaller the number of observations which are necessary.

Shortcomings. Several general problems and sources of error make it difficult to use dietary intake data without additional information when these methods are used to assess nutritional status.

Of particular concern in attempting to relate dietary intakes to anthropometric indices is the time frame which the dietary assessment covers. Even the most sensitive anthropometric indices such as weight or fatness take weeks or months of changes in dietary intake before they are measurable. If the time frame for dietary status is only a day or is unrepresentative of usual intake, correlations with anthropometric indices are likely to be low or nonexistent, especially in individuals. A second issue is what dietary constituents are being assessed. Changes in anthropometric measurements such as weight, fatness, and stature are closely associated in many situations with changes in energy and protein intakes; energy intakes are especially variable from day to day, and thus the assessment of habitual energy intakes requires weeks of observation. Even then changes in energy output due to physical activity or altered metabolism may affect the net energy available for weight or fat accumulation and growth. Moreover, in the very individuals who exhibit alterations in anthropometric measurements, such as patients suffering from anorexia nervosa or children who are failing to thrive, reported dietary intakes may be distorted. Finally, the focus of dietary status assessment may be inappropriate for exploring relationships of diet to anthropometry. Many dietary assessments focus not on energy but on obtaining rough estimates of intakes of protective nutrients such as vitamins and minerals which may be less highly associated with changes in anthropometric measurements, at least over the short term. The precision with which they are able to provide information on long-term intakes of specific micronutrients of interest, such as calcium and vitamin D and their associations with bone health in old age, may be poor unless specially designed dietary assessment tools are employed.

More general problems common to most dietary assessment methods include weak links to outcomes of interest, variability of dietary indices owing to inherent variation, as well as to other sources of error (sampling error, reporting error, coding error, and errors in food composition tables themselves). Also, in some cases habitual intakes may not be helpful. Inferences about diet in the causation of disease are also difficult to make if dietary information alone is collected.

Groups versus individuals. Dietary status assessment using food consumption surveys and population-based samples is becoming increasingly sophisticated (Pao et al. 1988; Subcommittee on Criteria for Dietary Evaluation, 1986; Beaton, 1988; Anderson, 1986; Mason et al., 1984). At the same time, the somewhat unique problems of dietary and nutritional assessment of individuals for counseling purposes are also receiving scrutiny (Bingham, 1987; Beaton, 1988; Dwyer, 1988). Many of the previously mentioned shortcomings are being overcome as newer methods and analytical techniques are becoming available.

Differing perspectives of assessors versus counselors. Those who are surveying the dietary intake of the population and those who are counseling individuals have very different perspectives and missions leading to different views and perspectives. Beaton (1988) has summarized these different perspectives well: "For the professional concerned about the health of the public as a whole, the problem he faces is . . . described by the estimated prevalence of inadequate intakes." This is a much smaller number of people than those of interest to "professionals who are counseling individuals, whose objective is to counsel each individual toward a situation that conveys a low risk to that person. To that professional, the proportion of women with intakes below the 'recommended intake' represents the magnitude of the problem he faces" (Beaton, 1988). Beaton suggests that the focus of the counselor should be on an acceptable level of risk for an individual, balancing between current consumption patterns and probability of harm stemming from dietary intake.

Computerized dietary analysis. In the past decade the widespread availability and low cost of computerized nutrient analysis systems has greatly increased the availability of dietary assessment analyses for both clinical and research applications (Thompson and Dwyer, 1987; Murphy, 1987). However, dietary and nutritional status analysis systems are unstandardized and vary widely in quality. Before they are used for dietary status assessment the quality control over data to be entered and the programs themselves need to be carefully evaluated (Frank and Pelican, 1986; Hoover, 1987).

Anthropometric Measurements

Rationale. The brief history of clinical nutritional status assessment provided earlier in this chapter suggests that the phase of uncritical acceptance of any and all biochemical and immunological indices which purport to measure nutritional status has passed, and investigators have returned to more abbreviated assessments. Many investigators have developed a new respect for simple anthropometric measurements because of their ability to provide early warnings of declines in nutritional status if such standardized monitoring techniques are employed on an ongoing basis.

Anthropometry. Anthropometric measurements are essential components of general nutritional status assessment. They measure the human body, its parts, and functional capacities. The most common anthropometric measurements are weight and changes in weight, stature, segmental lengths, fat folds, and various body circumferences and diameters. Additional measurements may be desirable for more specific purposes, such as weight gain and estimation of edema during pregnancy; head circumference during infancy; and serial estimates of weight for height, weight for age, and height for age during recuperation from failure to thrive.

Their utility is that they provide rough estimates of body composition or changes in body composition if they are taken serially. They have the advantages of being inexpensive, easy to carry out, and reproducible with a modicum of training. Their main disadvantage is their lack of precision. Since the rest of this volume is devoted to the role of anthropometric measurements in nutrition, this essential component of nutritional status assessment has been mentioned only briefly here.

Now that routine anthropometric measurements have found their way into clinical and public health practice, the next task is to improve the quality of measurements both in community and clinical studies. This will entail both the purchase of better equipment and more training and standardization of technique among those who take such measurements (Zerfas, 1985).

Excellent references on standard techniques are now available (Robbins and Trowbridge, 1984; Forbes, 1988; Abraham, 1988; Lohman et al., 1988; Roche, 1985; Himes et al., 1981; Chumlea et al., 1984; Cameron, 1978).

Other body composition assessment methods. Over the past two decades new methods of assessing body composition have become available, some of which offer great potential for clinical and nutritional survey use. These include methods for assessing lean body mass and fat-free mass by the use of total body water measurements with isotopes of hydrogen and oxygen, measures of total body potassium with radioactive tracers or stable isotopes such as K-40, measures of total body nitrogen by neutron activation, CAT scans, nuclear magnetic resonance, and whole body conductivity. Neutron activation of calcium and other elements such as sodium and phosphorus, and photon densitometry are being explored to measure bone mineral. The use of CAT scans, nuclear magnetic resonance, fat soluble gases, and carbon 14 to measure body fatness is also now being tested at the research level (Garrow, 1982; Forbes, 1987; Fallon, 1988; Watson, 1988). Applications of a more practical nature are likely once the validity and reliability of these procedures is better established and costs become more reasonable.

Shortcomings. The major difficulty with anthropometric measurements is that they are nonspecific and lack precision in estimating body composition. The newer methods are somewhat more precise in estimating body composition but are nonspecific, costly, and time-consuming.

History and Physical Examination

Medical and social history. One clinical nutrition expert claims that "the medical-social history of the patient provides 90% of the information necessary to arrive at a presumptive diagnosis of a medical condition, and the physical examination yields the remaining 10% "(Owen, 1984).

Several aspects of medical history suggest elevated risk of malnutrition. A recent loss of 10% or more of usual body weight in adults, failure to gain weight in children and pregnant women, and gradual losses or gains of large amounts of weight which have not been consciously intended signal possible malnutrition at all ages (Baker et al., 1988).

Those in certain age or physiological groups such as pregnant and lactating women, infants and growing children, adolescents during the pubertal growth spurt, those recovering from wasting diseases, and the very old and frail have elevated needs for nutrients in relation to their energy intakes, and are at increased risk of malnutrition. Others who are poor, unable to feed themselves, or who are mentally incapacitated are also especially vulnerable, especially if they are ill with conditions which may alter nutritional status or require dietary therapy.

The presence of long-standing chronic disease, especially if it has been untreated or unsuccessfully resolved, also increases probabilities of malnutrition. Such disorders include conditions affecting the gastrointestinal tract, such as vomiting, diarrhea, malabsorption syndromes, dumping syndrome, short gut syndrome, colitis, and ileitis.

Diseases of the liver and pancreas; conditions such as stroke which may affect ability to eat; emotional problems such as depression, grief and anorexia nervosa which may affect the desire to eat; and alcoholism, renal dialysis, burns, and draining wounds also may give rise to poor appetite, protracted loss of nutrients, and inadequate dietary intakes.

Acute conditions such as burns, trauma, and fever increase metabolic needs even in the face of otherwise inadequate intakes. Metabolic alterations in the terminal stages of cancer may result in cancer cachexia. Individuals who suffer from addictions, especially narcotics addicts and chronic alcoholics, are at high risk of malnutrition.

Iatrogenic malnutrition may also arise as a result of medical or surgical treatments (Young and Blass, 1982). While temporary nutritional complications may be the price of therapy, their persistence is often a sign of medical neglect rather than inevitable long-term sequelae of treatment.

Many surgical procedures give rise to malnutrition if potential complications are not anticipated and dealt with. These include small bowel bypass and gastrectomy. Hemodialysis may give rise to bone disease, hypovitaminosis, and depletion of several nutrients. Irradiation, apart from transient effects involving nausea and vomiting, may cause malabsorption due to radiation damage of the small bowel and to xerostomia or damage to the saliva-secreting cells of the mouth. Obesity treatment with very low calorie diets under 500 calories per day for many months accompanied by losses of large amounts of weight, and nonadherence to therapeutic diets after gastric resections or gastric stapling operations for massive obesity, may also result in malnutrition. Inadequate or misinterpreted dietary therapy, especially when several complex conditions requiring modified diets are present, or nonadherence to prescribed dietary modifications may also result in malnutrition.

Chronic use of prescription and over-the-counter drugs, especially when they occur in combination with each other, may also have adverse effects on nutritional status by altering intakes, synthesis, absorption, transport, storage, metabolism, or excretion of nutrients. (Roe, 1988; Young and Blass, 1982). This is especially likely to occur among the elderly, who often suffer from many chronic conditions and are taking many different drugs. Certain drugs may act as antinutrients, such as some of the anticonvulsants which are folic acid antagonists. Others such as corticosteroids may increase catabolism. Interactions of drugs with foods such as alcohol and nutrients may also give rise to problems (Mycek, 1989). And chemotherapy, radiation, and other procedures, especially when combined with multiple drug treatments, may decrease appetite (Owen, 1984). Other procedures such as extensive medical tests which involve going without food, and surgery with complications such as sepsis or development of abscesses, if without special nutritional support and especially if involving the gastrointestinal tract, adversely affect nutritional status.

Clinical signs and symptoms. There are two major groups of signs and symptoms associated with malnutrition: Those that are often associated with or related to deficiencies of one or more nutrients or malnutrition in general, and those that are unrelated to malnutrition but similar to them (Owen, 1984).

For example, koilonychia, or spoon-shaped fingernails, is sometimes present in severe iron-deficiency anemia, and transverse ridging of the nails is sometimes observed in protein-calorie malnutrition, but deformities of the fingernails are often due to other causes as well. The nonspecificity of most of these signs makes it difficult to make definitive diagnoses. Also, they usually occur late in the pathological process, so they are of little use in primary prevention of malnutrition.

Shortcomings of clinical methods. The observation and recognition of signs of malnutrition are among the most subjective aspects of nutritional status assessment. Standards for nutritional status assessment and training, especially if large populations are being surveyed, are therefore critical. Methods for standardizing observations are available which increase interobserver reliability and permit more definitive differential diagnosis (McLaren, 1988; McLaren, 1981; Zerfas, 1985; WHO/ECMANS, 1963). Only a few changes are specific for deficiencies of a single nutrient; most are nonspecific and may also reflect alterations in several nutrients or in some other aspects of health status. For this reason the current existence of clinical signs or symptoms of dietary deficiencies or stigmata which suggest past deficiencies, such as deformities, lesions, and scars, are only considered diagnostic when correlations with other components of nutritional history and current nutritional status are present (Alfin-Slater and Mirenda, 1980). Clinical signs and symptoms relate to long-term nutritonal status, e.g., many months in most cases. Therefore perfect correlations between them and dietary intake over the shorter term are not to be expected. Somewhat higher correlations may be expected when clusters of signs and symptoms occur together. For example, a patent Fontanelle, the varus or valgus deformity in the legs, and beading of the ribs (the rachitic rosary) all present together offer stronger support for the presence of rickets in a young child than does any sign by itself. Further support for such a diagnosis comes if dietary history and biochemical and radiologic studies are also suggestive of vitamin D deficiency.

Biochemical Measurements

Rationale. The concentration of essential nutrients and metabolites in body fluids, usually blood and urine, provides indicators of the nutrition of the cells and tissue stores of some nutrients. Patients and populations being surveyed to assess their nutritional status are understandably reluctant to submit to biopsies of tissues and organs to examine the function of cells directly. Biochemical measurements provide noninvasive means for assessing the nutritional status–related function of bodily cells by laboratory assessment of the fluids obtained. In some but not all instances these biochemical indicators provide earlier and more precise and reliable indicators of malnutrition than dietary intakes, medical history, clinical examination, and anthropometric measurements. They can also corroborate or refute presumptive diagnoses obtained by other means.

Methods. The number of biochemical measurements of nutritional status is expanding at an ever more rapid rate. Hematological indices include blood components such as cells or enzymes that can be related to nutrient intakes or body composition, the presence of abnormal metabolic products in blood, and abnormally high or low nutrient levels. Urine measures include urinary metabolites and excretion rates of the nutrient. Both blood and urine measurements may include responses to load, saturation, or isotopic tests (Pi-Sunyer and Woo, 1984).

Among the more common tests used to measure carbobydrate metabolism are fasting blood glucose and glucose tolerance tests. Serum lipids, including cholesterol and its subfractions in high-density lipoprotein and low-density lipoprotein, triglycerides, and abnormal lipid oxidation products such as ketone bodies are measured to assess lipid metabolism.

Biochemical measurements of proteins in the blood are used to assess the adequacy of dietary intake, metabolic changes due to tissue-protein malnutrition, and the depletion of body stores of protein. Serum albumin levels fall in severe protein-calorie malnutrition, but they are also altered if liver and kidney disease are present, in severe burns, and when the gut is chronically inflamed. Other plasma proteins with shorter half-lives such as transferrin, thyroxine-binding prealbumin, and retinol-binding protein fall more rapidly than serum albumin when protein nutriture is unsatisfactory, but they too are rather nonspecific. For example, in addition to protein-calorie malnutrition, serum transferrin levels are decreased in pernicious anemia, chronic infection, liver disease, iron overload, and protein-losing enteropathies. They are elevated in iron deficiency, pregnancy, hypoxia, and chronic blood loss. Prealbumin levels are depressed in protein malnutrition but may also be abnormal in patients with liver disease, such as hepatitis or cirrhosis, stress, inflammation, and surgical trauma, while they are maintained at abnormally high levels among patients on dialysis for chronic renal failure. Levels of retinol-binding protein are also low in vitamin A deficiency and liver disease, hyperthyroidism, and cystic fibrosis, as well as in protein-calorie malnutrition. Levels in blood and urine of metabolites of protein such as urea and the nitrogenous substance creatine, which is degraded to creatinine in the muscle, are used to measure kidney function and also serve as nonspecific indicators of deficient protein intake and muscle wasting.

A number of hematologic changes signal the presence of malnutrition from deficiencies of iron, folic acid, and vitamin B_{12}. Common measurements include hemoglobin, hematocrit, and observation of blood smears to assess the size, color, and shape of the blood cells. More sophisticated, sensitive, and expensive tests of iron deficiency include serum ferritin, which is an early sign of iron deficiency; plasma iron; transferrin, total iron-binding capacity, which assesses the ability of transferrin, the transport form of iron, to bind iron; and free erythrocyte protoporphyrin. The sequence of development of iron-deficiency anemia begins with depletion of bone marrow iron and of blood ferritin levels. An increase in total iron-binding capacity, free erythrocyte protoporphyrin, and decreased iron saturation is noted next. Then serum iron begins to decrease. Finally, the anemia becomes apparent. At this stage or possibly earlier than this functional changes may be apparent.

Anemias are also signs of vitamin B_{12} and folic acid deficiency. In this case, the anemia is megaloblastic in nature. Morphological examination and biochemical tests of serum B_{12} levels are helpful in distinguishing between the two causes. While serum folic acid is low in folic acid deficiency, it is so sensitive to dietary intakes that it only poorly reflects tissue stores and cellular function; for this purpose, red blood cell folic acid is more useful. An abnormal urinary metabolite, known as formiminoglutamic acid, is present and elevated in both vitamin B_{12} and folic acid deficiencies. Other, more complicated tests may also be needed to differentiate between the two deficiencies.

Dietary intakes of the water soluble vitamins thiamine, riboflavin, niacin, pyridoxine, pantothenic acid, and ascorbic acid are well reflected in blood and urinary levels of these nutrients, the preferred measures varying from one nutrient to another. However, they only reflect recent intake.

Blood levels of the fat soluble vitamins are kept under fairly tight control. Vitamin A nutriture is measured as serum retinol, and is a good measure of long-term intake but not of liver stores. Very low levels come somewhat earlier than do the clinical or functional signs of vitamin A deficiency. However, again, as with most of the biochemical indices of vitamin nutrition, they are also altered in a number of illnesses. Such conditions include chronic infection, liver disease, celiac disease, obstructive jaundice, and cystic fibrosis, and in these instances low levels are unrelated to poor nutrition. Biochemical indicators of vitamin D status include serum alkaline phosphatase, calcium, and inorganic phosphate, but none is very sensitive. Lately a test for the major circulating form of vitamin D, 25-hydroxyvitamin D, has become available. While it reflects both diet and solar exposure, it is far more specific and sensitive than the older indicators. Vitamin E is only poorly measured by present tests; blood levels of alpha-tocopherol do not always reflect either the level of intake or tissue stores. Vitamin K nutriture is measured by bleeding tendency as measured by prothrombin time. However, blood disorders and severe liver disease may also lead to abnormal measurements.

The biochemical indicators of nutritional status with respect to the mineral elements are mixed in their utility, since, like the electrolytes, their concentration is tightly controlled, and their levels are affected by numerous hormones. Serum calcium, phosphorus, magnesium, and zinc are poor indicators of dietary intake or of tissue stores, and are extremely nonspecific.

Other biochemical indicators which may be of interest include electrolytes in blood and liver function tests.

Other Components

Immunologic function. Tests of immune function are increasingly being included in clinical nutritional status assessments (Myrvik, 1988). They have the advantage of providing information which is functionally relevant. Their major disadvantage is their nonspecificity for malnutrition.

Foodways. When food-borne disease or food intoxication is suspected, a rigorous analysis of the entire food getting, storage, preparation, and consumption process may be necessary. Such data may be especially important in nutritional status surveys of unusual populations with unfamiliar diets (Wadsworth, 1984).

Demographic and economic information. Income, education, race, ethnicity, sex, age, socioeconomic status, living conditions, and other information on the sociology and culture of individuals being assessed are often relevant, especially if the purpose of the nutritional status assessment is to intervene to improve deficits.

CONCLUSIONS

The concept of nutritional status pervades the thinking of biomedical scientists with an interest in nutrition. To them it helps to make sense out of what otherwise appears to be a mass of contradictory information measuring many different levels and types of disturbances in nutritional status. Since nutrition is an applied science, the ultimate utility of the concept resides in its ability to simplify the complex, and it has met this test (Harper, 1987).

Shortcomings. Biochemical indicators of malnutrition for different nutrients vary in their specificity, sensitivity, validity, and reliability. Therefore they must be interpreted critically.

The potential causes of abnormal values include but are not limited to alterations in nutritional status. For example, blood levels of nutrients may be low because of dietary deficiency, poor absorption, impaired transport, abnormal utilization, or all of these causes, and the test itself is usually unable to differentiate between these. Additional biochemical tests and correlations with dietary, anthropometric, and clinical findings are often necessary to make definitive statements.

Some biochemical indicators are very sensitive and detect very early stages of dietary deficiency disease, while other indicators may remain within the normal range until very late in the pathological process of malnutrition's development.

The validity (accuracy) or the closeness of the value to the truth also varies from one indicator to the other. For example, one form of iron in the blood reflects stores of body iron poorly, whereas another reflects it well (Dallman, 1986). Obviously the ultimate biological and clinical sigificance of a given test will depend greatly on how well it measures what it is supposed to measure, and how closely this measurement relates to physiological function.

Differences are also apparent in the reliability (precision) or reproducibility of the various biochemical indicators of nutritional status.

Finally, appropriate standards against which biochemical indicators should be assessed are sometimes not available for those in certain age or physiological groups (Harper, 1987).

REFERENCES

Abraham S (1988): Height weight tables: Their sources and development In Shils ME, Young VR (ed): "Modern Nutrition in Health and Disease." Philadelphia: Lea & Febiger, pp 1509–1517.

Alfin-Slater RB, Mirenda R (1980): Nutrient requirements: What they are and basis for recommendations. In Alfin-Slater RB, Kritchevsky D (eds): "Nutrition and the Adult: Macronutrients." New York: Plenum Press, pp 1–48.

Anderson SA (1986): "Guidelines for the Use of Dietary Intake Data." Bethesda, Mol: Life Sciences Research Office, Federation of American Societies for Experimental Biology.

Annest JL (1983): Trends in the blood lead levels of the U.S. population: the second national health and nutrition examination survey (NHANES II) 1976–80. In Rutter U, Jones R (eds): "Lead Versus Health." London: Wiley, pp 33–48.

Baker JP, Barrocas A, Eliades J, George S, Hester DD, Jeejeebhoy KN, Kaminski MV, Kutsop A, Leider Z, Martin D, Matarese L, Szeluga DJ, Touger-Becker R (1988): Open forum: Nutritional assessment: Present and future. Nutritional Support Services 8: 7–11.

Beaton GH (1988): Criteria of an adequate diet. In Shils ME, Young V R (eds): "Modern Nutrition in Health & Disease." Philadelphia: Lea & Febiger, pp 650–666.

Bingham SA (1987): The dietary assessment of individuals: Methods, accuracy, new techniques and recommendations. Nutr Abstracts Rev (ser A) 57:705–741.

Block GA (1982): Review of validations of dietary assessment methods. Am J Epidemiol 115:492–505.

Bowman BB, Rosenberg IH (1982): Assessment of the nutritional status of the elderly Am J Clin Nutr 34:1142–1151.

Brooke OG (1987): Nutritional requirements of low and very low birthweight infants. Annu Rev Nutr 7:91–116.

Burt BA, Eklund SA, Landis J (1982): National Center for Health Statistics: Diet and dental health, a study of relationships: United States, 1971–74. Vital and Health Statistics Ser. 11, No. 225, DHHS Publ. No. (PHS) 82–1675, US Public Health Service. Washington, DC: GPO.

Buzby GP, Mullen JL (1988): Nutrition assessment. In Rombeau JL, Caldwell MD (eds): "Clinical Nutrition. Vol 1, Enteral Nutrition." Philadelphia: WB Saunders, pp 127–147.

Buzby GP, Mullen JL, Mattherws DL, Hobbs CL, Rosato EF (1980): Prognostic nutritional index in gastrointestinal surgery. Am J Surg 120:160–167.

Cameron N (1974): The methods of auxological anthropometry. In Falkner F Tanner JM (eds): "Human Growth. Vol 2, Postnatal Growth." New York: Plenum Press, pp 35–90.

Cassel J (1976): The contribution of the social environment to host resistance. Am J Epidemiol 104:107–111.

Chang RWS, Jacobs S, Lee B (1986): Use of APACHE II severity of disease classification to identify intensive care unit patients who would not benefit from total parenteral nutrition. Lancet 1:1483–1486.

Chernoff R (1987): Home nutrition support in elderly patients Clin Nutr 6:36–39.

Chumlea WC, Roche AF, Mukherjee D (1984): "Nutritional Assessment of the Elderly Through Anthropometry." Columbus, Ohio: Ross Laboratories.

Cox JH (1987): High-risk neonates and infants. In Lang CE (ed). "Nutritional Support in Critical Care." Rockville, Maryland: Aspen, pp 3–32.

Dallman PR (1986): Biochemical basis for the manifestations of iron deficiency. Annu Rev Nutr 6:13–40.

Detsky AS, Baker JP, O'Rourke KA. Metaanalysis of perioperative parenteral nutrition. Ann Intern Med (in press).

Devlin JT, Horton ES (1988): Hormone and nutrient interactions. In Shils ME, Young VR (eds): "Modern Nutrition in Health and Disease." Philadelphia: Lea & Febiger, pp 570–585.

Dwyer JT (1985): Nutritional aspects of anorexia nervosa and bulimia. In Emmett SW (ed): "Theory and Treatment of Anorexia Nervosa and Bulimia: Biomedical, Sociocultural, and Psychological Perspectives." New York: Brunner Mazel, pp 20–51.

Dwyer JT (1988): Assessment of dietary intake. In Shils ME, Young VR (eds): "Modern Nutrition in Health and Disease." Philadelphia: Lea & Febiger, pp 887–902.

Dwyer JT, Dietz WH, Andrews EM, Suskind RM (1982): Nutritional status of vegetarian children. Am J Clin Nutr 35:204–216.

Dwyer JT, Dietz WH, Hass G, Suskind R (1979): Risk of nutritional rickets among vegetarian children. Am J Dis Child 133:134–140.

Editorial (1986): TPN and APACHE. Lancet 1:1478.

Fallon MD (1988): Assessment of bone structure. In Shils ME, Young VR (eds): "Modern Nutrition in Health and disease." Philadelphia: Lea & Febiger. pp 861–886.

Forbes GB (1987): Influence of nutrition. In Forbes GB (ed): "Human Body composition: Growth, Aging, Nutrition and Activity." New York: Springer-Verlag, pp 209–247.

Forbes GB (1988): Body composition: Influence of nutrition, disease, growth and aging. In Shils ME, Young VR (eds): "Modern Nutrition in Health and Disease." Philadelphia: Lea & Febiger, pp 533–557.

Frank GC, Pelican S (1986): Guidelines for selecting a dietary analysis system. J Am Diet Assoc 86:72–75.

Garrow JS (1982): New approaches to body composition Am J Clin Nutr 35:1152–1158.

Greig PD, Baker JP, Jeejeebhoy KN (1982): Metabolic effects of total parenteral nutrition. Annu Rev Nutr 2:179–199.

Gruchow HW, Sobocinski KA, Barboriak JJ (1985): Alcohol, nutrient intake, and hypertension in US adults. JAMA 253:1567–1570.

Harlan WR, Hull AL, Schmouder RL, Landis JR, Thompson FE et al. (1984): Blood pressure and nutrition in adults: The national health and nutrition examination survey. Am J Epidemiol 120:17–28.

Harlan WR, Hull AL, Schmouder RP, Thompson FE, Larkin FA et al. (1983): National Center for Health Statistics: Dietary intake and cardiovascular risk factors. Part 1, Blood pressure correlates: United States 1971–75 Vital and Health Statistics. Ser. 11, No. 226 DHHS Publ. No. (PHS) 83-1676, US Public Health Service. Washington, DC: GPO.

Harper AE (1987): Evolution of recommended dietary allowances—new directions? Annu Rev Nutr 7:509–537.

Harvey KB, Ruggiero JA, Regan CS, Bistrian BR, Blackburn GL (1978): Hospital morbidity and mortality risk factors using nutritional assessment. Clin Res 26:581 Aa.

Heymsfield SB, Williams RJ (1988): Nutritional assessment by clinical and biochemical methods. In Shils ME, Young VR (eds): "Modern Nutrition in Health and Disease." Philadelphia: Lea & Febiger. pp 817–860.

Himes JH, Roche AF, Thissen D (1981): Parent specific adjustments for assessment of recumbent length and stature. "Monographs in Paediatrics." Basel, Switzerland: Karger, vol 13.

Hobbiss JH, Buston A, Gallagher P, Roberts C, Tweedle DEF (1984): A comparison of the Sheffield prognostic index, serum albumin, and age in the prediction of surgical complication. Clin Nutr 3:227–230.

Hohenbrink K (1987): The pediatric patient. In Lang CE (ed): "Nutritional Support in Critical Care." Rockville, Md: Aspen, pp 33–60.

Hoover LW (1987): Nutrient data bases: Choosing wisely. Clin Nutr 6:198–207.

Howard L, Heaphey LL, Timchalk M (1986): A review of the current national status of home parenteral and enteral nutrition from the provider and consumer perspective. J Parenter Enteral Nutr 10:416–424.

Jeejeebhoy KN, Baker JP, Wolman SL, Wesson DE, Langer B, Harrison JE, McNeill KG (1982): Critical evaluation of the role of clinical assessment and body composition studies in patients with malnutrition and after total parenteral nutrition. Am J Clin Nutr 35:1117–1127.

Jelliffe DB (1966): "The Assessment of the Nutritional Status of the Community." Geneva: WHO. WHO Monograph Ser. No. 53.

Jelliffe EFP, Gurney M (1973): Definition of the problem. In Roche AF, Falkner F (eds): "Nutrition and Malnutrition: Identification and Measurement." New York: Plenum Press, pp 1–14.

Jequier E, Acheson K, Schutz Y (1987): Assessment of energy expenditure and fuel utilization in man. Annu Rev Nutr 7:187–208.

Kaminski MV, Fitzgerald MJ, Murphy RJ, Payast P, Hoppe MC, Winborn AL, Pluta J (1977): Correlation of mortality with serum transferrin and anergy. J Parenter Enteral Nutr 1:27a.

Kennedy EM (1988): Dietary assessment. In Paige DM (ed): "Clinical Nutrition." St. Louis: CV Mosby, pp 148–164.

Knaus WA, Draper EA, Wagner DP, Zimmerman JE (1985): APACHE II: A severity of disease classification system. Crit Care Med 13:818–829.

Lang CE, Shulte CV (1987): The adult patient. In Lang CE (ed): "Nutritional Support in Critical Care." Rockville, Md: Aspen, p 61–90.

Lawson DH, Richmond A, Nixon DW, Rudman D (1982): Metabolic approaches to cancer cachexia. Annu Rev Nutr 2:277–230.

Lifshitz JZ (1987): Home parenteral nutrition. Clin Nutr 6:7–16.

Lohman TG, Roche AF, Martorell R (1988): "Anthropometric Standardization Reference Manual." Champaign, Ill: Human Kinetics.

McLaren DS (1981). "A Colour Atlas of Nutritional Disorders." London: Wolfe.

McLaren DS (1988): Clinical manifestations of nutritional disorders. In Shils ME Young VR (eds): "Modern Nutrition in Health and Disease." Philadelphia: Lea & Febiger, 733–745.

Mahaffey KR, Annest HL (1986): Association of erythrocyte protoporphyrin with blood lead level and iron status in the second national health and nutrition examination survey 1976–1980: Association with selected demographic and socioeconomic factors. Environ Res 41:327–338.

Marr JW, Heady JA (1986): Within and between person variation in dietary surveys: Number of days needed to classify individuals. Hum Nutr Appl Nutr 40A: 347–364.

Mason JB, Habicht JP, Tabatabai H, Valverde V (1984): "Nutritional Surveillance." Geneva: WHO.

Mullen JL, Buzby GP, Waldman MT, Getner MH, Hobbs CL, Rosato EF (1979a): Prediction of operative morbidity and mortality by preoperative nutritional assessment. Surg Forum 30:80–82.

Mullen JL, Gertner MH, Buzby GP, Goodhart SL, Rosato EF (1979b): Implications of malnutrition in surgical patients. Arch Surg 114:121–125.

Munro HN, Suter PM, Russell RM (1987): Nutritional requirements of the elderly. Annu Rev Nutr 7:23–49.

Murphy SP (1987): Use of national survey data bases for nutrition research. Clin Nutr 6:208–219.

Mycek MJ (1989): Interaction of drugs with foods and nutrients. In Simko MD, Cowell C, Gilbride JA (eds): "Nutrition Assessment: A Comprehensive Guide for Planning Intervention." Rockville, Md: Aspen, pp 93–118.

Myrvik QN (1988): Nutrition and immunology. In Shils ME, Young VR (eds): "Modern Nutrition in Health and Disease." Philadelphia: Lea & Febiger, pp 585–616.

Owen GM (1984): Physical examination as an assessment tool, Section 1: Medical history and physical signs of malnutrition. In Simko MD, Cowell C, Gilbride JA (eds):" Nutrition Assessment: A Comprehensive Guide for Planning Intervention." Rockville, Md: Aspen, pp 57–58.

Pao E, Sykes K, Cypel Y (in press): "Methodological Research for Large Scale Dietary Intake Surveys 1975–1988." Human Nutrition Information Service, Home Economics Research Report U.S. Department of Agriculture.

Pilch SM, Senti FR (1984a): "Assessment of the Zinc Nutritional Status for the U.S Population Based on Data Collected in the Second National Health and Nutrition Examination Survey 1976–1980." Bethesda, Md: Life Sciences Research Office, Federated Societies for Experimental Biology. Available from National Technical Information Service No. PB 84-218544, Springfield, Va.

Pilch SM, Senti FR (1984b): "Assessment of the Iron Nutritional Status for the U.S. Population Based on Data Collected in the Second National Health and Nutrition Examination Survey 1976–1980." Bethesda, Md: Life Science Research Office, Federation of American Societies for Experimental Biology. Available from National Technical Information Service No. PB 85-115418, Springfield, Va.

Pi-Sunyer FX, Woo R (1984): Laboratory assessment of nutritional status. In Simko MD, Cowell C, Gilbride JA (eds): "Nutrition Assessment: A Comprehensive Guide for Planning Intervention." Rockville, Md: Aspen, pp 139–174.

Robbins GE, Trowbridge FL (1984): Anthropometric techniques and their applications. In Simko MD, Cowell C, Gilbride JA (eds): "Nutrition Assessment: A Comprehensive Guide for Planning Intervention." Rockville, Md: Aspen, pp 69–92.

Roberts J (1978): National Center for Health Statistics: Cardiovascular conditions of children 6–11 years, United States, 1963–65 and 1966–70. Vital and Health Statistics, Ser. 11, No. 166, DHEW Publ. No. (PHS) 78–1653 U.S. Public Health Service. Washington, DC: GPO.

Roberts D, Thelin D, Weinstein S (1982): Parenteral and enteral nutrition. A cost benefit audit. Minn Med 20:707–710.

Roche AF (ed) (1985): "Body Composition Assessments in Youth and Adults: Report of the Sixth Ross Conference on Medical Research." Columbus, Ohio: Ross Laboratories.

Roe DA (1988): Diet, nutrition and drug reactions. In Shils ME, Young VR (eds): "Modern Nutrition in Health and Disease." Philadelphia: Lea & Febiger, pp 630–648.

Russell RM Sayhoun NR (1988): Adults. In Paige DM (ed): "Clinical Nutrition." St. Louis: CV Mosby, pp 137–147.

Seltzer MH, Bstidas JA, Cooper DM, Engler P, Slocum B, Fletcher HS (1980): Instant nutritional assessment. J Parenter Enteral Nutr 3:157–159.

Sempos C, Cooper R, Kovar MG, Johnson C, Drizd T et al. (1986): Dietary calcium and blood pressure in national health and nutrition examination surveys I and II. Hypertension 8:1067–1074.

Senti FR, Pilch SM (1984): "Assessment of the Folate Nutritional Status of the US Population Based on Data Collected in the Second National Health and Nutrition Examination Survey 1976–1980. Bethesda, Md: Life Sciences Research Office, Federated American Societies for Experimental Biology. Available from National Technical Information Service No. PB 85-164051/AS, Springield, Va.

Shils ME (1988): Enteral (tube) and parenteral nutrition support. In Shils ME, Young VR (eds): "Modern Nutrition in Health and Disease." Philadelphia: Lea & Febiger, pp 1023–1068.

Simms JM, Smith JAR, Woods HF (1982): A modified prognostic index based upon nutritional measurements. Clin Nutr 1:71–79.

Smickilas-Wright H, Guthrie HA (1984): Dietary methodologies: Their uses, analyses, interpretations and implications. In Simko MD, Cowell C, Gilbride JA (eds): "Nutrition Assessment: A Comprehensive Guide for Planning Intervention." Rockville Md: Aspen, pp 119–138.

Solomon NW (1988): Non-nutrient factors in metabolism. In Paige DM (ed): "Clinical Nutrition." St. Louis: CV Mosby, pp 36–48.

Subcommittee on Criteria for Dietary Evaluation, Coordinating Committee on Evaluation of Food Consumption Surveys, Food and Nutrition Board, Commission on the Life Sciences, National Research Council (1986): "Nutritient Adequacy: Assessment Using Food Consumption Surveys." Washington, DC: National Academy Press.

Swan PS (1983): Food consumption by individuals in the United States: Two major surveys. Annu Rev Nutr 3:413–432.

Thompson JK, Dwyer JT (1987): Computer applications in outpatient nutrition services: Fostering the computer connection. Clin Nutr 6:185–191.

Twomey PL, Patching SC (1985): Cost effectiveness of nutritional support. J Parenter Enteral Nutr 9:3–10.

Trowbridge FL (1988): Infants and children. In Paige DM (ed): "Clinical Nutrition." St. Louis: CV Mosby, pp 119–136.

U.S. Department of Health and Human Services and U.S. Department of Agriculture (1986): "Nutrition Monitoring in the United States: A Progress Report from the Joint Nutrition Monitoring Evaluation Committee." DHHS Publ. No. (PHS) 86-1255, US Public Health Service. Washington, DC: GPO.

Wadsworth G. (1984): Health and disease. In Wadsworth GA (ed): "The Diet and Health of Isolated Populations." Boca Raton, Fla: CRC Press, pp 4–11.

Ward MWN, Danzi M, Lewin MR, Rennie MJ, Clark CG (1982): The effects of subclinical malnutrition and refeeding on the healing of experimental colonic anastomoses. Br J Surg 69:308–310.

Waterlow JC (1986): Metabolic adaptation of low intakes of energy and protein. Annu Rev Nutr 6: 495–526.

Watson RC, Grossman H, Meyers MA (1988): Radiological findings in nutritional disturbances. In Shils ME, Young VR (eds): "Modern Nutrition in Health and Disease." Philadelphia: Lea & Febiger, pp 906–930.

Widdowson FM (1988): Nutrition and cell and organ growth. In Shils ME, Young VR (eds): "Modern Nutrition in Health and Disease." Philadelphia: Lea & Febiger, pp 617–629.

WHO/ECMANS (World Health Organization, Expert Committee on Medical Assessment of Nutritional Status) (1963): "Medical Assessment of Nutritional Status" WHO Technical Report Services No. 258.

World Health Organization, Food and Agricultural Organization and International Union of Nutritional Sciences (1973): "Food and Nutrition Terminology: Definitions of Selected Terms and Expressions in Current Use." Geneva: WHO pp 8, 30.

Yetley E, Johnson C (1987): Nutritional applications of the health and nutrition examination survey (HANES). Annu Rev Nutr 7:441–463.

Young RC, Blass JP (1982): Iatrogenic nutritional deficiencies. Annu Rev Nutr 2:201–227.

Zerfas AJ (1985): Manual for Examiners; Checking Selected Clinical Features. "Los Angeles, Calif: Division of Epidemiology, School of Public Health, University of California at Los Angeles.

Anthropometric Assessment
of Nutritional Status, pages 29–49

3
Nutrition and Physical Growth

MICHAEL GRACEY
Health Department of Western Australia, East Perth 6004, Australia

INTRODUCTION

It is accepted, almost unchallenged, that nutrition is the major determinant of growth patterns in infants and children. But how strong is the evidence for this? What is the true place of nutrition in determining the patterns of growth in infancy and childhood? And how does this affect nutritional anthropometry in nutritional assessment in early life? These important questions can be approached more rationally if we consider the nutritional requirements which are believed to be needed to sustain growth in "normal" circumstances and how physical growth patterns are influenced by conditions in which nutrient intakes are enhanced or compromised. In discussing these issues, we will question the basis on which growth "standards" in childhood exist.

In this chapter we will consider situations where undernutrition and overnutrition have significant effects on the growth of infants and young children. "Optimal" nutrition is almost impossible to define, and it will be argued that measurable outcomes which involve the growth and nutrition of infants and children must be assessed on reliable data for the population and age group involved.

WHAT IS SOMATIC GROWTH?

Growth is a major physiological feature of infancy, childhood, and adolescence which results from the interplay of various factors, genetic and environmental, which affect everyone and which are dependent on the availability of dietary energy and nutritients. Growth is a measurable characteristic which can be assessed in relation to the attained sizes of children and to the rates and patterns which precede their attained sizes at given ages and when growth ceases after adolescence.

Growth is a complex process which involves a wide spectrum of metabolic processes. Cellular aspects of growth have been discussed in detail elsewhere (e.g., Cheek, 1968) and aspects of body composition of infants and children and the growth of bodily organs have been summarized recently (Widdowson,

1985; Gracey, 1987). Those aspects of growth will not be discussed here—we will confine our attention to somatic growth of the whole child, after birth, and how this relates to nutritional status and its assessment by anthropometry.

VARIATIONS IN GROWTH

It is often not appreciated that growth is not a continuous, simple, steady, linear process of accumulation of body tissues. When examined over short intervals, somatic growth is sporadic, with periods when increments cannot be discerned being interspersed with others when growth is much more rapid and measurable. Furthermore, growth "spurts" are characteristic of different periods of growth; the most rapid periods of postnatal growth are in the first few months of life and during adolescence. Another important, and sometimes overlooked, feature of growth is the wide variation in growth rates which occurs in different, normal individuals. These variations in normal growth patterns are important for clinicians and others who work with growing children to appreciate because the "average" patterns of growth which are illustrated in growth charts can, misleadingly, suggest that growth is a smoother process than it really is. An example of this (Fig. 1) is the fitted velocity curves (light lines) of five different girls plotted against chronological age compared with the average values calculated at each age and fitted by the same function (thick line); quite obviously, the "average" curve gives a misleading idea of what occurs in different individuals at different ages during their adolescent growth spurts (Marubini, 1978). If the five velocity curves are plotted according to their time of maximal velocity (right), the resultant mean constant curve (broken line) gives a better idea of the pattern of growth which occurred in those five individuals.

THE MAIN PHASES OF POSTNATAL GROWTH AND CHANGE IN BODILY PROPORTIONS

Birth occurs when weight gain is more rapid than at any time of postnatal life and, remarkably, this process of weight gain normally continues virtually without interruption (Widdowson, 1985; Thomson et al., 1968; Tanner et al., 1966). The first few months of postnatal life are characterized by very rapid growth in weight and in length. This is more apparent if growth is expressed as *velocity* of gain in weight and length over this period rather than as attained weight and length over the same period of time (Fig. 2).

Infancy (the first 12 months of life) is characterized by very rapid growth, fastest immediately after birth and slowing sharply by 12 months of age. Different anthropometric dimensions change at different rates; breadth of the hips and shoulders, for example, increases by 55% in boys in the first year and by 54% in infant girls, while the crown–rump length increases by 45% (boys) and 42% (girls). During that time the head circumference measurements increase by 39% and 35% (Hansman, 1970).

In early childhood most bodily dimensions grow in a more or less linear fashion, as do height and weight, although rates of growth of these dimensions

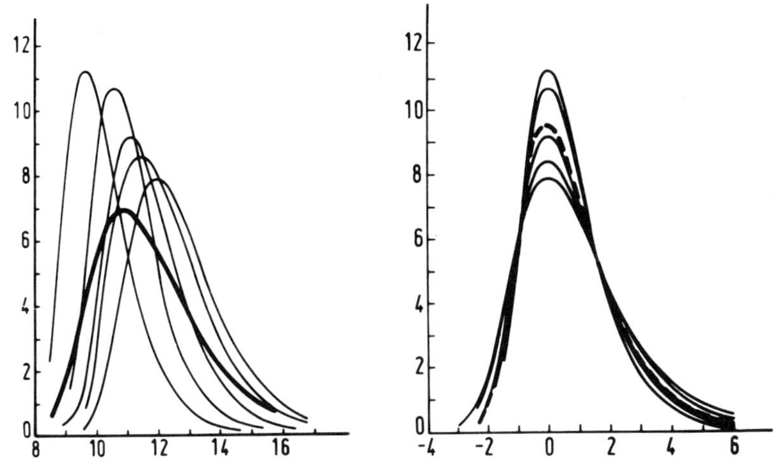

Fig. 1. Five individual velocity curves **(left)** and the velocity curve fitted to average values (thick line). In the figure on the **right** the same velocity curves are plotted not by chronological age (as on the left) but according to their time of maximum velocity. The mean constant curve (interrupted line) gives a better idea of the velocity of growth which the individuals experienced. (Reproduced from Marubini, 1978, with permission of the publisher.)

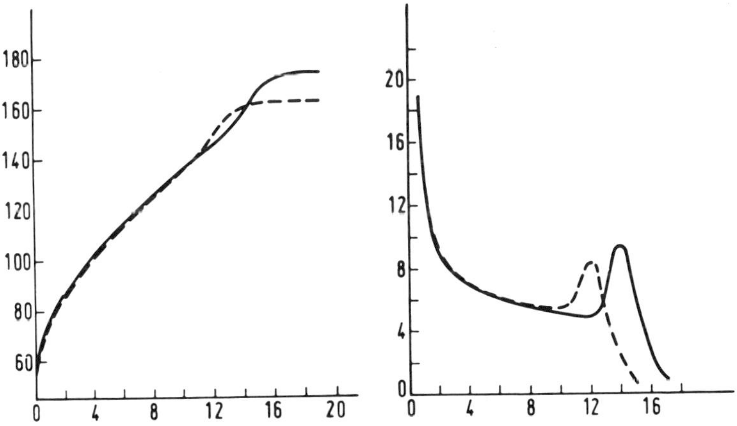

Fig. 2. Attained growth in supine length and height (cm) of boys (continuous line) and girls (interrupted line) by years is shown on the **left.** Their rate of growth (growth velocity) in cm/y is shown on the **right.** (Reproduced from Tanner et al., 1966, with permission of the publisher.)

are not necessarily the same. Despite these differences in rates of growth, they tend to be related by an exponential function such as $y = \chi^a$, where y and χ are the bodily dimensions and a the exponential relationship between them. This constant relationship between growth dimensions is referred to as allometry.

Through infancy, childhood, and adolescence, there is a characteristic change in bodily proportions. At all stages of growth the dimensions of the head are relatively advanced and closer to adult size than are those of the trunk, which in turn is in advance of the limbs. The advanced relative size of the head and skull is due partly to the relatively mature size of the brain in infancy and early childhood. These differences are reflected by the ratio of vertical head height to total length (stature), which in the normal neonate is 1 : 4, while in the normal adult this ratio of vertical head height to total height (erect stature) is almost double that (about 1 : 7.5).

During the adolescent growth spurt, the major skeletal differences between males and females emerge; the shoulders become relatively wider than the pelvis in males and the reverse occurs in females. These differences are accentuated by the relative increase in deposition of fat around the pelvic girdle in females and by deposition of fat in the breast tissue and upper arms in adolescent girls. A rapid increase in height also occurs in adolescence—this begins at about 10.5–11 years in girls and at about 12.5–13 years in boys (Fig. 2). There are also major sex differences in the rate of acquisition of lean body weight in adolescence. Boys have a fast and sustained increase in growth of lean weight with a slight increase in fat in early puberty, followed by a decline. On the other hand, girls acquire less lean weight and develop more body fat. The increase in lean weight in adolescent males coincides with the most rapid increase in height (Parizkova, 1977) and continues into the early part of the third decade (Forbes, 1978; Burmeister and Bingert, 1967); in females the increase in lean weight ceases by about 18 years of age, by which time gain in height has declined remarkably (Tanner, 1962). The overall gain in lean body weight in males during the second decade is about 100%; in females the increase is only about 50%. When considering the eventual, overall proportions of "average" males and females, it is useful to remember that boys and girls are approximately the same height when the pubertal growth spurt starts in girls; boys then have a bigger growth in height and have approximately two years more of preadolescent growth than girls—when their growth spurt commences they are, on average, 10 cm taller than the average girl was at the start of her adolescent growth spurt.

NUTRITIONAL AND ENERGY REQUIREMENTS

Growth involves nutritional and energy costs, and estimation of the individual infant's or child's requirements must include this as well as the needs for physical activity, basal metabolism, and the repair of damaged or diseased tissues. The nutritional requirements of infants and children are calculated based on these general principles. Recommendations about these requirements are given by the Ministry of Health (1968), FAO/WHO (1973), FAO/WHO/UNU (1985), the Food and Nutrition Board (1980), and the American Academy of Pediatrics (1985). Recommendations about dietary requirements are largely based on a combination of results of animal experimental studies and small numbers of metabolic balance studies which have been done on humans in controlled environments, and on epidemiological data from well-nourished and undernourished populations. To some extent, published recommendations are arbitrary, and recent alterations (mostly downwards) to recommended energy intakes for infants help illustrate this point well (Table 1). The alterations which were made recently to dietary intake requirements for infants and preschool children were based to some extent on an analysis by Whitehead et al. (1981) of 16 studies carried out in Canada, Sweden, the United Kingdom, and the United States using a variety of methods to document dietary intakes in infants and children who were considered to be growing normally in relation to internationally used (NCHS) reference values for growth (NCHS, 1976). This brings us to the dilemmas involved in deciding what is normal growth in infancy and childhood as well as assessing different methods which are used to estimate energy intakes in infants and children.

Dietary methods used in the studies analysed by Whitehead et al. (1981) to assess energy intakes included test weighing of breast-fed infants (Wallgren, 1944–1945; Hofvander et al., 1979; Chandra, 1981); 24-hour recall diet histories (Ferris et al., 1980); three- to five-day records of food consumption (Yeung et al., 1980; Morgan et al., 1976; Morgan and Mumford., 1977); weighed records over several days (Black et al., 1976; DHSS, 1975); and delivering of measured supplies of all foods delivered to the mothers' homes (Fomon et al., 1971). Another dilemma which this involves is the impact of different patterns of infant- and child-feeding practices on the growth of healthy youngsters.

PATTERNS OF NORMAL GROWTH

The pioneering studies by Fomon et al. (1971) in the United States carefully documented the patterns of growth in 142 "normal" white infants in Iowa

TABLE 1. Energy Requirements for Infants: Comparison of FAO/WHO (1973) Figures With Updated Recommendations of FAO/WHO/UNU (1985)

	kcal/kg		kJ/kg	
Age (months)	1973	1985	1973	1985
0–3	120	116	500	485
3–6	115	99	480	415
6–9	110	95	460	400
9–12	105	101	440	420
Average over first year	112	103	470	430

whose mothers chose not to breast-feed their babies. The mothers agreed to take part in studies of dietary patterns, nutrient intakes, and growth of their infants and were given nine artificial formulas each providing 67 kcal/dL. More than 90% of subjects enrolled in the study completed the planned period of observation to 112 days (16 weeks). The results were presented as 10th, 25th, 50th, 75th, and 90th centile values for gain in weight and length for each sex. It was found that average gains in weight and length were greater in formula-fed infants than in a group of breast-fed infants studied previously but that the differences were not statistically significant. The investigators did comment, however, that the breast-fed infants were "a highly selected group." The work of Fomon and his colleagues, based largely on studies in bottle-fed infants, has been used extensively to help estimate the dietary intakes required by infants to sustain normal growth.

Other workers have found that breast-fed babies grow more slowly during infancy than do those who are bottle-fed. These include studies from the United States (Owen et al., 1984; Ferris et al., 1980; Duncan et al., 1984); Europe (Salmenperä et al., 1985); and Australia (Hitchcock et al., 1986). Our Australian study included prospectively collected data from 394 infants who were attending metropolitan and rural child health centres within 400 km of Perth (Hitchcock et al., 1982a, 1985). From birth to 3 months, weight gains were similar for boys (2.5 kg) and for girls (2.3 kg) whether they were breast-fed or bottle-fed. From 3 to 6 months weight gains were greater in infants who were bottle-fed from birth (2.0 kg for each sex) or breast-fed for only a short time (1.9 kg) than in those who were exclusively breast-fed for 6 months (1.6 kg) or longer (1.7 kg). Weight gains continued to be greater in the bottle-fed infants after the age of 6 months. Over the first 12 months of life, bottle-fed boys gained 410 g more and girls gained 750 g more than those who were breast-fed from birth (Hitchcock et al., 1985). Differences in growth rates between breast-fed and formula-fed infants (Taitz, 1971) appear to have lessened over recent years with the introduction of low-solute, so-called "humanized" milks (Holly and Cullen, 1977; Evans, 1978), and not all studies have shown these differences in growth between breast-fed and bottle-fed infants. Underwood and Hofvander (1982) reviewed the literature about this subject several years ago.

Our own studies of healthy, breast-fed Australian infants (Hitchock et al., 1981a) showed that they had weight gains in the second 3 months of infancy which were well below those reported from Britain (Ministry of Health, 1959): 1.70 kg for boys in Perth and 2.13 kg in the United Kingdom, and 1.71 kg for girls in Perth and 2.13 kg in Britain. The increments of our subjects in Perth, in fact, more closely resembled those reported by Waterlow (1979) for infants from 13 collated studies in less-developed countries than those reported from Britain. It should be emphasized that the Australian figures quoted came from healthy, well-nourished infants of healthy, well-nourished Australian mothers, mostly of British origins. Apart from the possibility that those British reference values used in that study are inappropriate for healthy, breast-fed infants, it is possible that the apparent decline in somatic growth or weight gain in the second quarter of infancy is a normal physiological phenomenon (Hitchcock et al., 1981a). Finnish infants who were breast-fed have also been shown to have slower length velocity after the age of 3 months than a group of infants who were weaned early and given bottle feeds plus solids (Salmenperä et al., 1985). The Finnish workers found that their breast-fed subjects had a protein intake of 0.9 g/kg/d, which was less than half the then-recommended daily allowance (2g/kg/d), and questioned whether their slower growth was physiological or if it might be due to nutritional deficiency.

More recently, Whitehead et al. (1986) showed that infants in Cambridge (England) had slower rates of growth than the NCHS (American) values and the Tanner (British) weight curves (Tanner et al., 1966), and that for most of infancy triceps and subscapular skinfold thicknesses stayed around the 10th centile of the corresponding Tanner reference children (Tanner and Whitehouse, 1975). Those workers concluded that babies grow differently now that infant feeding patterns have changed. One of their main concerns was that mothers who choose to use current growth charts to monitor the growth of their babies may be concerned that their babies' growth is slipping backwards across the percentiles.

Such studies call into question the use of well-established growth charts and their application in ethnically disparate populations, but, before this can be discussed, we must consider what growth charts are, how they are derived, and how they should be used. The use and misuse of growth charts has been discussed recently by Tanner (1986).

GROWTH CHARTS

Cross-Sectional Data

Most growth charts that are in widespread use are based on data from cross-sectional studies of apparently healthy infants and children. Cross-sectional studies are widely used for this purpose because they generate data quickly, are relatively easy to perform, and are inexpensive. If sufficient individuals are measured over a particular age range, say 0–5 years, the data can be expressed as centiles which give a good idea of the distribution of various anthropometric measurements at different ages.

Waterlow et al. (1977) have discussed the use and presentation of cross-sectional height and weight data for comparing the nutritional status of groups of children under the age of 10 years. These and other aspects about growth charts are discussed in Chapter 10, this volume.

Longitudinal Data

Longitudinal studies of growth have the major advantage of *continuity* over cross-sectional studies. Longitudinal data help demonstrate the *dynamic*, sequential nature of growth, which can then be expressed as growth *velocity* (e.g., length, height, or weight per month) over measured time periods. This shows quite clearly that growth in infancy and childhood is not a steady, simple process between two time points. Longitudinal studies involve measurements of the same individuals at different ages over a period of time (Meredith, 1955) and, therefore, take months or years to perform. This, and difficulties in retaining study subjects for repeated, regular physical measurements over long periods of time, limits the numbers of adequate longitudinal growth studies which have been performed.

Growth Velocity Charts

Growth velocity is demonstrably much more rapid during infancy and adolescence than at other times (Fig. 2). Measurement of growth velocity (i.e., weight/time or height/time) gives a much clearer indication of the peaking of the *rate* of growth during these growth spurts. This emphasizes the dynamic nature of growth which is nowhere near so evident if charts of attained (or "distance") weight or height are used (Fig. 2). This has led to the development of velocity growth standards (Roche and Himes, 1980) whose use is discussed elsewhere (Chapter 10, this volume; Tanner et al., 1966; Marshall, 1977, Roche and Himes, 1980).

REFERENCE VALUE FOR GROWTH

Reference values for growth in childhood are sometimes referred to as growth "standards." This term should be avoided because it implies the use of reference measurements like a gold standard or as goals which children should be expected to reach at different ages. International reference values, like the NCHS growth charts (Hamill et al., 1977) or the World Health Organization growth charts (WHO, 1978), are appropriate sources of references for expected growth at different ages and for international comparisons of growth of different groups of children. They can be used in clinical paediatrics to show alterations in an individual child's pattern of growth and response to therapy; minor differences of national median values and centile distributions from international reference values are, in general, unimportant in the clinical context. The NCHS charts (Hamill et al., 1977) were prepared from nationally representative American samples, and it has been suggested that they will be applicable for many years because of the documented cessation of secular trends in growth in the United States (Roche and Himes, 1980).

Locally derived reference values for growth are used in many countries and should be useful if the samples on which they are based are sufficiently large and representative of the whole population. This is often not possible, and there is disagreement about which reference values to use when adequate, locally representative references are not available. These issues are discussed in more detail in Chapter 10, this volume. The potential difficulties with using international reference values, such as the NCHS values, are most evident in developing countries where undernutrition is prevalent. The strong impact of environmental factors, which can overwhelm the genetic factors in the growth of young children growing up in developing countries, has been well demonstrated by Martorell (1984). He showed that median heights of 7-year-old boys from the highest socioeconomic backgrounds in several developing countries were not vastly different and were of the same order as the 50th centile value for the NCHS growth charts (Fig. 3); on the other hand, significant stunting occurred in boys of the same age from the lowest socioeconomic backgrounds in the same countries. This raises issues central to our theme because of the widespread impact of undernutrition and the adverse nutritional effects of high rates of infections on the growth patterns of children growing up in developing countries. This is considered in more detail below.

SECULAR TRENDS IN GROWTH

The earlier physical maturation and larger attained sizes of succeeding generations of children in industrialized societies is referred to as the "secular trend" in growth (Tanner et al., 1982) and is generally attributed to improved standards of living and health and better nutrition, in particular (van Wier-

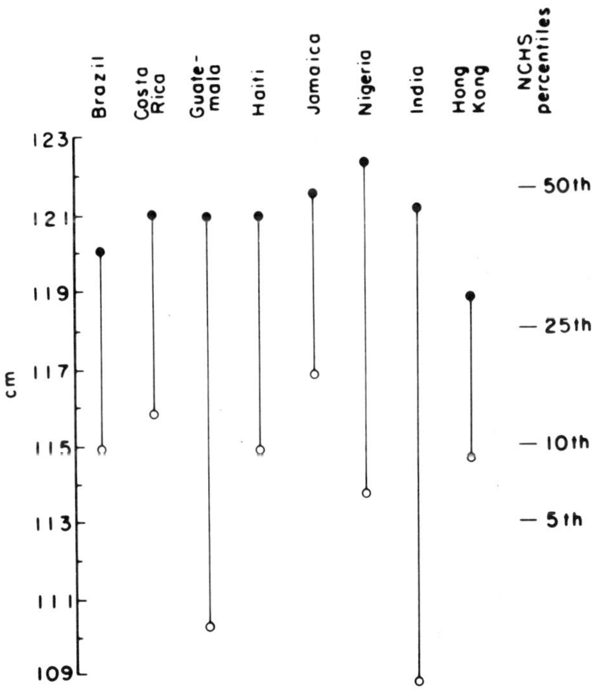

Fig. 3. Median heights of 7-year-old boys from the highest socioeconomic backgrounds (●) from several countries compared with boys of the same age from the lowest socioeconomic backgrounds (○) in the same countries. The NCHS 5th, 10th, 25th, and 50th centiles are shown on the right for comparison. (Reproduced from Martorell, 1984, with permission of the publisher.)

ingen, 1986). The rapidity of this trend is shown by the experience in Norway over the six decades from 1920 to 1975 (Brundtland et al., 1980); this also shows that environmental influences can have an acute, negative impact on growth as well as the usual upward progression of growth rates and sizes of children which occurs with improved standards of living and health.

This trend for modern children in the West to be larger than previous generations cannot be relentlessly progressive, and there is evidence that secular trends in growth in the United States have reached a "plateau" and have ceased (NCHS, 1978), so much so that in populations of high socioeconomic levels, the secular move to tall height and early maturation appear to have lost their discriminative usefulness as a health indicator (van Wieringen, 1986). Perhaps children in such countries have already reached their optimal size. Meanwhile, in countries where industrialization is proceeding rapidly, secular trends in growth are occurring; the industrializing nations of Southeast Asia demonstrate this.

Singapore is an urban Asian republic with a predominantly Chinese population, and its recent rapid socioeconomic development has been accompanied by improved health and a significant increase in the height of its children (Wong et al., 1972). The local approach there is to produce their own cross-sectional growth charts and to update them every 5–10 years (Wong, 1985). A recent study of ethnic Chinese children aged 5 years and under living in London showed that they were taller and heavier than Chinese children in Hong Kong (Wheeler and Tan, 1983) and in terms of percentage height for age were taller than their own mothers. A secular trend in growth of Japanese children living in the United States has also been well documented (Eveleth and Tanner, 1976). Korean children born and raised in Japan were shown to be taller, heavier, and relatively longer legged than Korean children living in their own country (Kim, 1982); these differences have been attributed to improved living conditions and food consumption patterns (Lee et al., 1981). This evidence for the ability of Asian children to alter their growth patterns in response to altered living circumstances should, perhaps, urge caution about suggestions that their growth patterns are "different" (Falkner, 1985). Where industrial and social development are occurring rapidly, it can be expected that secular trends in growth are also taking place—this strengthens the desire to have locally relevant growth references, if possible.

ETHNIC DIFFERENCES IN GROWTH

Ethnic differences in growth patterns, which to some extent involve genetic factors, accentuate the complexities of selecting the "right" growth references. Our own work with Australian Aboriginal children illustrates this point well. In a large, cross-sectional survey of young Aborigines in Western Australia, we were faced with the dilemma of which growth references to choose since no growth charts for Aboriginal children, based on sufficiently large numbers representative of healthy Aborigines, are available (Gracey et al.,

1983). Selection of appropriate reference values for Aborigines is complicated by their skeletal differences from Europeans (Abbie, 1974), which include relatively higher limb-to-trunk ratios (Abbie, 1976). However, this is also complicated by the high incidence of infectious diseases, and unsatisfactory dietary practices and their consequences in young Australian Aborigines (Kettle, 1966; Gracey et al., 1983). When our survey data (Fig. 4) are compared visually against three sets of reference values, it can be seen that more of the Aboriginal subjects would be considered to be "undernourished" if they were compared with the then Australian national growth charts (NHMRC, 1975), However, those Australian figures were not representative of the Australian population, and their use has recently been replaced by the NCHS growth charts (NHMRC, 1986). We chose to compare our survey data to the NCHS reference values. This showed that 14% of infants (0–12 months) and 22% of older children (12–30 months) were underweight, i.e., <80% of standard weight for age. Twelve percent of all subjects were stunted but, by weight-for-

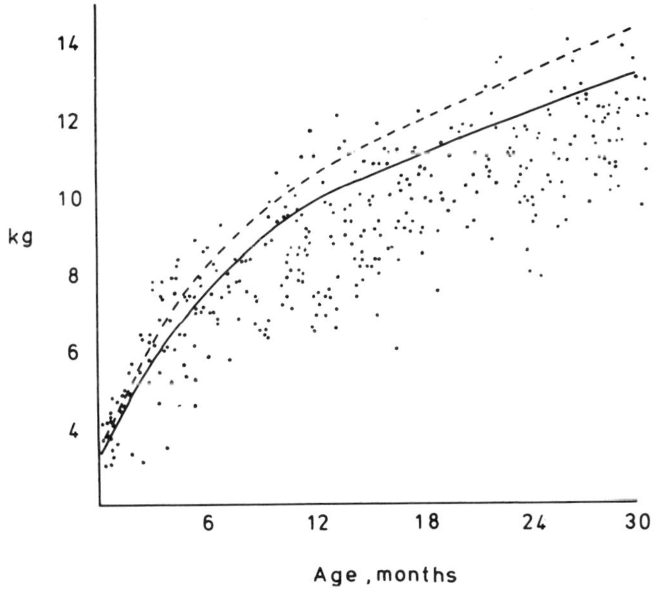

Fig. 4. Weight-for-age distribution of Australian Aboriginal children aged up to 30 months in or around rural towns in Western Australia. Each dot represents an individual child's weight at the age shown. The interrupted line (top) is the 50th centile of the 1975 Australian National Health and Medical Research Council reference value. The continuous line (bottom) is the 50th centile of the NCHS reference values. (Reproduced from Gracey et al., 1983, with permission of the publisher.)

length analysis, only 2.5% of subjects were moderately malnourished (<80% standard weight for length). Use of the then-recommended Australian growth standards (NHMRC, 1975) would have given a much less favourable view of the nutritional status of these Aboriginal children. The information available with the NCHS tables allows statistical comparisons to be made with other sets of data such as ours. Although the NCHS growth charts may not be entirely appropriate for comparisons with the growth of Australian Aboriginal infants and children, they at least provide a very well documented, independent set of reference values against which these comparisons can be made. This will permit valid comparisons (through the independent reference values) against other groups of children in other parts of the world and will enable monitoring of the nutritional status of Aboriginal children, over time, against interventions aimed at improving their standards of health and nutrition.

Assessment of the nutritional status of ethnic minorities, such as Asian children, in countries like Australia, Britain, and the United States presents similar difficulties in selecting appropriate growth references for comparisons. Furthermore, it should be anticipated that children in these minority groups will show secular trends in growth while this growth may have slowed or ceased in most of the population in their countries of adoption.

INFLUENCE OF UNDERNUTRITION ON GROWTH

Globally, undernutrition in developing countries and overnutrition in industrialized societies are the most common nutritional disorders of infants and children. Malnutrition in children in developing countries has repeatedly been linked with impaired growth (Mata, 1978), but the well-documented synergism of nutrition and infection (Scrimshaw et al., 1959) is so complex that the adverse nutritional impacts of repeated infections cannot be neatly separated from the impact of undernutrition itself.

Two clinical examples are given which illustrate how undernutrition in children can retard growth and how these children respond with catch-up growth when they are successfully treated. The first example is anorexia nervosa, in which undernutrition is clearly attributable to impaired nutrient and energy intakes. Although this condition is rare in young children, it does occur from time to time, and Prader et al. (1963) have shown how this can retard weight and length velocity, attained weight and length, and skeletal maturation even in the first few years of life. Catch-up growth occurs during phases of dietary and nutritional recovery. A very similar pattern has been shown repeatedly in children with untreated coeliac disease (Prader et al., 1963; Anderson, 1987) where malnutrition and growth failure occur because of intestinal malabsorption; catch-up growth occurs quickly in response to a gluten-free diet (Fig. 5).

This is clearly associated with histological repair of the intestinal mucosal damage, recovery of intestinal digestive and absorptive functions, and improved appetite and nutrient and energy intake. Other malabsorptive diseases

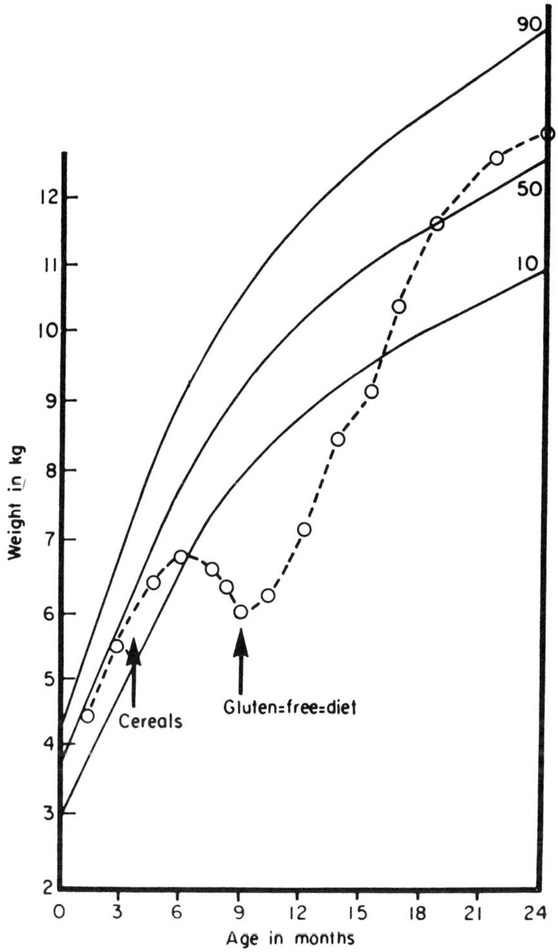

Fig. 5. Growth chart of a child with coeliac disease. Introduction of gluten containing cereals in the diet was followed by slowing of growth and failure to thrive. After diagnosis and the introduction of a gluten-free diet, there was a rapid gain in weight and recovery to the child's normal growth pattern. (Reproduced from Anderson et al., 1987, with permission of the publisher.)

in children show similar nutritional responses and catch-up growth, but in many patients, e.g., in cystic fibrosis, clinical and nutritional recovery may be delayed by complicating features such as chronic respiratory tract infections.

Causes of impaired intestinal function and malabsorption in malnutrition are complex and are often accompanied by deficiencies of multiple dietary nutrients, such as zinc. Major factors include repeated gastrointestinal infections and parasitic infestations and the extensive mucosal injury which they produce, leading to impaired mucosal digestion and transmucosal transport of nutrients (Gracey, 1981). Bacterial contamination of intestinal secretions in malnourished children is associated with altered bile salt metabolism which, in turn, interferes with the handling of nutrients, including fat. Bacterial toxin–induced malabsorption of carbohydrates is another possible complication with nutritional consequences (Thelen et al., 1978). Apart from the intestinal lesion in malnutrition, there can be significant impairment of hepatic and exocrine pancreatic function which can compromise nutritional status. Collectively, these gastrointestinal features illustrate the contribution of the vicious circle of *malnutrition-malabsorption-malnutrition* to impaired nutrition and growth in children in developing countries (Gracey, 1985). These gastrointestinal aspects of nutrition and growth are often subclinical, and it is very likely that a significant proportion of such children have unrecognized chronic diarrhoea and malabsorption (Gracey, 1988).

There are gastrointestinal diseases of children in which deficiences of specific nutrients are involved (Anderson et al., 1987). These include 1) isolated lipase deficiency, a specific defect in fat digestion, 2) trypsinogen deficiency, in which protein digestion is affected, 3) the rare disease acrodermatitis enteropathica, which is associated with zinc deficiency, and 4) inborn errors of metabolism such as chloride-losing diarrhoea, glucose-galactose malabsorption, and sucrase-isomaltase deficiency, which involve specific defects of intestinal absorption and digestion. Malabsorption of nutrients is often secondary to underlying gastrointestinal diseases, such as gastroenteritis; examples include secondary lactose intolerance and protein-losing enteropathy. All these gastrointestinal diseases have nutritional implications and can cause impaired growth and failure to thrive. Growth can, of course, be adversely affected by a wide range of diseases, and impaired growth is a sensitive indicator of organic disease in infants and young children (Kristianson et al., 1981).

INFANT FEEDING PRACTICES AND THE INFLUENCE OF OVERNUTRITION ON GROWTH

In Western industrialized countries, including Australia (Lawson et al., 1978; Hitchcock et al., 1986); the United States (Martinez and Dodd, 1983; Martinez and Nalezienski, 1979, 1981); Britain (Sloper et al., 1977; Wharton, 1982; Whitehead et al., 1986); and Scandinavia (Hofvander and Petros-Barvazian, 1978; Vahlquist, 1975; Verkasalo, 1980; Biering-Sorenson et al., 1980) there has been a revival in breast-feeding in recent years accompanied by a delay in the introduction of solids. This return to more natural infant feeding practices is most marked in the higher socioeconomic classes (Hitchcock et al., 1986). Another important recent change in infant feeding practices is the now widespread use of so-called humanized infant formulas. These new commercial preparations are made to resemble the chemical composition of human milk.

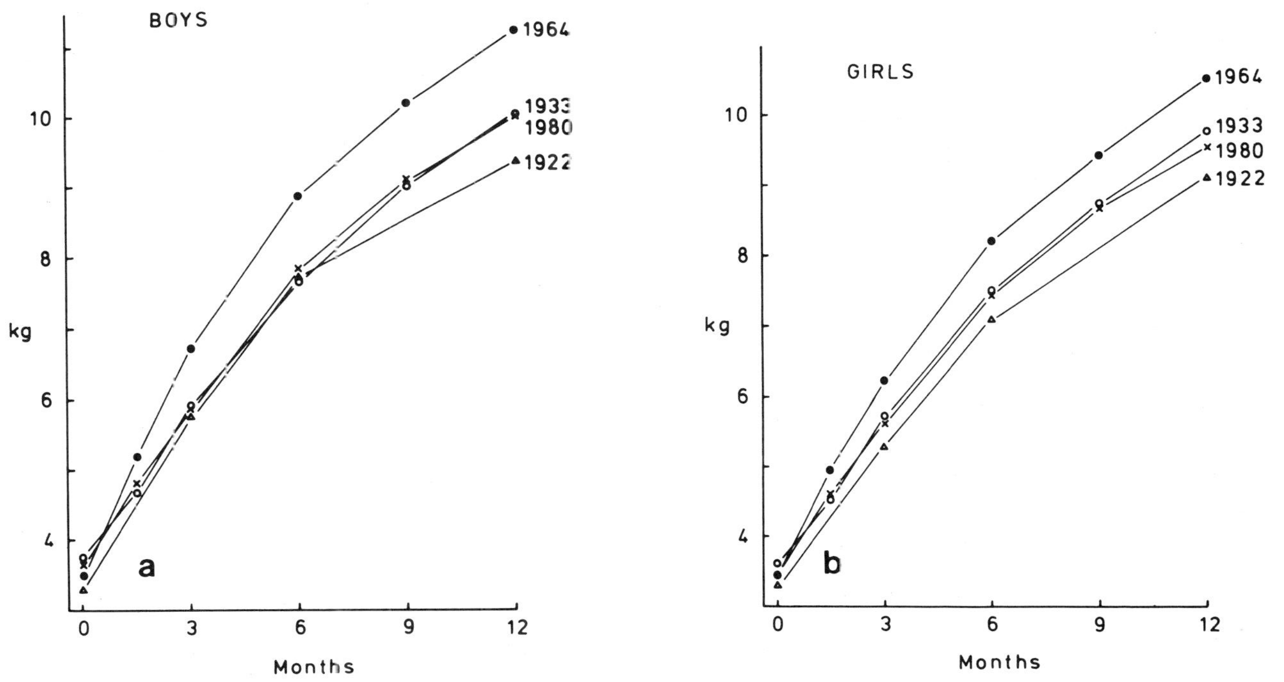

Fig. 6. Mean weights of Australian boys **(a)** and girls **(b)** in studies published from the 1920s to the 1980s. Weight gains in infancy were highest in the mid-1960s. (Redrawn from Hitchcock et al., 1981b.)

At 12 months of age, 35% of food energy in Australian infants came from milk and formula (Owles et al., 1982). At 2 years this proportion had dropped to 20% (Hitchcock et al., 1982b) and then to 14%, 13%, and 11% at 3, 4, and 5 years of age. Other features to emerge from our study were that there was little increase in the absolute weight of food consumed between the ages of 1 and 5 years and the fact that eating patterns seemed to be well established by the age of 2–3 years.

The changes in patterns of infant feeding practices in Australia over the past 50 years seem to have been accompanied by quite remarkable changes in weight gains in Australian infants over that time. Average birth weights of the subjects in our prospective Perth Child Growth Study who were born in 1979 were 3.56 kg for boys and 3.47 kg for girls; this is similar to those found by Bell and Lay (1968) in the mid-1960s, by Boulton (1981) in the late 1970s, and slightly less than by Clements in 1933. Figure 6 shows that median weight gains at 3, 6, 9, and 12 months of age were much greater in the 1964 sample than in the other studies.

It is tempting to suggest that the increased weight gains of infants which occurred in Australia and other Western countries in the 1960s and early 1970s were due to the widespread early introduction of solids, such as cereals (Shukla et al., 1972; Oakley, 1977), and the use of cow's milk formulas, often made up too concentrated (Fomon, 1971; Taitz, 1976) and with sugar added. This is important because that pattern of infant feeding practices was common in Western countries at that time and many of the growth charts still in use in some countries were based on measurements made of children in the 1960s and early 1970s.

The recent return to breast-feeding has been accompanied by significant changes in nutrient intake patterns in these infants. Protein intakes were much less in Perth in the first 6 months of life than in earlier studies of predominantly bottle-fed infants. The mean daily protein intake of infants aged 6 months in the mid-1960s, for example, (Hankin, 1965) was 36 g, compared to the estimated 18.4 g for boys and 15.1 g for girls in our study which was done more than 10 year later. By 1 year of age, when mixed feeding had become well established, these differences were much less. A similar trend has been found also in the United States (USDA, 1980).

The increased popularity of breast-feeding which has occurred also in Britain was commented on by Wharton (1982), who showed that in 1980 one-third more babies were breast-fed at birth while at 4 months of age the number being breast-fed was twice that in 1975. At the same time the median age for introduction of solids had moved from 8 to 12 months of age; as many others, including ourselves, have found, solids were introduced into the diet in breast-fed babies later than in bottle-fed babies. Another interesting facet of Wharton's commentary of an official British document (Martin and Monk, 1982) about breast-feeding in 1980 was that nearly all the bottle-fed babied were being given a satisfactory infant formula—98% at 6 weeks and 94% at 4 months.

SUMMARY

Growth is a fundamental physical feature of infancy and childhood which can be used to advantage to assess the physical well-being of individuals and groups of youngsters in different circumstances around the world. In order to do this, we need to understand normal patterns of growth in infants and children and their wide, normal variations and how growth is influenced by genetic and environmental factors.

Growth imposes nutritional demands which have been much better defined in recent years. Environmental influences, particularly infections and inadequate nutrition, adversely affect patterns of growth in children in underdeveloped countries and other disadvantaged circumstances, and these are crucial considerations in assessing the growth patterns of different groups of children. Infant feeding practices and the composition of milks fed to infants and young children can also have strong influences on patterns of growth.

Assessment of the growth and nutritional status of individuals and groups of children by use of anthropometry must be based on sound and appropriate reference charts and tables and should take into account the numerous normal variables and disease states which affect growth and nutritional status.

REFERENCES

Abbie AA (1974): Physical standards of nomadic Aboriginal children. Med J Aust 1:470–471.

Abbie AA 1976): Morphological variation in the adult Australian Aboriginal. In Kirk RL, Thorne AG (eds): "The Origins of the Australians." Atlantic City, NJ: Humanities Press, pp 211–214.

American Academy of Pediatrics, Committee on Nutrition (1985): "Pediatric Nutrition Handbook." Forbes CB, Woodruff CW (eds): Elk Grove Village, Ill: American Academy of Pediatrics.

Anderson CM (1987): Coeliac Disease. In Anderson CM, Burke V, Gracey M (eds): "Paediatric Gastroenterology." 2nd ed Oxford: Blackwell Scientific, pp 375–400.

Anderson CM, Burke V, Gracey M (1987): "Paediatric Gastroenterology." 2nd edn. Oxford. Blackwell Scientific.

Bell JW, Lay PM (1968): The growth of Australian infants during the first year of life: A comparison, 1933 and 1964. Med J Aust i:541–544.

Biering-Sørensen F, Hilden J, Biering-Sørensen K (1980): Breast feeding on the increase (editorial). J Trop Pediatr 26:ii–iii.

Black AE, Billewicz WZ, Thomson AM (1976): The diets of preschool children in Newcastle upon Tyne 1968–71. Br J Nutr 35:105–113.

Boulton J (1981): Nutrition in childhood and its relationships to early somatic growth, body fat, blood pressure, and physical fitness. Acta Paediatr Scand Suppl 284.

Brundtland GH, Liestol K, Walloe L (1980): Height, weight, and menarcheal age of Oslo schoolchildren during the last 60 years. Ann Hum Biol 7:307–322.

Burmeister W, Bingert A (1967): Die quantitativen Veränderungen der menschlichen Zellmasse zwischen dem 8 und 90 Lebensjahr. Klin Wochenschr 45:409–416.

Chandra RK (1981): Breast feeding, growth and morbidity. Nutr Res 1:25–31.

Cheek DB (1968): "Human Growth." Philadelphia: Lea & Febiger.

Clements FW (1933): The growth curve of Australian infants during the first year of age. Med J Aust 1:543–549.
Department of Health and Social Security (DHSS) (1975): A nutrition survey of preschool children 1967–8. Rep Health Soc Subj No. 10. London: Her Majesty's Stationery Office.
Duncan B, Schaefer C, Sibley B, Fonseca NM (1984): Reduced growth velocity in exclusively breast-fed infants. Am J Dis Child 138:309–313.
Evans TJ (1978): Growth and milk intake of normal infants. Arch Dis Child 53:749–751.
Eveleth PB, Tanner JM (1976): "Worldwide Variations in Human Growth." Cambridge: Cambridge University Press.
Falkner F (1985): "Monitoring Growth." In Gracey M, Falkner F (eds): "Nutritional Needs and Assessment of Normal Growth." New York: Raven Press, pp 123–137.
FAO/WHO (1973): "Energy and Protein Requirements." Report of a joint FAO/WHO Ad hoc Expert Committee, World Health Organization Technical Report Series, No. 522. Geneva: WHO.
FAO/WHO/UNU (1985): "Energy and Protein Requirements." World Health Organization Technical Report Series, No. 724. Geneva: WHO.
Ferris AG, Laus MM, Hosmer DW, Beal VA (1980): The effect of diet on weight gain in infancy. Am J Clin Nutr 33:2635–2642.
Fomon SJ (1971): A pediatrician looks at early nutrition. Bull NY Acad Med 47:569–578.
Fomon SJ, Thomas LN, Filer LJ, Ziegler EE, Leonard MT (1971): Food consumption and growth of normal infants fed milk-based formulas. Acta Paediatr Scand, Suppl 223.
Food and Nutrition Board, National Reasearch Council (1980): "Recommended Dietary Allowances." 9th rev ed. Washington, DC: National Academy of Sciences.
Forbes GB (1978): Body composition in adolescence. In Falkner F, Tanner JM (eds): "Human Growth. Vol 2." New York: Plenum Press, pp 234–272.
Gracey MS (1981): Nutrition, bacteria and the gut. Br Med Bull 37:71–75.
Gracey M (1985): "Diarrhoeal Disease and Malnutrition: A Clinical Update." Edinburgh: Churchill Livingstone.
Gracey M (1987): Normal growth and nutrition. World Rev Nutr Diet 49:160–210.
Gracey M (1988): Bacterial causes of acute and chronic diarrhea in children. In Lebenthal E (ed): "Textbook of Gastroenterology and Nutrition in Early Childhood." 2nd ed. New York: Raven Press.
Gracey M, Murray H, Hitchcock NE, Owles EN, Murphy BP (1983): The nutrition of Australian Aboriginal infants and young children. Nutr Res 3:133–147.
Hamill PVV, Drizd TA, Johnson CL, Reed RB, Roche AF (1977): Growth curves for children birth–18 years, United States. DHEW Publ. No. (PHS) 78-1650, Vital and Health Statistics, Ser. 2, No. 165. Washington, DC: GPO.
Hankin ME (1965): Infant feeding. Food Nutr Notes Rev 22:47–55.
Hansman C (1970): Anthropometry and related data, anthropometry skinfold thickness measurements. In McCammon RW (ed): "Human Growth and Development." Springfield, Ill: CC Thomas, pp 103–154.
Hitchcock NE, Gracey M, Gilmour AI (1985): The growth of breast fed and artificially fed infants from birth to twelve months. Acta Paediatr Scand 74:240–245.
Hitchcock NE, Gracey M. Gilmour AI, Owles EN (1986): "Nutrition and Growth in Infancy and Early Childhood. A Longitudinal Study from Birth to 5 Years." Monographs in Paediatrics. Basel: Karger.
Hitchcock NE, Gracey M, Owles EN (1981a): Growth of healthy breast-fed infants in the first six months. Lancet 2:64–65.

Hitchcock NE, McGuiness D, Gracey M (1982a): Growth and feeding practices of Western Australian infants. Med J Aust 2:64–65.
Hitchcock NE, Owles EN, Gracey M (1981b): Breast feeding and growth of healthy infants. Med J Aust 2:536–537.
Hitchcock NE, Owles EN, Gracey M (1982b): Dietary energy and nutrient intakes and growth of healthy Australian infants in the first year of life. Nutr Res 2:13–19.
Hofvander Y, Hagman S, Sjolin S (1979): Breast milk consumption in healthy Swedish infants. Var F da 31 (suppl 3): 192.
Hofvander Y, Petros-Barvazian A (1978): WHO collaborative study on breast feeding. Acta Paediatr Scand 67:556–560.
Holly D, Cullen D (1977): A comparison of weight gain in breast fed and bottle fed babies. Public Health London 91:113–116.
Kettle ES (1966): Weight and height curves for Australian Aboriginal infants and children. Med J Aust 1:972–977.
Kim YS (1982): Growth status of Korean schoolchildren in Japan. Ann Hum Biol 9:453–458.
Kristianson B, Karlberg J, Fallströuc SP (1981): Infants with low rate of weight gain. Acta Paediatr Scand 70:665–663, 663–668.
Lawson JS, Mays CA, Oliver TI (1978): The return to breast feeding. Med J Aust 2:229–230.
Lee SK, Kimura J, Toyokawa H (1981): Food consumption in Koreans living in Tokyo. Hum Ecol Race Hyg 47:162–163.
Marshall WA (1977): "Human Growth and Its Disorders." New York: Academic Press.
Martin J, Monk J (1982): "Infant Feeding 1980." Office of Population Censuses and Surveys. London: Her Majesty's Stationery Office.
Martinez GA, Dodd DA (1983): 1981 milk feeding patterns in the United States during the first 12 months of life. Pediatrics 71:166–170.
Martinez GA, Nalezienski JP (1979): The recent trend in breast feeding. Pediatrics 64:686–692.
Martinez GA, Nalezienski JP (1981): 1980 update : The recent trend in breast feeding. Pediatrics 667:260–263.
Martorell R (1984): Genetics, environment and growth : Issues in the assessment of nutritional status. In Velasquez A, Bourges H. (eds): "Genetic Factors in Nutrition." New York: Academic Press.
Marubini E (1978). Mathematical handling of long-term longitudinal data. In Falkner F, Tanner JM (eds): "Human Growth." London: Ballière Tindall.
Mata L (1978): "The Children of Santa Maria Cauqué. A prospective field study of health and growth." Cambridge, Mass: MIT Press.
Meredith HV (1955): Longitudinal anthropometric data in the study of individual growth. Ann NY Acad Sci 63:510–527.
Ministry of Health (1959): "Standards of Normal Weight in Infancy." Rep Public Health Med Subj No. 99. London: Her Majesty's Stationery Office.
Ministry of Health (1968): "A Pilot Study of Nutrition in Young Children in 1963." Rep Public Health Med Subj No. 118. London: Her Majesty's Stationery Office.
Morgan J, Mumford P (1977): Feeding practices and food intake of children under two years of age. Proc Nutr Soc 36:47A.
Morgan J, Mumford P, Evans E, Wells JKC (1976): Food intake and anthropometric data on children under 4 years old living in the south of England. Proc Nutr Soc 35:74A.
National Health and Medical Research Council (NHMRC) (1975): "Charts and Tables

of Heights, Masses and Head Circumferences of Infants and Children." Canberra: Australian Government Publishing Service.
National Health and Medical Research Council (NHMRC) (1986): "Report of the 101st Session." Canberra: Australian Government Publishing Service.
National Center for Health Statistics (NCHS) (1976): National Center for Health Statistics, growth charts 1976. Monthly Vital Statistics Report 25, No. 3 (suppl). DHEW Publ. No. (HRA) 76-1120. Rockville, Md: U.S. Department of Health, Education, and Welfare.
National Center for Health Statistics (NCHS) (1978): NCHS growth curves for children, birth to 18 years. DHEW Publ. No. (PHS) 78-1650 (Vital and health statistics; series 11; no. 165). Hyattsville, Md: U.S. Department of Health, Education and Welfare, 1977.
Oakley JR (1977): Differences in subcutaneous fat in breast- and formula-fed infants. Arch Dis Child 52:79–80.
Owen GM, Garry PJ, Hooper EM (1984): Feeding and growth of infants. Nutr Res 4:727–731.
Owles EN, Hitchcock NE, Gracey M (1982): Feeding patterns of Australian infants. Birth to one year. Hum Nutr Appl Nutr 36A:202–207.
Parizkova J (1977): "Body Fat and Physical Fitness." The Hague: Martinus Nijhoff.
Prader A, Tanner JM, Von Harnack GA (1963): Catch-up growth following illness of starvation. J Pediatr 62:646–659.
Roche AF, Himes JH (1980): Incremental growth charts. Am J Clin Nutr 33:2041–2052.
Salmenperä L, Perheentupa J, Sumes MA (1985): Exclusively breast-fed healthy infants grow slower than reference infants. Pediatr Res 19:307–312.
Scrimshaw NS, Taylor CE, Gordon JE (1959): Interactions of nutrition and infection. Am J Med Sci 237:367–403.
Shukla A, Forsyth HA, Anderson CM, Marwah SM (1972): Infantile overnutrition in the first year of life: A field study in Dudley, Worcestershire. Br Med J 4:507–515.
Sloper KS, Elsden E, Baum JD (1977): Increasing breast feeding in a community. Arch Dis Child 52:700–702.
Taitz LS (1971): Infantile overnutrition among artificially fed infants in the Sheffield region. Br Med J 1:315–316.
Taitz LS (1976): Relationship of infant feeding patterns to weight gain in the first weeks of life. In Laron Z (ed): "Pediatric and Adolescent Endocrinology. Vol 1, The Adipose Child." Basel: Karger, pp 60–65.
Tanner JM (1962): "Growth at Adolescence." 2nd ed. Oxford: Blackwell Scientific, Oxford.
Tanner JM (1986): Use and abuse of growth standards. In Falkner F, Tanner JM (eds): "Human Growth." 2nd ed. New York: Plenum Press, pp 95–109.
Tanner JM, Hayashi T, Preece MA, Cameron N (1982): Increase in length of leg relative to trunk in Japanese children and adults from 1957 to 1977; comparison with British and with Japanese Americana. Ann Hum Biol 9:411–424.
Tanner JM, Whitehouse RH (1975): Revised standards for triceps and subscapular skinfolds in British children. Arch Dis Child 50:142–145.
Tanner JM, Whitehouse RH, Takaishi M (1966): Standards from birth to maturity for height, weight, height velocity and weight velocity: British children, 1965. Arch Dis Child 41(pt 2):454–472; 613–635.
Thelen P, Burke V, Gracey M (1978): Effects of intestinal microorganisms on fluid and electrolyte transport in the jejunum of the rat. J Med Microbiol 11:463–470.
Thomson AM, Billewicz WZ, Hytten FE (1968): The assessment of fetal growth. J Obstet Gynaecol Br Commonwealth 75:903–916.

Underwood BA, Hofvander Y (1982): Appropriate timing for complementary feeding of the breast-fed infant. A review. Acta Paediatr Scand 294(suppl):1–32.

U.S. Department of Agriculture (USDA) (1980): Nationwide food consumption survey, 1977–78. Food Nutr Notes Rev 37:34–35. Abstract.

Vahlquist B (1975): Evolution of breast feeding in Europe. J Trop Pediatr Environ Child Health 21:11–18.

van Wieringen JC (1986): Secular growth changes. In Falkner F, Tanner JM (eds): "Human Growth." 2nd ed. New York: Plenum Press, pp 307–331.

Verkasalo M (1980): Recent trends in breast feeding in Southern Finland. Acta Paediat Scand 69:89–91.

Wallgren A (1944–1945): Breast milk consumption of healthy full-term infants. Acta Paediat Scand 32:778–790.

Waterlow JC (1979): Adequacy of breast feeding. Lancet 2:897–898.

Waterlow JC, Buzina R, Keller W, Lane JM, Nichaman MZ, Tanner JM (1977): The presentation and use of height and weight data for comparing the nutritional status of groups of children under the age of 10 years. Bull WHO 55:489–498.

Wharton B (1982): A quinquennium in infant feeding. Arch Dis Child 57:895–897.

Wheeler E, Tan SP (1983): Trends in the growth of ethnic Chinese children living in London. Ann Hum Biol 5:441–446.

Whitehead RG, Paul AA, Ahmed EA (1986): Weaning practices in the United Kingdom and variations in anthropometric development. Acta Paediat Scand 323(suppl):14–23.

Whitehead RG, Paul AA, Cole TJ (1981): A critical analysis of measured food energy intakes during infancy and early childhood in comparison with current international recommendations. J Hum Nutr 35:339–348.

Widdowson EM (1985): Growth and body composition in childhood. In Brunser O, Carrazza F, Gracey M, Nichols B, Senterre J (eds): "Clinical Nutrition of the Young Child." New York: Raven Press, pp 1–14.

Wong HB (1985): Growth monitoring. In Brunser O, Carrazza F, Gracey M, Nichols B, Senterre J (eds): "Clinical Nutrition of the Young Child." New York: Raven Press, pp 45–47.

Wong HB, Tye CY, Quek KM (1972): Anthropometric studies on Singapore children. J Singapore Paediatr Soc 14:68–89.

World Health Organization (WHO) (1978): A growth chart for international use in maternal and child health care. Guidelines for Primary Health Care Personnel. Geneva: WHO.

Yeung DL, Hall J, Leung M (1980): Adequacy of energy intake of infants. J Can Diet Assoc 41:48–52.

Anthropometric Assessment
of Nutritional Status, pages 51–82

4
Theoretical Considerations in the Measurement and Interpretation of Change in Adult Dimensions

STEPHEN M. BAILEY
Department of Anthropology, Tufts University, Medford, Massachusetts 02155

INTRODUCTION: WHAT IS IT THAT WE MEASURE?

When an English settler pointed and asked his companion the name of that large hopping animal, so goes the tale, the indigenous Australian's reply, "I don't know what you're asking," sounded to the settler like "Kan-gar-oo." This play on the hazards of linguistic referral holds a lesson for those who estimate adult nutritional status using physical dimensions. In a theoretical sense, our challenge also is one of referral. We point dimensional observations at biological referents and trust the line of sight is clear.

Like the tale's protagonists, we can generate ambiguous referrals. Unlike them, our referrals go well beyond ostension, or linking observation to object by pointing. A dimensional datum aims at several targets, ranging from its immediate referent to more distant biological correlates. What we measure, in other words, is always relational. The route, moreover, is indirect and often poorly described. Adults in particular are likely to present unmeasured or unmeasurable variables, such as age-related loss of tissue density or occult pathology, that intervene between measurement and referent. Further ambiguity is created by serial measurements. Time-dependent effects range from nonnutritional changes in subject and genotype–environmental interactions to cohort effects and drift in observer technique. They can be especially problematic when measurement occasions may span decades.

Given the complications, one might question the premise. Why not rely, for instance, on more "direct" observations from radiographs or serum biochemistries? One response is theoretical: All data, however straightforward they may appear, are signs pointing at objects, and none are immune from the hazards of referral. A second response is pragmatic: Anthropometric data meet the mandate of most clinical or epidemiological designs for estimates of adult nutritional status that are technically simple, noninvasive, inexpensive, and easily comparable. This need is particularly salient in the developing world, but it applies also to many arenas of health care in complex societies. A third response is institutional: Adult anthropometric data are required by basic research venues in human biology, nutrition, and medicine in order to quantify human physique, including shape. Accordingly, the relevant question becomes, which adult dimensional measurements offer the soundest biological interpretation?

Words, Maps, and Measurements

Answering this requires a venture into theory. The tale of kangaroo and settler signals the choice of an approach called "linguistic pragmatism" to how we acquire, represent, and interpret facts (Wartofsky, 1968). Application of this model to measurement activities is based on the assumption that instruments represent extensions of our senses (Ackermann, 1985), and that measurement outcomes represent extensions of our everyday significations; an anthropometric datum is an arbitrary numerical sign referring to the magnitude of a nutritional object. Rules analogous to semantic and syntactic transformations assign "meaning" to this sign by linking it to a specific biological referent and ordering the relations between this sign and others in the biological system. To take an example. "35 cm" has no nutritional meaning until it is assigned to "arm circumference." This datum, in turn, has no explanatory significance until incorporated into a map—we may consider it a sentence of sorts—that causally relates the magnitude of datum to others such as kilograms of body fat. Relating magnitudes also introduces the problem of precision, which will be covered in the section on Measuring True Referent Change.

Of course, the map of a dimensional referral cannot be perfect; if it were, it would cease to be a map and become the body itself. Rather, key elements of the map approach isomorphism, or the same form, as the "real" biological objects or processes. Other elements, most in fact, are ignored. The map, moreover, remains operable only through empirical confirmation, and intelligible only in the context of higher-order nutritional theories about how we decipher it. If such a process seems tortuous, it is no more so than that used by an astronomer to judge stellar evolution from bands on a spectrograph, or by a geneticist to discriminate molecular variation from fluorescent gels. As with everyday language, moreover, the complexity of scientific maps is masked by routinism.

It can be seen, then, that like words, dimensional measurements do not "speak for themselves." They exist only in relation to other biological objects and a map, often implicit or poorly filled in, that relates the two. The degree to which we are able to specify this map can be called a measurement's interpretability. The map linking chest circumference to lean body mass (LBM), for instance, does not adequately discriminate the relation of dimensional datum to intermediate objects, including subcutaneous fat, pectoral and latissimus muscle, skeletal breadth, and lung volume, each of which could act as a referent. In practical terms, this may not represent a problem for simple comparisons at extremes of a distribution; a male with a 106 cm chest girth will have a greater LBM than his peer of 91 cm. But it is problematic for applications requiring finer discriminations; an increase of 5 cm could implicate breathing cycle, push-ups, nascent obstructive lung disease, or excess calories. Hence, we can say that chest circumference is difficult to interpret. Finally, since no one carries exactly the same map, whether of nutritional status or ordinary language, competing theories emerge regarding these maps' relevance. Scientific interpretation thus becomes a consensual social activity subject to nonscientific influences (Kuhn, 1970; Holton, 1978).

The task, then, is not straightforward. Changes in the datum will reflect real changes in the referent, changes in associated biological objects, and changes attributable to nonbiological sources, including chance. How do we apportion these? This model can be roughly operationalized through the concept of sensitivity. Broadly speaking, this is the degree to which a measurement can detect change in a biological state such as nutriture. There are varying approaches to quantifying and decomposing sensitivity that will be considered shortly. To best sort the issues in context of adult dimensional change, this chapter will proceed from quantification of datum error, through problems of placing changes in datum in biological perspective, to the validity of referents. Further, the data under scrutiny will begin with comparatively simple anthropometric indicators of caloric status and progress to multivariate composites that characterize shape, which is more complexly related to nutriture. Throughout, in the spirit of maps and marsupial apocrypha, we would do well to question at what we are pointing.

SENSITIVITY IN THEORY AND PRACTICE

Although popularly considered a quality, sensitivity is more accurately viewed as a composite quantity; any one of several constructed scales or ratios that summarize how much of datum change is attributable to change in nutritional referent. There is surprising latitude in how to define and operationalize this scale. Following Habicht et al. (1979), variance in total measurement sensitivity can be decomposed into variance in consistency (also termed reproducibility and by Habicht, precision); accuracy (also termed bias); and dependability (a less familiar entity discussed in the section on Measuring True Referent Change). On the other hand, many epidemiological sources treat sensitivity as a subspecies of accuracy, since it postulates a "true" change in referent that is related to measured change (Kelsey et al., 1986). In this context, sensitivity is usually contrasted with specificity. The most familiar scale of measurement error, reliability, ignores accuracy altogether and conflates consistency with dependability. However a scale apportions changes in the datum, it is dependent on the datum's map for its own meaning; indeed, the definition of what constitutes error changes according to both the hypothesis under scrutiny and the instrument under hand (Ackermann, 1985; Feyerabend, 1975). The rationale for attending to error, moreover, is not encompassed by the F-statistic. It is better understood by examining the role of precision in science.

The mission of science is to develop explanations for natural phenomena. These explanations require direct, unambiguous comparisons of natural qualities such as hotness and coldness or largeness and smallness that can be termed "fundamental magnitudes" (Wartofsky, 1968). These comparisons are achieved by imposition of arbitrary scales. "Massness," for instance, becomes redefined as weight, or a ratio of scalar mass to scalar gravitational acceleration, which can be compared with other weights. From this and volume, a ratio of scalar lengths, we further derive density. It is the invariant relations among derived measurements, then, and not the natural phenomena underlying them, that populate scientific models. Put more simply, "we explain by pointing to a relationship" (Holton, 1973).

Because they are scalar, the utility of derived measurements can depend on the fineness of their intervals. In this sense, precision is a form of information. The narrower the range within which we cannot discriminate one measurement from another, the more empirical information is at hand to test competing hypotheses (cf. Popper, 1959; also see Stevens, 1946).

Straightforward enough, but for two problems. First, the assumed relation between derived scale and fundamental magnitude may not be linear or even regular. Consider skinfolds: Thirty mm at the subscapular site is three times 10 mm. Is it three times as much "fatness"? By convention, yes, but biological events suggest otherwise. The obese owner of a 30 mm subscapular skinfold may have crossed some metabolic threshold on the way to sudden death from myocardial infarction, while his lean counterpart with a 10 mm skinfold has not. This is a problem of referral for which there is no easy solution. The most common strategies are purely statistical: Transformation of nonlinear variables into forms closer to the strictures of a linear model, or building the model itself on nonlinear assumptions, for instance using orthogonal polynomials (Draper and Smith, 1981). It is even possible, although rarely done, to construct nonlinear models with variables that have irregular intervals (Myers, 1979). All of these approaches, however, depend on empirical confirmation that the scales, raw or transformed, correspond well to natural magnitudes. In the case of nutritional status, such confirmation is sparser than we would wish.

A second problem arises because precision is bound to goals of prediction. Some hypotheses, such as daily pulsatile growth, require precision beyond that currently obtainable, so effort focuses on developing more sensitive instruments with finer scalar intervals. Other hypotheses, such as functional dichotomization of subcutaneous fat into upper and lower segments, require far less precision than currently obtainable. In either case, it is useful to ask if the precision sought is allied with the predictive requirements of the hypothesis. In practice, however, maximum precision tends to be sought regardless of hypothesis. Indeed, inadequate precision, rather than an incorrect hypothesis, often is indicted as the source of disagreement between prediction and outcome.

Such concern is statistically justifiable in that lack of precision can contribute sufficient error that disparate outcomes become indiscernable (Snedecor and Cochran, 1967). Biological observations, moreover, generally carry less precision than those in fields such as experimental physics that have provided science with most of its measurement theory (Kuhn, 1970). On the other hand, the preponderance of nutritional designs with measurements of high reproducibility but marginal interpretability suggests our concern for precision may have grown beyond purely objective grounds. Ironically, as we emphasize measurement error, explanation in the physical sciences increasingly is viewed as driven as much by serendipity and salesmanship as by precision (cf. Kuhn, 1970; Feyerabend, 1975; Lakatos, 1976; Ackermann, 1985).

Operationalizing Precision

Precision, then, concerns measurement intervals, and perfect precision implies infinitely small intervals unlikely to be realized in a quantum world. A better term for nonepistomological usage is consistency, which can be defined as reproduction of a measurement within arbitrarily defined scalar intervals; a skinfold is twice found to be 18 mm thick using a 1 mm interval and thus deemed consistent. Errors in consistency are theoretically and statistically attributable only to the observer of record, but in a causal sense they encompass all sins from worn caliper gears to misrecorded data sheets. Obviously, each of these media will support different types of error. Worn gears may introduce systematic nonlinear error still an order of magnitude smaller than sloppy and nonsystematic observer technique, while recording error will be discontinuous and of unpredictable magnitude. Moreover, subjects influence consistency. Older subjects, for instance, appear to be associated with reduced consistency (cf. Chumlea et al., 1984a; Wormersly and Durnin, 1977) because of greater lability in skin elasticity and soft tissue compressibility. Similarly, obese subjects present great difficulties in landmark location and delineation of fat and muscle tissue. In this causal sense, then, all consistency error represents a triadic interaction of instrument, technique, and subject. This view of error also suggests several betterments. Routine calibration of instruments is vital. Using training models of like age, sex, and body composition to the sample is useful, as is willingness to admit defeat when subjects are patently unmeasurable. The major solution, however, is routine repeat measurements. Figure 1 demonstrates that for largely independent remeasurements, correlations between some "true" value X and the mean of the remeasured values X_1, X_2 ... X_n rises dramatically. Even comparatively correlated remeasurements, such as those taken at very close time intervals or without completely repeating a technique, still improve the overall association substantially.

If a design includes more than one observer, then total error also includes between-observer errors, and subject–observer interaction errors. The former can be thought of as an extension of single-observer errors in consistency, while the latter is related to the concept of accuracy, albeit divorced from any standard.

A great deal of interobserver error stems from implicit disagreements over landmark location. Indeed, definitions of landmarks vary sufficiently from one study to another that most comparisons of reliability are problematic even if

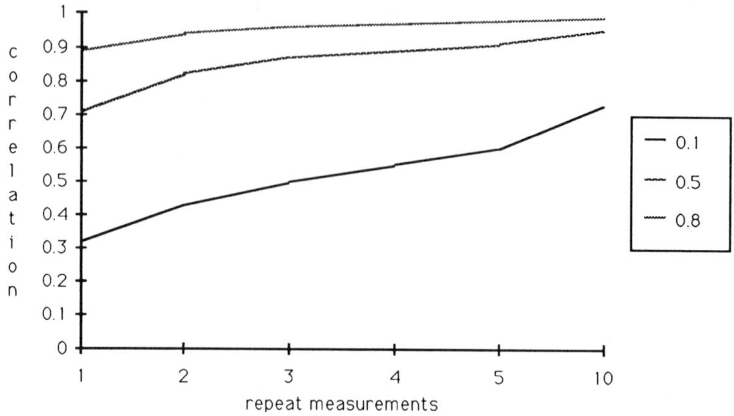

Fig. 1. As the number of independent remeasurements increases from 1 to 10, correlations between a variable and its "true" value rise markedly. The magnitude of the rise will depend on the correlation, here shown for three cases of 0.1, 0.5, and 0.8, between "true" value and an initial measurement. (Data adapted from Kelsey et al., 1986.)

we disregard the magnitude dependence (and thus population specificity) of much anthropometric error. In lieu of millennial agreement over methodology, it is the responsibility of project leaders to scrupulously define landmarks and technique from initial observer training through publication. Useful illustrated definitions are found in Cameron (1986); Zerfas (1979) has an excellent discussion of sources of technical error in the field; the most thorough review of conflicting methodologies, with recommendations, is contained in the first five chapters of Lohman et al. (1988).

Observer accuracy relates datum to referent through the concept of a "true" measurement assumed to be congruent with the actual referent. Of course, a standard does not produce a "true" value; for the theoretical reasons discussed earlier, such a value is fundamental and cannot be directly measured. More practically, even experienced investigators acting as standards have off days. For these reasons, measurements of bias based on subject–observer interaction may be more useful. In either case, it appears worthwhile to differentiate accuracy from bias, two terms often used synonymously. The former best refers to all discrepancies between observer and standard, while the latter best refers to a systematic trend in observer measurements, be it above or below a standard, or in relation to a specific subject. Thus a measurement could be highly inaccurate, but if the signs balance, nonbiased. This redefinition also removes the current necessity of employing a redundancy, "systematic bias," to describe trend inaccuracy.

Test–Retest Algorithms

The classic quantification of reliability is for one observer to measure the same subjects twice within a brief period. If we assume there is some "true" measurement X, then the test–retest difference is simply a difference between the total errors associated with each measurement occasion EX_1 and EX_2. The statistical analysis of choice here is a simple matched pairs t-test (Snedecor and Cochran, 1967). A related, if oddly named, consistency measure is the technical error of measurement, r, which is basically the standard deviation of the differences between X_1 and X_2:

$$r = \sqrt{\frac{\sum_1^N Z_i^2}{2N}}$$

(NCHS, 1973). When squared and divided by between-subject variance, it has the advantage of being comparable across measurement scales.

Some investigators prefer a product-moment correlation coefficient between measurement occasions, rx_1X_2, which is termed the coefficient of reproducibility or reliability. A product-moment correlation, however, is insensitive to mean differences between test and retest; the intraclass correlation coefficient is preferable here because it permits partitioning (Snedecor and Cochran, 1967). Bias can be related to either correlation: If we assume that errors are independent, then $rx_1X_2 = (rx_1X)\ (rx_2X)$, where X = some "true" value. The fundamental hazard with any test–retest correlation is being lulled by the gratifyingly high coefficient. Nearly any data will produce an r well above 0.9, however large the systematic inaccuracy.

Inaccuracy can be measured using a matched pairs t-test in which the observer is compared with an experienced standard (Woolf, 1968), while bias can be quantified with a simple chi squares sign test (Siegel, 1956). Alternatively, a Z-score can be generated in which the numerator is an observer's measurement subtracted from the mean of the "true" or standard's measurements, and the denominator is the standard deviation of the standard's values (Kelsey et al., 1986).

When designs require multiple observers, the statistical test of choice for interobserver error is two-way analysis of variance (Snedecor and Cochran, 1967; Hall, 1980). It permits sorting of the two main and the interaction effects, as well as testing for nonlinearity of error between observers. As stated above, the interaction term is a useful test for bias related to subject, rather than to standard.

Finally, it is worthwhile to realize that consistency error is more than "noise" that widens confidence intervals. It also can create spurious associations or attenuate legitimate ones. This is the case if measurement error for one variable is correlated with the actual magnitude of another variable (Greenland, 1980). Regression of the variables in question for the purpose of residual analysis is particularly relevant if this problem is anticipated (Mosteller and Tukey, 1977).

Longitudinal Reliability

Longitudinal, or multiple occasion, data require a somewhat different approach to reliability. In general, there is opportunity for greater interobserver error due to personnel turnover and drift in technique; this necessitates ongoing monitoring of reliability. Moreover, unless the measurement intervals are very close, rather like a test–retest situation, the true values X_1 and X_2 change along with the errors E_{X1} and E_{X2}. Intervening physiological variables also can change significantly. Thus, calculation of reliability becomes problematic. For instance, longitudinal reliability is often thought of as the correlation between sequential measurements, assuming independence of error, or $r = V_X/(V_X + V_E)$, where V_X = between-occasion variance of the true measurements, and V_E = between-occasion variance of the errors (Goldstein, 1979). If multiple observers are used, a superior approach for reasons analogous to those cited for a single occasion is repeated measures two-way analysis of variance (Draper and Smith, 1981). This algorithm, moreover, permits testing for nonlinearity of time effects, which can be important in extended adult longitudinal designs.

In any case, it is necessary to sort out components of change attributable to true measurement change from those related to regression toward the mean and measurement error. James (1973) has shown that when reliability is low, most regression to the mean is attributable to error, and provides guidelines for partitioning these three effects. Another approach is to simply subtract variance in observer consistency obtained using a brief test–retest from variance obtained over a longer, empirically defined interval that is still too brief to include major change in nutriture; the remainder is considered due to nonnutritional physiological fluctuation (Habicht et al., 1979; Mueller and Martorell, 1988). There are two theoretical difficulties with this approach. The first resides in the assumption that a brief test–retest will capture all consistency variance and no physiological fluctuation, while a somewhat longer remeasurement interval will capture all physiological fluctuation and no consistency change other than that already detected. The second is the assumption that remaining between-subject biological variance is nutritionally driven; this may be invalid for better nourished or older populations in which genetic variance becomes significant. Nevertheless, the approach is markedly preferable to simple test–retests of consistency applied to longitudinal data.

MEASURING TRUE REFERENT CHANGE

Thus far, the datum referent map has been considered from the point of view of the datum's consistency and accuracy. It is equally important to reverse the perspective: How well is change in the true referent reflected by change in the datum? As Himes points out (1987), failure to consider this can lead to confusion of measurements appropriate for evaluating nutritional status with measurements appropriate for evaluating nutritional outcomes. The capability of a measurement to discriminate true change in its referent can be operationalized variously as its dependability (Habicht et al., 1979) or its sensitivity and specificity (Kelsey et al., 1986). Both approaches presume separate quantification of consistency, so that remaining datum change can be attributed to either nutritional referent or nonnutritional fluctuation. The epidemiological approach, which best lends itself to clinically definable disease or risk states, scales the ability of a measurement to capture true cases or true change (sensitivity), and reject false cases or nonnutritional change (specificity). Either discrete or continuous criteria can be accommodated. Alternatively, Habicht et al. quantify dependability along lines similar to those described earlier for sorting real longitudinal change from regression toward the mean and nonnutritional fluctuation. That is, continuous variance attributable to inconsistency, together with variance attributable to real mean change, is subtracted from total within-subject variance based on two measurement occasions separated by a period likely to be small relative to real change and large relative to nonnutritional fluctuations (Habicht et al., 1979, p 371).

By these lights, weight or BMI are highly precise, but not particularly dependable (Fig. 2). Their variance can be attributed to hydration level, gastrointestinal status, and underwear choice, in addition to true nutritional perturbation. Triceps skinfold, by contrast, is less precise but more dependable. Other measures, such as chest circumference, offer neither quality.

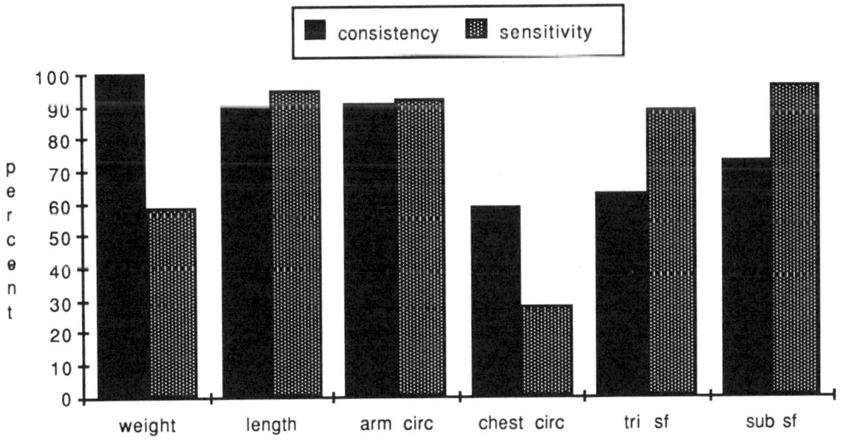

Fig. 2. Incremental consistency and sensitivity can differ substantially in a single measurement and across measurements. Generally, both scales are higher for data from cross-sectional designs. (Data adapted from Habicht et al., 1979.)

These data are based on comparatively brief intervals. The trends also appear to hold for longer periods. Rookus et al. (1987a), for example, found that over 4 years, short-term within-subject fluctuations of BMI, measured as standard deviations corrected for trend, were nearly 3 times the rate of yearly change. Data from longer-term studies, such as 2-year increments of the Framingham sample over a total of 18 years, indicate even greater within-subject variance, approaching 3.5 kg STD (Gordon and Shurtleff, 1973). The results of such large within-subject fluctuations can include a swamping of smaller weight or BMI changes caused by real gain or loss of fat, with a resulting inability of either clinician or patient to detect biologically significant changes. On the other hand, some skinfolds such as the anterior thigh or triceps are sufficiently imprecise that for incremental purposes the benefits of their superior dependability are lost.

Finally, little is known about the degree to which sensitivity may be affected by the subject's genotype. Any biological trait represents the outcome of genotype expressed through multiple environments. Both genetic theory and recent studies suggest that traits with marked genetic variability—this includes most dimensional and many physiological referents—include significant variance contributed by genotype interaction with the environment (Poehlman et al., 1986; Bouchard and Tremblay, 1985). That is, the characteristic expressed by a given genotype may respond nonlinearly to two disparate nutritional environments, and the type of nonlinearity may vary between genotypes. An interaction particularly could influence serial measurements of nutritional status involving systematic treatment effects such as caloric manipulation or physical training.

These genetic data bring out a theoretical caveat to dependability. It concerns how nutritional, or "true" effects, and nonnutritional, or "false" effects, are partitioned. Of mathematical necessity, "nonnutritional" comes to encompass all change not directly attributable to a specific disease or risk state. This wastebasket holds not only fluctuations related to hydration, gastrointestinal contents, occult pathology, and clothing, but also those related to genetic expression, and to metabolic or anatomical elements that are acceptable nutritional referents in other analyses. Put in terms of our linguistic model, the breadth of definition assigned to "nonnutritional" makes its biological discrimination vague, and the dichotomous map so formed, less interpretable.

This loss of interpretability indicates the need for more sophisticated measures of sensitivity or dependability. In the interim, it appears wisest to choose anthropometric measurements with attention to both sensitivity and consistency, rather than to a conflation of the two provided by reliability.

THE USE AND ABUSE OF RATIOS

Weight–Height Ratios

The most common anthropometric estimators of nutritional status are those that relate weight to height. All serve as proxies for total body fat, itself estimated from measurements such as body density or lean body mass. Typically, weight and height are related through an index, which is a ratio having one or both terms expressed as exponential powers: W/H^P or $H/W^{1/P}$. The quest for ever higher correlations to body fatness has produced a fabulous variety of ratios and indices, from the simple subject *W*/reference *W* (relative weight); to the more sophisticated W/H^2 (Quetelet's index, or the body mass index); W/H^3 (Rohrer's index); or $H/W^{1/3}$ (the ponderal index). Moreover, as Benn notes (1971), there is no intrinsic reason to avoid fractional powers and much to gain. Micozzi and his coworkers, for instance, have found height powers of 2 for males and 1.5 for females to best characterize the National Health and Nutrition Examination Survey. Khosla and Lowe found powers of 1.94 best for both sexes, while Abel-Malek et al. argue for $W^{1.2}/H^{3.3}$ to best correlate with body density in male and female Fels subjects (Micozzi et al., 1986; Khosla and Lowe, 1967; Abdel-Malek et al., 1985).

Why are there so many indices? Primarily because in attempting to meet an assumption of statistical independence from height, each becomes population specific. The dilemma develops as follows: Maximizing such independence by adjusting powers also tends to strengthen correlations—typically on the order of .80—to the real biological referent, body fat. However, optimal correlations to total fat and independence from height are necessarily congruent only if there is no statistical association between total fat and height. This would appear so; variance in body fat per se is independently distributed from and uncorrelated with variance in the axial skeleton (Khosla and Lowe, 1967; Bilewicz et al., 1962; also see Tanner, 1951).

A difficulty arises, however: Fat may be effectively uncorrelated to the axial skeleton, but it is not uncorrelated to that skeleton's breadth. This is because of the latter's strong correlations to the lean body or fat-free mass. The obese, in turn, average more muscle mass and skeletal breadth than the lean of a similar height (cf. Himes and Bouchard, 1985; Garn et al., 1983, 1986; Frisancho and Flegel, 1983). Thus the central assumption of the height term's independence from body fat comes to depend on exact biological referent: Is variance in height pointing solely at variance in the axial skeleton, or in the entire skeleton, or in the total lean body mass? The height term in fact serves as proxy for all variance in weight not attributable to fat, that is, to variance in muscle, viscera, bone, extracellular water, and so forth. By doing so, it frees the weight term to point directly at variance in fat. This is why weight–height indices tend to be trustworthy only across about two standard deviations of height; beyond that range, allometric relationships of lean to axial skeleton change too much (Benn, 1971).

Further complications are introduced by aging. After the 1930s, height losses in both sexes due to bone loss and intervertebral compression proceed at a slower rate than loss of lean body mass (Forbes and Reina, 1970). In addition, nongenetic components of variance in stature appear to diminish from childhood onward (Byard et al., 1988). As a result, the height term in an adult index is a different species of proxy at 60 than at 30.

In sum, these difficulties, taken with disparate initial populational distributions of variance in body composition and stature (cf. Schmitt and Harrison, 1988; Mukherjee and Roche, 1984; Floury, 1970; Goldbourt and Medalie, 1974), produce weight–height indices that are specific to the population distribution from which they were generated (Garn et al., 1986). The problem can be ameliorated by construction of indices based on correlation to an independent measure of body fat, such as density, rather than to weight (Roche, 1984). Further cross-validation studies are needed to clarify the impact of index specificity—it is a species of compromised interpretability—but they are unlikely to uncover a universal index.

The shortcomings of weight—height indices should not obscure their value. Their terms are straightforward to learn, highly consistent, and comparative standards abound. Moreover, weight–height indices are uniquely cost-effective, in that we gain a sizable amount of nutritional information for a comparatively modest investment in equipment and training. Such indices are highly useful tools for single-occasion epidemiological screening and for intrapopulational comparisons of reasonably similar groups. They are less sure as clinical proxies for individual body fat or for comparisons between dissimilar populations. Finally, they should be interpreted with caution when applied to special adult groups such as the lean, the chronically ill, the athletic, or the elderly, and when used in any longitudinal analysis.

Other Ratios

Ratios or composites other than weight for height have become popular as estimators of shape. The waist–hip circumference ratio, for instance, is currently much used to represent subcutaneous fat distribution (cf. White et al., 1986; Hartz et al., 1984; Jones et al., 1986). There are difficulties with determining the referent of this ratio. Hip circumference is partly determined by pelvic breadth and trochanteric conformation, highly heritable traits, and partly by gluteal development and fat stores over those gluteal muscles, rather less heritable traits (Susanne, 1977; Bouchard and Tremblay, 1985). The only mapping rule with which single occasion measurements can discriminate these referents—that gluteal fat variance is greater than pelvic breadth variance—is inadequate to the task.

Waist circumference, by contrast, directly involves no skeletal girth but is influenced by tone and development of the abdominal and lower back muscles, largely nonheritable traits, and by subcutaneous and omental stores of fat, traits of intermediate heritability (Susanne, 1977; Bouchard and Tremblay, 1985). Posture and gastrointestinal status also affect waist circumference. The mapping rule here—that variance in circumference refers to variance in these fat stores—appears more empirically defensible, although we know little about populational variability in the ratio of subcutaneous to omental fat (see the section on Relating Surface Dimensions to Function). Landmarks for both circumferences, finally, vary widely (Lohman et al., 1988), suggesting noncomparability across studies. An alternative circumference ratio, using the waist and thigh, has both theoretical and empirical advantages. It combines the technical ease of taking circumferences with a somewhat clearer mapping to the biological referent, subcutaneous fat contour (Mueller et al., 1987). Neither ratio, however, permits fine enough resolution of referents to detail the transition from normal to abnormal contour.

Finally, there is theoretical justification for the stance that geometric constructs such as fat area or volume that are derived from dimensions should bear a closer relation to biological referents than do simple linear measurements (cf. Himes et al., 1980; Baker et al., 1958; Gurney and Jelliffe, 1973). This follows from the fact that an anulus of fat of constant thickness will contain more fat cells. i.e., more area and volume, as its diameter increases. Thus, a 184 cm male of 16 mm triceps skinfold has a good deal more actively metabolizing fat cells in his 34 cm upper arm than his 168 cm counterpart of identical skinfold thickness but 29 cm arm circumference. The shorter man is "fatter" relative to his height, but the taller man is "fatter" in a net physiological sense that may be closer to our intentions in making the measurement. Empirical validation of this hypothesis has been equivocal, however; in adults, fat areas are better correlated to weight of total body fat, probably because of the correspondence of measurement units and their patterns of error, but not to percent body fat, which is divorced from linear dimension (Himes et al., 1980). Thus, if geometric areas or volumes can be accurately estimated (in itself not a trivial task, cf. Heymsfeld et al., 1982; Gurney and Jelliffe, 1973; Forbes et al., 1988), they seem to provide a clearer pathway to biological referent and therefore may be preferable for research purposes.

CHANGE IN ANTHROPOMETRIC MEASURES WITH AGE

Much of our understanding of adult dimensional change relies on large, cross-sectional samples that characterize adult nutritional status using simple summary measures such as weight, weight for height, skinfold thicknesses, or circumferences. Such data have been presented in well-known sources such as the U.S. Health and Nutrition Examination Surveys (NCHS, 1965, 1979, 1987), and the Ten-State Nutritional Survey (CDC, 1972).

The numbers demonstrate, in sum, that the most common dimensional change in adults is gain of weight and fat through the fifth decade of adult life. This is reflected in increases in most girths and related diameters as well. Thus in the HANES II data (NCHS, 1987), we find an increase from a median of 72.0 kg at 18–24 years in males to 79.0 kg at 45–54 years; females increase from 58.0 kg to 65.5 kg over the same time span. As shown in Figure 3, BMI increases from 23.0 in males and 21.6 in females 18–24 years to 25.9 in males 45–55 years of age, and to 25.9 in females 65–74 years of age. More direct measures of subcutaneous fatness, such as the triceps and subscapular skinfolds, show similar trends, with a nearly 15% increase in male upper limb fatness and 39% increase in male trunk fatness over three decades. These latter data also suggest a greater acquisition of trunk fat with age. Such findings have

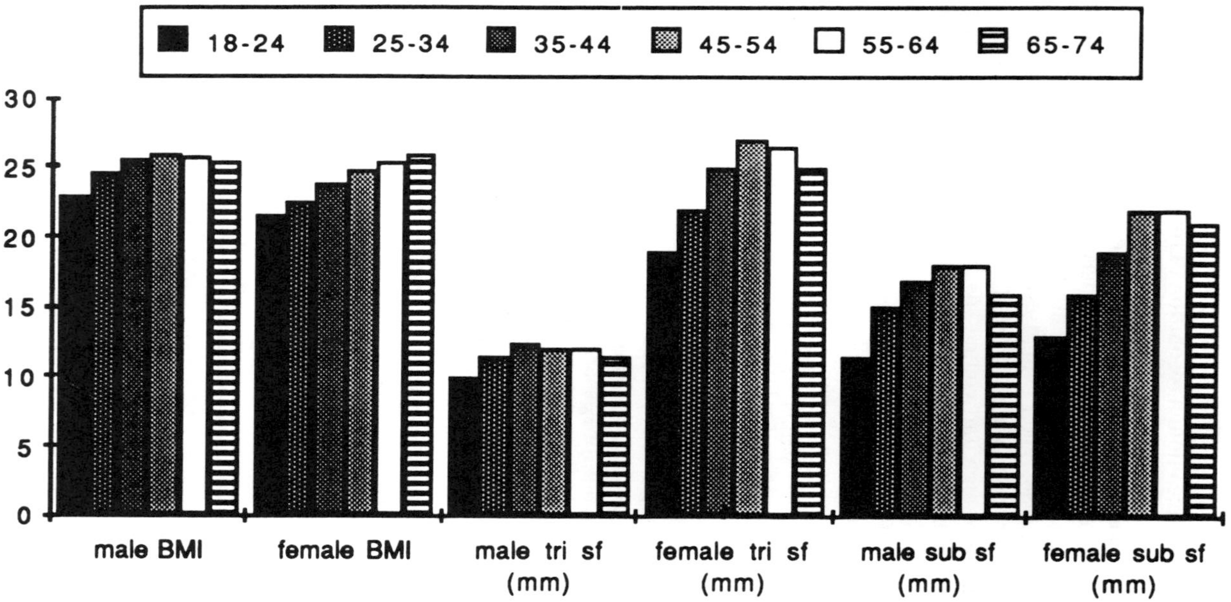

Fig. 3. Fatness, as represented by BMI, and triceps and subscapular skinfolds, increases through the fifth decade of life in males and the sixth decade of life in females. Females' greater fatness varies according to dimensional site, and is not clearly distinguishable using BMI because weight has sex-specific referents. (Data adapted from NCHS, 1987.)

been corroborated by studies of various designs, including total communities (Montoye et al., 1965) and large cross-sectional samples of specific-age cohorts (Steen et al., 1977; Masters et al., 1960).

Cross-sectional studies of human body composition, moreover, demonstrate increases with age in total fat by weight, on the order of 10 kg, and more substantial gain in percent body fat, on the order of 15%, as lean is lost simultaneously (cf. Lesser et al., 1963; Young et al., 1963; Durnin and Wormersly, 1974; Noppa et al., 1979; but see Norris et al., 1963). The effect is more pronounced in females, and in middle age. These data also suggest a second type of fat redistribution with age, such that fat associated with surface dimensions increases less rapidly than internal fat depots. Both types of redistribution have been confirmed by more sophisticated measures discussed in the section on Relating Surface Dimensions to Function.

Unfortunately, such cross-sectional, or single measurement occasion data do not present a particularly accurate picture of change. Increments defined by cross-sectional data represent differences between the averages of two or more groups composed of separate individuals, rather than averaged differences between the same individuals at two or more measurement occasions. As a result, cross-sectional data necessarily conflate true changes in individual biological parameters over time with changes attributable to cohort membership. These cohort effects include secular change in dimensions or underlying physiology, disparate sampling frames, and in the older age categories, differential survivorship (Goldstein, 1979; Damon, 1965). Put in theoretical context, mapping changes in datum and referent using more than one person introduces an untenable number of possible pathways and intervening elements.

Norris's early cross-sectional findings on the Baltimore aging sample, for instance, indicated older males neither weighed more nor possessed more body fat (Norris et al., 1963). Subsequent longitudinal data from the same population showed otherwise (Borkan and Norris, 1977). Clearly the cross-sectional sample included both cohort effects (older groups were significantly shorter) and differential survival (heavier and fatter men tended to die earlier and thus be underrepresented at later ages). Cross-sectional data, moreover, are particularly ill-suited for examining velocity, or incremental change per unit time, whether in pubertal heights or middle-aged waists. Despite these problems, a great many statements about adult dimensional change with age are based on large cross-sectional studies. In large part, this reflects the measurement intervals necessary to demonstrate significant individual change; an adult longitudinal design can absorb the attention of its investigators over much of their active research careers and across several federal funding regimes.

Even if the designs were facile, however, it would not follow that adult longitudinal data are a pancea. Unless more than one cohort is tracked, multiple occasion measurements are insensitive to secular trend, and thus over time may cease to adequately represent current populations. Moreover, pure longitudinal data can be insensitive to time of measurement effects such as seasonality. This can be ameliorated by mixing. Through original intent or redesign, some subjects drop out while others are newly recruited, and two or more cohorts become represented, or mixed, in one study. If done in a rational manner, mixing permits examination of both longitudinal and cohort effects simultaneously, and it markedly reduces the net time required to demonstrate significant change or treatment effects. Useful theoretical discussions of mixed model data analysis can by found in Schaie, 1965; Baltes, 1968; Goldstein, 1979; and van't Hof et al., 1977.

Partitioning Effects

Relatively little work has been done on partitioning longitudinal and cross-sectional effects in adults. It is clear that weight and fat deposition increase until early middle age, but the rate of increase, the point of deflection, and its variance relatable to age seem population specific (cf. Forbes and Reina, 1970; Cronk et al., 1982; Friedlaender et al., 1977; Borkan et al., 1983; Noppa et al., 1979; Khoury et al., 1983; Rookus et al., 1987b). Data from the largest adult longitudinal study, the Boston Veteran's Administration Study (Friedlander et al., 1977; Borkan et al., 1983), indicates that weight in men increases both longitudinally and by cohort (secular trend) into the sixth decade, while weight-for-height increases slightly into the fifth decade and then wanes to adolescent values by the ninth decade of life (Fig. 4). Further, although abdominal circumference increases into the seventh decade and hip breadth to life's end, the nature of the change differs; velocity of abdominal breadth appears to diminish with age while hip breadth velocity is remarkably constant. Height diminishes some 1.5 cm between the third decade and the end of life; interestingly, most nonaxial, nonweight-bearing skeletal dimensions, including biacromial diameter and arm span, also decline significantly after the fifth decade. Yet with the exception of arm span, these same variables increase by like-aged cohort (secular trend).

The Boston data do not directly address the problems of differential survivorship or representativeness, although the population appears to be taller and healthier than those in U.S. probability samples. Nevertheless, the results suggest that the dramatic increases and decreases in adult dimensions derived cross-sectionally are colored by cohort effects. In addition, they reflect marked changes in allometric relationships between soft tissue and surface dimensions with age.

An underutilized strategy for longitudinal data analysis is principal components or factor analysis (cf. Cronk et al., 1982; Baumgartner et al., 1986; Szczotka, 1981). Each component or factor is a statistically distinct weighted linear combination distilled from a large set of primary variables; each represents latent structure, so to speak. The relative weighting of individual variables within these components or factors affords interpretation of structure, while individual scores can be calculated from the component or factor for subsequent use in regression or analysis of variance. For instance, Cronk, using principal components analysis of longitudinal data, found that high or in-

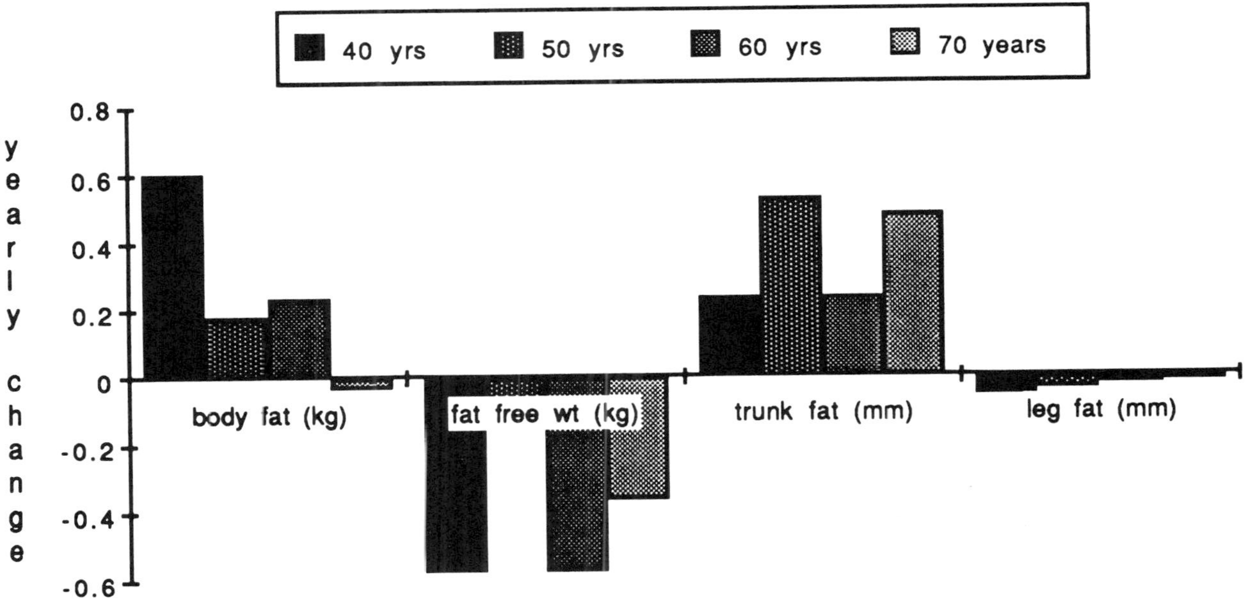

Fig. 4. Longitudinal medians on Boston males demonstrates that total fat incremental velocity remains positive until the eighth decade of life, while lean is lost from the fourth decade onward. Radiographic measurements from the axilla and lateral calf indicate positive velocity for subcutaneous trunk fat but little change in leg fat. These data can be compared with the cross-sectional medians in Figure 3. (Data adapted from Borkan and Norris, 1977.)

creasing body mass indices in childhood could explain between 35% and 60% of variance in adult percent body fat, body mass index, and total body fat, and about 10%–15% of variance in fat cell number (Cronk et al., 1982).

Another source of data on adult dimensional change is the prospective or follow-up studies of health risk factors, particularly for coronary artery disease and sudden death (Feinleib et al., 1977; Garn et al., 1980; Hsu et al., 1977; Stokes et al., 1985; Khoury et al., 1983). Garn and his coworkers, for instance, have shown continuities in adult subcutaneous fatness over 15 years, with correlations on the order of 0.4–0.6. These data further demonstrate that much of the existing lability in mean fatness is provided by the obese, some 50% of whom fall out of such a category over two decades. Although these data probably overestimate actual canalization because of failure to correct for regression to the mean, they still suggest the existence of subpopulations with differing propensities toward acquisition of fat; the relative tracking tendencies of such groups can be better understood by analyzing percentiles rather than simple mean or medians.

A third source of information on dimensional change is the numerous short-term studies of weight gain or loss, usually in highly selected populations such as the obese in weight loss programs or athletes in training (cf. Bray et al., 1978; Belko et al., 1987; Buono et al., 1985; Butts et al., 1985). The most useful of these studies relates change in anthropometric measurement to independent measures of the biological referent (cf. King and Katch, 1986; Belko et al., 1987). It is less desirable to correlate change in one dimensional measurement, such as skinfold thickness, to another, such as BMI (Bray et al., 1978; Garn et al., 1987) because this introduces a triangular structure of intervening variables: those between the independent dimensional variable and its referent, and those between the dependent dimensional construct and that same referent.

King and Katch (1986) deserve note for measuring changes in surface anthropometry and density at constant increments of weight loss rather than of time. Such a labor intensive design is useful in that it permits precise testing of hypotheses regarding linearity of effect over naturally defined intervals of the referent. In this case, the investigators found that while all anthropometries changed in response to caloric deprivation, the pattern of change was not uniform. Triceps, abdominal, and thigh skinfolds lost substantially more thickness than did suprailiac or subscapular sites, while biiliac and waist circumferences lost more than the upper trunk or arm. A consonant finding has been shown for uncontrolled increments of weight gain, without data on density, from a large sample over five years (Garn et al., 1987)

PREDICTION OF BODY COMPARTMENTS

Since Robertson bribed "ten middling-sized men" to immerse themselves in the village cistern in 1757 (cited in Boyd, 1933), there has been active interest in applying Archemedean principles to the quantification of physique. The quest for convenient surface indicators of biological parameters became systematized with Matiegka (1921) and McCloy (1936). Anthropometric measurements lacked a satisfactory biological referent, however, until Behnke specified the two-compartment model of body composition corrected for lung volume in 1942. Subsequent refinements, particularly those by Rathbun and Pace (1945), and Keys and Brozek (1953), linked anthropometry to this model of internal architecture. However, it will be seen that these linkages have not been without difficulties.

One approach has beeen to link body composition to body configuration or shape. This is chiefly associated with Behnke and his students (Behnke et al., 1959; Behnke and Wilmore, 1972). The system's underlying assumption is that "in healthy adults whose body form is not distorted by excessive fat, there is an organized body structure or pattern characterized by anthropometric relationships obtainable on a few individuals and applicable to many" (Behnke et al., 1959, p 214). To achieve this characterization, ratios of circumferences and diameters to constants produce quotients that can be singly or in groups associated with body fat, muscularity, and skeletal robusticity. In addition, percent deviations of selected quotients from a reference standard can be displayed in a graphic profile called a *somatogram.* The model recently has been modified to better differentiate muscular and nonmuscular body regions (Katch et al., 1987).

Multiple Regression

A more common strategy uses multiple regression. In this approach, total body fat becomes an outcome variable predicted by independent anthropometric variables. Once performed on a small, labor intensive sample, the resultant equation can be used to "plug in" anthropometries and predict percent fat.

The dilemma of regression approaches has been poor external validity; prediction equations are population specific (Lohman, 1981). This specificity springs from a number of causes. Measurement error is comparatively high, and apparently population specific, for many anthropometric measures. Thus, equations derived from populations with one pattern of measurement error may be particularly ineffective in using similar measurements from a dissimilar population (Flint et al., 1977). This is particularly true for dissimilar age distributions, since the predictive relationship of surface dimensions to internal body architecture changes with age (Noppa et al., 1979; Flint et al., 1977; Chumlea et al., 1984b; Ward et al., 1975; Young et al., 1963). Moreover, simple adjustments for age and sex are inadequate because populations may yet differ in sample distribution of body composition (Mukherje and Roche, 1984; Roche, 1984).

In addition, although most regression users are now sensitized to the hazards of using colinear independent *(X)* variables in a stepwise algorithm (Draper and Smith, 1981), the dependent *(Y)* variable receives less care. It is often assumed erroneously that a regression's independent variables will provide an equally precise prediction of several different expressions of the biological referent represented by the dependent *(Y)* variable. Thus body density, percent body fat, or weight of lean and fat mass are shuffled in search of higher R^2's. However, each *Y* reexpression carries with it different distributions of error relative to *X*, and thus has different impacts on equation robusticity (cf. Draper and Smith, 1981; Neter and Wasserman, 1974). In addition, assumptions of regression linearity tend to be more sensitive to nonnormality in *Y* than in *X* (cf. Neter and Wasserman, 1974; Mosteller and Tukey, 1977).

Of course, the most nutritionally meaningful variance in *Y* may well be that *not* explained by variance in *X*. Fatter people, for instance, usually weigh more. But what is of greater interest is how some people come to be fatter than others of the same weight. If the sample has a typically skewed and wide-tailed distribution of weights, most of the variance in *Y* will be explained by variance in weight; in a multiple stepwise regression model, smaller effects may be swamped. If other independent variables are available, partial correlations or supressor variables can circumvent this problem (Pedhazur, 1982).

Inconstant Constants

Most significantly, assumptions about a regression's biological referent may be invalid. The two-compartment model postulates lean and fat of constant density: "The choice of compartments into which a body is divided," Brozek stated, "is dictated first, by the constancy of their composition, and second, by the availability of suitable methods for estimating their size in different individuals and in the same individual in different nutritional states" (Brozek et al., 1963:115).

This assumption has not gone unchallenged. There are broad theoretical objections best summarized by Garn's quip: "In biological systems, constants have a way of not being very constant" (Garn, 1963; also Siri, 1956). There are even greater empirical difficulties. The supposed constants were based on a remarkably small sample that severely underrepresented density variance attributable to race, sex, and age (cf. Wedgewood, 1963; Brozek et al., 1963; Siri, 1956; Fidanza et al., 1953; Trotter et al., 1960; Bakker and Struikenkamp, 1977; Sheng and Huggins, 1979); to pathology (Cohn et al., 1981); and even to species model (cf. Kodama, 1971; Rathbun and Pace, 1945). Moreover, it has been clear for some time that fat and lean do not behave metabolically as if they are unitary compartments (cf. Bolinder et al., 1983; Krotkiewski et al., 1983). But supporters and detractors alike have been swayed by the obvious utility of Archemedean assumptions for estimating caloric status, and the apparently modest predictive error, on the order of 2.5% associated with these falsifications of constancy assumptions.

Recent findings, however, suggest deficiencies so grave as to call into question the model's scientific value. As shown by Clarys and Martin (1987), muscle mass in seven female cadavers ranged from 45% to nearly 54.8% of total adipose-free tissue, while bone ranged from 17.4% to 25.7%. In six male cadavers, the same ranges were 48.8%–58.6% and 16.3%–22.7% of adipose-free tissue, respectively. Variation in these and other components of lean produce a total adipose-free tissue standard deviation of about .02 g/mL. This in turn translates to a remarkable 15% range of estimation of percent body fat. Such a range explains the phenomenon, usually unnoted in final drafts, of negative body fat predictions for lean subjects (and in the popular press, of anomalously low estimates, on the order of 1%–3% body fat, for some male athletes). Unfortunately, the same degree of error may pass undetected in fatter subjects. If replicated, these data may force us to reject the Archemedean basis of the two-component model; lean is not gold and fat is not silver.

If we do so, we are left without a scientifically adequate means of using surface dimensions to predict body composition. This is scarcely a catastrophy. For nutritional purposes, there are adequate alternatives using simple ordinal comparisons; a subject with an 85th percentile subscapular skinfold or BMI has significantly more body fat than a subject in the 70th percentile. Moreover, if acknowledged, this shortfall could stimulate development of more realistic models of body architecture that ultimately would allow secure prediction.

RELATING SURFACE DIMENSIONS TO FUNCTION

A large literature now describes the correspondence of adult dimension, including both size and shape, to underlying metabolic dysfunction and morbidity. Reviews of these correspondences have been published elsewhere (Bailey, 1985; Kissebah et al., 1988; Depres et al., 1988). In sum, it has been shown that elevated body fat or weight is independently associated with risk factors of diabetes, gall bladder disease, cancer of the endometrium and breast, coronary artery disease including hypertension, angina pectoris, and miocardial infarction. Subcutaneous fat distribution, moreover, may play a stronger role in the etiology of some disease states than does obesity or overweight per se (cf. Vague, 1956; Feldman et al., 1969; Foster et al., 1987; Weinsier et al., 1985). Indeed, so fundamental is the association of fat distribution with glucose metabolism that it may hold for all primates (Shively et al., 1987).

Increasing evidence indicates that both fat distribution and its impact on physiological parameters are population specific (Bailey et al., 1987; Fried and Kral, 1987; Ramirez and Mueller, 1980; Szathmary and Holt, 1983; Haffner et al., 1986; Bogin and MacVean, 1981). Mestizo, Native American, and Oceanic populations, in particular, may have dysfunctionally prone adipose tissue located higher on the anterior trunk than do Anglo groups. There are no comparable data on African or central/south Asian populations.

Males and females, moreover, seem to differ significantly in regional adipocyte size and metabolism (cf. Krotkiewski et al., 1983; Rebuffe-Scrive et al., 1985; Bolinder et al., 1983). Men have relatively more internal fat mass, and larger internal adipocytes, while women have relatively larger subcutaneous adipocytes, particularly in the femoral and gluteal regions. These sex differences appear to be androgen sensitive (Evans et al., 1984).

Regional variation in adipocyte metabolism also is well established. In general, female adipocyte triglyceride metabolism is higher except perhaps in the omental region (Fried and Kral, 1987; Gurr et al., 1982; Rebuffe-Scrive et al., 1985). This sex difference, taken with the ambiguous referents of the waist–hip ratio, may be responsible for conflicting findings regarding which skinfold or circumference is best correlated to internal fat. Seidell et al. (1987) found, for instance, that intra-abdominal deposits were better correlated to waist–hip ratio in men and waist–thigh ratio in women. By contrast, Baumgartner et al. (1988) found that CAT scan sections analogous to waist–hip ratios were positively correlated to areas of subcutaneous fat and intra-abdominal fat in women, but not in men.

Quantifying Shape

A consistent challenge in many of these studies has been adequate quantification of surface contour or shape. Early attempts included Edwards's factor analyses of raw value skinfolds (1951), Skerlj's characterization of female shape (1953), Howell's use of factor analysis to compare dimensional measurements with Sheldonian somatotypes (1951), and Garn's development of skinfold "pattern profiles" (1955). More recent approaches have tended to utilize multivariate analysis of a number of normalized skinfolds (Mueller and Reid, 1979; Bailey et al., 1982) or circumferences (Johnston et al., 1988). As an illustration, Table 1 shows an analytic approach, principal components analysis, using young adult skinfold data. The second principal component indicates a systematic contrast of upper and lower body skinfold thicknesses; a subject strongly characterized by this component would be expected to display elevated serum insulin and glucose. A related synthetic approach, cluster analysis, groups individuals on the basis of their similarities in skinfold thicknesses. The first cluster of subjects in Figure 5 thus demonstrates a pattern of fat deposition characteristic of the second principal component. Other multivariate techniques such as discriminate analysis or canonical correlation permit

TABLE 1. Principal Components Analysis of Young Adult Skinfold Data

	Components		
Skinfold	1	2	3
Mandibular	0.116	0.363	−0.421
Acromial	0.273	0.204	0.403
Biceps	0.299	−0.273	0.097
Triceps	0.287	−0.301	−0.011
Anterior forearm	0.291	−0.191	−0.041
Subscapular	0.287	0.216	0.392
Umbilical	0.263	0.356	0.045
Suprailiac	0.265	0.328	0.162
Anterior thigh	0.299	−0.182	−0.198
Medial calf	0.286	−0.159	−0.103

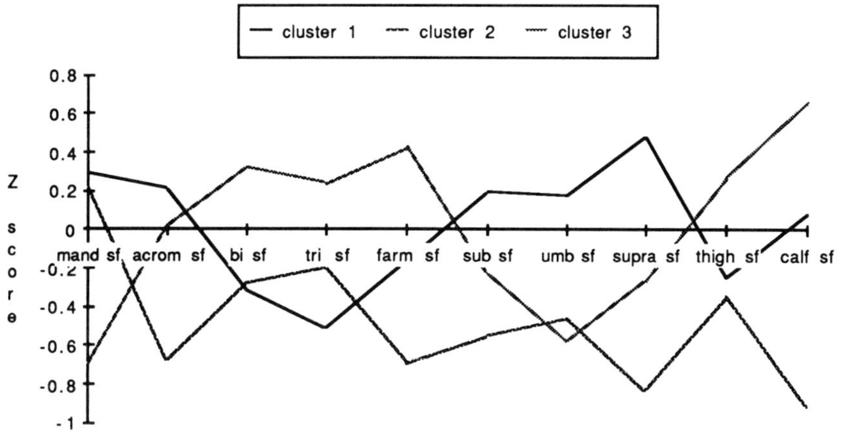

Fig. 5. *Z*-scored skinfolds can be clustered or grouped on the basis of their intrasubject similarities. In this sample of young adult males, the first cluster represents trunkal fat patterning, and the third, peripheral fat patterning.

simultaneous analysis of two or more dependent variables (Cooley and Lohnes, 1971). Canonical correlation is particularly useful when associating two sets of biological observations that each display natural internal structure, such as serum lipid fractions with fat distribution (Bailey et al., 1987).

An alternative approach has been the construction of simple ratios that adequately characterize the contrast initially identified by multivariate techniques; this strategy somewhat alleviates the poor interpretability associated with most ratios. They also are the method of choice for large-scale screening (Norgan and Ferro-Luzzi, 1986). The most popular of these has been the hip–waist circumference ratio noted earlier. A skinfold ratio using a trunk site such as the subscapular and a lower limb site such as the anterior thigh or the calf appears somewhat more effective than an upper limb–trunk contrast in characterizing overall subcutaneous fat distribution (cf. Mueller and Stallones, 1981; Kaplowitz et al., 1987). On the negative side, use of skinfold ratios tends to cull out fatter subjects with unmeasurable folds (Mueller et al., 1987); in this case, a waist–thigh circumference ratio may be preferable. Finally, some evidence suggests the most relevant ratios, whether skinfolds or circumferences, are those that effectively contrast subcutaneous fat on the anterior trunk with omental or mesenteric fat beneath (cf. Ashwell et al., 1985; Sparrow et al., 1986; Davis et al., 1986). This is a different referent than those considered to date using multivariate approaches, and it is unclear if the same contrasts or ratios apply.

There are fewer data on shape change and its relation to physiological change. Mueller, using cross-sectional data, has demonstrated that trunkal fatness increases with age (1982). Trunkal fat patterns defined by circumferences also have been found to resist change in the face of weight loss (Lanska et al., 1985; Johnston et al., 1988; Wadden et al., 1988). There is ample cross-sectional corroboration of trunkal fat increase with age in adults (Garn and Young, 1956; Garn, 1960; Skerlj et al., 1953; Malina and Bouchard, 1988), with longitudinal evidence the trend begins in late infancy (Bailey et al., 1982; Roche and Baumgartner, 1988; Johnston, 1988) and continues into middle age (Chien et al., 1975). Moreover, increased trunkal fatness in middle age has been associated with increased serum lipid levels, and elevated risk of subsequent cardiovascular disease and sudden death (Larsson et al., 1984; Baumgartner et al., 1987). Finally, we know less than we would like about the relations between dimensional changes and adipocyte function; Bjorntorp et al. (1975) have reported that weight reduction through nutritional intervention increases adipocyte triglyceride turnover differentially according to anatomic site.

CONCLUSIONS

I have advanced two major arguments. The first is that theoretical models exist that permit reconceptualization of problems of measurement. Interpretability represents such a reconception. The second is that there is ample empirical justification for concern with interpretability. Indices such as sensitivity or dependability provide a means of quantification, but more sophisticated scales must be developed to test more specific maps of datum and referent.

In this light, recent technology such as nuclear magnetic resonance imaging (NMRI) and single photon emission computed tomography (SPECT) present an unusual opportunity. By visualizing the metabolical activity of local anatomical structures, they force scrutiny of our decades-old models of body architecture. The biological object ceases to be a reified "compartment," such as body fat, or a systemic function, such as serum triglyceride level, and becomes a local phenomenon such as the differential loss of insulin receptor activity on the membrane of large omental adipocytes, or neurotransmitter binding patterns in the limbic system of the brain. We thus face unusual gains in both precision and our ability to map datum to referent.

The most fruitful use of these novel technologies in nutritional assessment may be to invoke a stringent reductionist paradigm. This strategy would target the local: We would analyze the relation of histological events to their metabolic correlates, and then refer local dimensions to their underlying tissue morphology. This is not a novel proposal; Bjorntorp has called for current research in obesity to follow the successful reductionist strategies of hematology a century ago (Bjorntorp, 1984), with an emphasis on examining the local unit, the cell, associated with particular symptoms; and Borkan et al. (1982) have called for association of localized CAT scan data with disease states. Reviving such a research agenda achieves two useful ends: We maximize our use of these technologies enhanced precision, and we generate a far richer map linking observation to referent. It may yet be possible to point out the kangaroo.

REFERENCES

Abdel-Malek AK, Mukherjee D, Roche AF (1985): A method of constructing an index of obesity. Hum Biol 57:415–430.

Ackermann RJ (1985): Data, instruments, and theory Princeton, NJ: Princeton University Press.

Ashwell M, Cole TJ, Dixon AK (1985): Obesity: New Insight into the anthropometric classification of fat distribution shown by computed tomography. Br. Med J 290:1692–1694.

Bailey SM (1985): Human physique and susceptibility to noninfectious disease. Yearbook Phys Anthropol 28:149–173.

Bailey SM, Campos HC, Schosinski K, Mata L (1987): Relationship of upper body fat distribution to serum glucose and lipids in a Costa Rican population. Am J Phys Anthropol 73:111–117.

Bailey SM, Garn SM, Katch VM, Guire, KE (1982): Taxonomic identification of human fat patterns. Am J Phys Anthropol 59:361–366.

Bailey SM, Gershoff SN, McGandy RB, Nondatsuta A, Tantiwongse P (1985): Subcutaneous fat remodelling in Southeast Asian infants and children. Am J Phys Anthropol 68:123–130.

Baker PT, Hunt EE, Sen T (1958): The growth and interrelationships of skinfold and brachial tissues in man. Am J Phys Anthropol 16:39–48.

Bakker HK, Struikenkamp RS (1977): Biological variability and lean body estimates. Hum Biol 53:181–225.

Baltes PB (1968): Longitudinal and cross-sectional sequences in the study of age and generation effects. Hum Dev 11:145–171.

Baumgartner RN, Heymsfield SB, Roche AF, Bernardino M (1988): Abdominal composition quantified by computed tomography. Am J Clin Nutr 48:936–945.

Baumgartner RN, Roche AF, Chumlea WC, Siervogel RM, Glueck CJ (1987): Fatness and fat patterns: Associations with plasma lipids and blood pressures in adults, 18 to 57 years of age. Am J Epidemiol 126:614–628.

Baumgartner RN, Roche AF, Guo S, Lohman T, Boileau RA, Slaughter MH (1986): Adipose tissue distribution: The stability of principal components by sex, ethnicity, and maturation stage. Hum Biol 58:719–735.

Behnke AR (1942): Specific gravity of healthy men. JAMA 118:495–497.

Behnke AR, Guttentag OE, Brodsky C (1959): Quantification of body weight and configuration from anthropometric measurements. Hum Biol 31:213–234.

Behnke AR, Wilmore JH (1972): The evaluation and regulation of body build and composition. Englewood Cliffs, NJ: Prentice-Hall.

Belko AZ, Van Loan M, Barbieri TF, Mayclin. P (1987): Diet, exercise, weight loss, and energy expenditure in moderately overweight women. Int J Obes 11:93–104.

Benn RT (1971): Some mathematical properties of weight for height indices used as measures of adiposity. Br J Prev Soc Med 25:42–50.

Billewicz WZ, Kemsley WFF, Thomson AM (1962): Indices of adiposity. Br. J Prev Soc Med 16:183–187.

Bjorntorp P (1975): Efect of an energy reduced dietary regimen in relation to adipose tissue cellularity in obese women. Am J Clin Nutr 28:450–452.

Bjorntorp P (1984): Morphological classifications of obesity: What they tell us, what they don't. Int J Obes 8:525–533.

Bogin B MacVean RB (1981): Nutritional and biological determinants of body fat patterning in urban Guatemalan children. Hum Biol 53:259–268.

Bolinder J, Kager L, Ostman J, Arner P (1983): Differences at the receptor and postreceptor levels between human omental and subcutaneous adipose tissue in the action of insulin on lipolysis. Diabetes 32:117–122.

Borkan GA, Gersoff SG, Robbins AH (1982): Assessment of abdominal fat content by computed tomography. Am J Clin Nutr 36:172–177.

Borkan GA, Hults DE, Glynn RJ (1983): Role of longitudinal change and secular trend in age differences in male body dimensions. Hum Biol 55:629–641.

Borkan GA Norris AH (1977): Fat redistribution and the changing body dimensions of the adult male. Hum Biol 49:495–514.

Bouchard C, Norgan NG (ed): Tremblay A (1985): Genetics of body composition and fat distribution. In "Human Body Composition and Fat Distribution." Euro-Nut. Report No. 8. Den Haag: CIP-Gegevens Koninklijke Bibliotheek.

Boyd E (1933): The specific gravity of the human body. Hum Biol 5:646–672.

Bray GA, Greenway FL, Molitch ME, Dahms WT, Atkinson RL, Hamilton K (1978): Use of anthropometric measures to assess weight loss. Am J Clin Nutr 31:769–773.

Brozek J, Grande F, Anderson JT, Keys A (1963): Densitometric analysis of body composition: Revision of some quantitative assumptions. Ann NY Acad Sci 110:113–139.

Buono MJ, McKenzie TL, McKenzie RE (1985): Effects of a diet and exercise progrm on blood lipids, cardiovascular function and body composition in obese women. Med Sci Sports 17:189–194.

Butts NK, Bewster E, Van Ossbree P, Price S (1985): Effects of a 12 week weight training program on the body composition of women over and under 40 years of age. Med Sci Sports 17:267–276.

Byard PJ, Siervogel RM, Roche AF (1988): Age trends in transmissible and non-transmissible components of family resemblance for stature. Ann Hum Biol 15:111–118.

Cameron N (1986): The methods of auxological anthropology. In Falkvier F, Tanner JM (eds): "Growth. Vol. 3." New York: Plenum Press.

Centers for Disease Control 2nd ed. (CDC) (1972): "Ten-State Nutritional Survey in the United States, 1968–70. Vol III: Clinical, Anthropometry, Dental." DHEW Publ. No. (HSM) 72–8131.

Chien S, Peng MT, Chen KP, Huang TF, Chang C, Fang HS (1975): Longitudinal studies on adipose tissue and fat distribution in human subjects. J Appl Physiol 39:825–830.

Chumlea WC, Roche AF, Rogers E (1984a): Replicability for anthropometry in the elderly. Hum Biol 56:329–337.

Chumlea WC, Roche AF, Webb P (1984b): Body size, sucutaneous fatness and total body fat in older adults. Int J Obes 8:311–317.

Clarys JP, Martin AD (1987): The concept of the adipose tissue-free mass. In Norgan NG (ed): "Human Body Composition and Fat Distribution." Den Haag: CIP-Gegevens Koninklijke Bibliotheek.

Cohn SH, Ellis KJ, Vartsky D, Sawitsky K, Gartenhaus W, Yasumura S, Vaswani AN (1981): Comparison of methods of estimating body fat in normal subjects and cancer patients. Am J Clin Nutr 34:2839–2847.

Cooley WW, Lohnes PR (1971): Multivariate data analysis. New York: Wiley.

Cronk CE, Roche AF, Chumlea WC Kent R (1982): Longitudinal trends of weight/stature^2 in childhood in relationship to adulthood body fatness measures. Hum Biol 54:751–764.

Damon A, (1965): Discrepancies between findings of longitudinal and cross-sectional studies in adult life: Physique and physiology. Hum Dev 8:16–22.

Davis PSW, Jones PRM, Norgan NG (1986): The distribution of subcutaneous and internal fat in man. Ann Hum Biol 13:189–192.

Depres J-P, Tremblay A, Bouchard C (1988): Regional adipose tissue distribution and plasma lipoproteins. In C Bouchard C, Johnston F (eds): "Fat Distribution During Growth and Later Health Outcomes." New York: Liss.
Draper N, Smith H (1981): "Applied Regression Analysis." 2nd ed. New York: Wiley.
Durnin JVGA, Wormersley J (1974): Body fat assessed from total body density and its estimation from skinfold thickness: Measurements on 481 men and women aged 16 to 72 years. Br J Nutr 32:77–97.
Edwards DAW (1951): Differences in the distribution of subcutaneous fat with sex and maturity. Clin Sci 10:305.
Evans DJ, Hoffman RG, Kalkhoff RK, Kissebah AH (1984): Relation of androgenic activity to body fat topography, fat cell morphology and metabolic aberrations in premenopausal women. J Clin Endo. Metabol 57:304–310.
Feinleib M, Garrison RJ, Fabsitz R, Christian JC, Hrubec Z, Borhani NO, Kannel WB, Roseman R, Schwartz JT, Wagner JO (1977): The NHLBI twin study of cardiovascular disease risk factors: Methodology and summary of results. Am J Epidemiol 106:284–295.
Feldman R, Sender AJ, Siegelaub AB (1969): Difference in diabetic and nondiabetic fat distribution patterns by skinfold measurements. Diabetes 18:478–485.
Feyerabend PK (1975): "Against Method. New York: Humanities Press.
Fidanza F, Keys A, Anderson JT (1953): Density of body fat in man and other animals. J Appl Physiol 6:252–256.
Flint MM, Drinkwater BL, Wells CL, Horvath SM (1977): Validity of estimating body fat of females: Effect of age and fitness. Hum Biol: 49:559–572.
Florey C du V (1970): The use and interpretation of ponderal index and other weight–height ratios in epidemiological studies. J Chronic Dis 23:99–103.
Forbes GB, Brown MRB, Griffiths HJL (1988): Arm muscle plus bone area: Anthropometry and CAT scan compared. Am J Clin Nutr 47:929–931.
Forbes GB, Reina JC (1970) Adult lean body mass declines with age: Some longitudinal observations. Metabol 19:653–663.
Foster CJ, Weinsier RL, Birch R, Norris DJ, Bernstein RS, Wang JW, Pierson RN, Van Itallie TB (1987): Obesity and serum lipids: An evaluation of the relative contribution of body fat and fat distribution to lipid levels. Int J Obes 11:151–161.
Fried SK, Kral JG (1987): Sex differences in regional distribution of fat cell size and lipoprotein lipase activity in morbidly obese patients. Int J Obes 11:129–140.
Freidlander JS, Costa PT, Bosse R, Ellis E, Rhoads JG, Stroudt HW (1977): Longitudinal physique changes among healthy white veterans at Boston. Hum Biol 49:541–558.
Frisancho AR, Flegel PN (1983): Elbow breadth as a measure of frame size. Am J Clin Nutr 37:311–314.
Garn SM (1955): Relative fat patterning: An individual characteristic. Hum Biol 27:75–89.
Garn SM (1960): Fat accumulation and aging in males and females. In "The Biology of Aging." American Institute of Biological Sciences Symposium No. 6.
Garn SM (1963): Some pitfalls in the quantification of body composition. Ann NY Acad Sci 110:172–174.
Garn SM, Bailey SM, Cole PE (1980): Continuities and changes in fatness and obesity. In Schemmel R (ed): "Nutrition, Physiology and Obesity." Boca Raton, Fla: CRC Press.
Garn SM, Leonard WR, Hawthorne VM (1986): Three limitations of the body mass index. Am J Clin Nutr 44:996–997.

Garn SM, Pesick SD, Hawthorne VM (1983): The boney chest breadth as a frame size standard in nutritional assessment. Am J Clin Nutr 37:315–318.

Garn SM, Sullivan TV, Hawthorne VM (1987): Differential rates of fat change relative to weight change a different body sites. Int J Obes 11:519–525.

Garn SM, Young RW (1956): Concurrently fat loss and fat gain. Am J Phys Anthropol 14:497–504.

Goldbourt U, Medalie JH (1974): Weight–height indices: Choice of the most suitable index and its association with selected variables among 10,000 adult males of heterogeneous origin. Br J Soc Prev Med 25:42–50.

Goldstein H (1979): "The Design and Analysis of Longitudinal Studies." New York: Academic Press.

Gordon T, Shurtleff D (1973): Means at each examination and interexamination variation of specified characteristics: Framingham Study, exam 1 to 10. In Kannel W, Gordon T (eds): "The Framingham Study. DHEW No. 74-478: Washington, DC: GPO.

Greenland S (1980): The effect of misclassification in the presence of covariates. Am J Epidemiol 112:564–569.

Gurney JM, Jelliffe DB (1973): Arm anthropometry in nutritional assessment: Nongram for rapid calculation of muscle circumference and cross-sectional muscle and fat areas. Am J Clin Nutr 26:912–916.

Gurr MI, Jung RT, Robinson MP, James WPT (1982): Adipose tissue cellularity in men: The relationship between fat cell size and number, the mass and distribution of body fat, and the history of weight gain. Int J Obes 6:419–436.

Habicht JP, Yarbrough C, Martorell R (1979): Anthropometric field methods: Criteria for selection. In "Jelliffe DB, Jelliffe EFP (eds): "Human Nutrition. Vol 2." New York: Plenum Press.

Haffner SM, Stern MP, Hazuda HP, Rosenthal M, Knapp A (1986): The role of behavioral variables and fat patterning in explaining ethnic differences in serum lipids and lipoproteins. Am J Epidemiol 123:830–839.

Hall JC, O'Quigley J, Giles GR, Appleton N, Stocks H (1980): Upper limb anthropometry: The value of measurement variance studies. Am J Clin Nutr 33:1846–1851.

Hartz AJ, Rupley DC, Rimm AA (1984): The association of girth measurements with disease in 32,856 women. Am J Epidemiol 119:71–80.

Heymsfield S, McManus C, Smith J, Stevens V, Nixon DW (1982): Anthropometric measurement of muscle mass: Revised equations for calculation of bone free arm muscle area. Am J Clin Nutr 36:680–690.

Himes J (1987): Purposeful assessment of nutritional status. In Johnston F (ed): "Nutritional Anthropology." New York: Liss.

Himes JH, Bouchard C (1985): Do the new Metropolitan Life Insurance weight–height tables correctly assess body frame and body fat relationships? Am J Public Health 75:1076–1079.

Himes JH, Roche AF, Webb P (1980): Fat areas as estimates of total body fat. Am J Clin Nutr 33:2093–2100.

Holton G (1973): "Introduction to Concepts and Theories in Physical Science." Reading, Mass: Addison-Wesley.

Holton G (1978): "The Scientific Imagination: Case Studies." Cambridge, Mass: Harvard University Press.

Howells WW (1951): Factors of human physique. Am J Phys Anthropol 9:159–192.

Hsu P-H, Mathewson FAL, Rabkin SW (1977): Blood pressure and body mass index patterns—a longitudinal study. J Chronic Dis 30:93–113.

James KE (1973): Regression toward the mean in uncontrolled clinical studies. Biometrics 29:121–130.

Johnston FE (1988): Sex differences in fat patterning in children and youth. In Bouchard C, Johnston F (eds): "Fat Distribution During Growth and Later Health Outcomes." New York: Liss.

Johnston FE, Wadden TA, Stunkard AJ, Pena M, Pierson RN, Van Itallie TB (1988): Body fat distribution in obese women, I: Patterns of fat distribution. Am J Clin Nutr 47:225–228.

Jones PRM, Hunt MJ, Brown TP, Norgan NG (1986): Waist–hip circumference ratio and its relation to age and overweight in British men. Hum Nutr 40C: 239–247.

Kaplowitz HJ, Mueller WH, Selwyn BJ, Malina RM, Bailey D, Mirwald RL (1987): Sensitivities, specificities, and positive predictive value of simple indices of body fat distribution. Hum Biol 59:809–825.

Katch FI, Behnke AR, Katch VL (1987): The ponderal somatogram: Evaluation of body size and shape from anthropometric girths and stature. Hum Biol 59:439–458.

Kelsey JL, Thompson WD Evans AS (1986): Methods in observational epidemiology. New York: Oxford University Press.

Keys A, Brozek J (1953): Body fat in adult man. Physiol Rev 33:245–325.

Khosla T, Lowe CR (1967): Indices of obesity derived from body weight and height. Br J Prev Soc Med 21:122–128.

Khoury P, Morrison JA, Mellies MJ, Glueck CJ (1983): Weight change since age 18 years in 30–55 year-old whites and blacks. JAMA 250:3179–3187.

King MA, Katch F (1986): Changes in body density, fatfolds and girths at 2.3 kg increments of weight loss. Hum Biol 58:709–718.

Kissebah AH, Peiris A, Evans DJ (1988): Mechanisms associating body fat distribution to glucose intolerance and diabetes mellitus. In Bouchard C, Johnston F (eds): "Fat Distribution During Growth and Later Health Outcomes." New York: Liss.

Kodama AM (1971): In vivo and in vitro determination of body fat and body water in the hamster. J Appl Physiol 31:218–222.

Krotkiewski M, Bjorntorp P, Sjostrum L, Smith P (1983): Impact of obesity on metabolism in men and women: Importance of regional adipose tissue distribution. J Clin Invest 72:1150–1162.

Kuhn TS (1970): "The Structure of Scientific Revolutions." Chicago: University of Chicago Press.

Lakatos I (1976): "Proofs and Refutations." Cambridge: Cambridge University Press.

Lanska DJ, Lanska MJ, Hartz AJ, Kalkhoff RK, Ripley D, Rimm AA (1985): A prospective study of body fat distribution and weight loss. Int J Obes 9:241–246.

Larsson B, Svardsudd K, Welin L, Wilhelmsen L, Bjorntorp P, Tibblin G (1984): Abdominal adipose tissue distribution, obesity and risk of cardiovascular disease and death: 13 year follow up of participants in the study of men born in 1913. Br Med J 288:1401–1404.

Lesser GT, Kumar I, Steele M (1963): Chnages in body composition with age. Ann NY Acad Sci 110:578–587.

Lohman TG (1981): Skinfolds and body density and their relation to body fatness: A review. Hum Biol 53:181–225.

Lohman TG, Roche AF, Martorell R (1988): "Anthropometric Standardization Reference Manual." Champaign, Ill: Human Kinetics.

Malina RM, Bouchard C (1988): Subcutaneous fat distribution during growth. In Bouchard C, Johnston F (eds): "Fat Distribution During Growth and Later Health Outcomes." New York: Liss.

McCloy CH (1936): Appraising physical status: The selection of measurements. University of Iowa Studies in Child Welfare 12, No. 2. Iowa City: University of Iowa Press.

Masters AM, Lesser RP, Beckman G (1960): Tables of average weight and height of Americans 65 to 95 years. JAMA 1972:658–662.

Matiegka J (1921): The testing of physical efficiency. Am J. Phys Anthropol 4:223–230.

Micozzi MS, Albanes D, Jones Y, Chumlea C (1986): Correlations of body mass index with weight, stature, and body composition in men and women in NHANES I and II. Am J Clin Nutr 44:725–731.

Montoye HJ, Epstein FH, Kjelsberg MO (1965): The measurement of body fatness: A study in a total community. Am J Clin Nutr 16:417–427.

Mosteller F, Tukey JW (1977): "Data Analysis and Regression." Reading, Mass: Addison-Wesley, pp 135–162.

Mueller WH (1982): The changes with age of the anatomical distribution of fat. Soc Sci Med 16:191–196.

Mueller WH, Martorell R (1988): Reliability and accuracy of measurement. In Lohman TG, Roch AF, Martorell, R (eds): Anthropometric Standardization Manual." Champaign, Ill: Human Kinetics.

Mueller WH Reid RM (1979): A multivariate analysis of fatness and relative fat patterning. Am J Phys Anthropol 199–208.

Mueller WH, Stallones L (1981): Anatomical distribution of sucutaneous fat: Skinfold choice and construction of indices. Hum Biol 53:321–335.

Mueller WH, Wear ML, Hanis CL, Barton SA, Schull WJ (1987): Body circumferences as alternatives to skinfold measurements of body fat distribution in Mexican-Americans. Int J Obes 11:309–318.

Mukherjee D, Roche AF (1984): The estimation of percent body fat, body density and total body fat by maximum regression equations. Hum Biol 56:79–109.

Myers JL (1979): "Fundamentals of Experimental Design." 3rd ed. Boston: Allyn and Bacon.

National Center for Health Statistics (NCHS) (1965): Weight, height, and selected body dimensions of adults, United States, 1960–62 Ser. 11, No. 8. DHEW Publ. No. (HRA) 76–1074. Washington, DC: GPO.

National Center for Health Statistics (NCHS) (1973): Selected measurements of children 6–11 years, United States. Ser. 11, No. 123. DHHS Publ. Washington, DC: GPO.

National Center for Health Statistics (NCHS) (1979): Weight and height of adults, 18–74 years of age, United States 1971–74. Series 11, No. 211. DHEW Publ. No. 79–1659. Washington, DC: GPO.

National Center for Health Statistics (NCHS) (1981): Plan and operation of the second national health and nutrition examination survey, 1976–80. Ser. 1, No. 15. DHHS Publ. No. (PHS) 81–1317. Washington, DC: GPO.

National Center for Health Statistics (NCHS) (1987): Anthropometric reference data and prevalence of overweight, United States, 1976–80. Ser. 11, No. 238. DHHS Publ. No. (PHS) 87–1688. Washington, DC GPO.

Neter J, Wasserman W (1974): "Applied Linear Statistical Models." Homewood, Ill: RD Irwin.

Noppa H, Anderson M, Bengtsson C, Bruce A, Isaksson B (1979): Body composition in middle-aged women with special reference to correlation between body fat mass and anthropometric data. Am J Clin Nutr 32:1388–1395.

Norgan NG, Ferro-Luzzi A (1986): Simple indices of subcutaneous fat patterning. Ecol Food Nutr 18:117–123.

Norris AH, Lundy T, Shock NW (1963): Trends in selected indices of body composition in men between the ages 30 and 80 years. Ann NY Acad Sci 110:623–639.

Pedhazur EJ (1982): "Multiple Regression in Behavioral Research." 2nd ed. New York: Holt, Rinehart and Winston.

Poehlmann ET, Tremblay A, Depres JP, Fontaine E, Perusse L, Theriault G, Bouchard C (1986): Genotype - controlled changes in body composition and fat morphology following overfeeding in twins. Am. J Clin Nutr 43:723–731.

Popper K (1959): "The Logic of Scientific Discovery." London: Hutchinson.

Ramirez ME, Mueller WH (1980): The development of obesity and fat patterning in Tokelau children. Hum Biol 52:675–687.

Rathbun EN, Pace N (1945): Studies on body composition, 1: Determination of body fat by means of specific gravity. J Biol Chem 158:667–671.

Rebuffe-Scrive M, Enk L, Crona N, Lonnroth P, Abrahamsson L, Smith U, Bjorntorp P (1985): Fat cell metabolism in different regions of women. Effect of menstrual cycle, pregnancy and lactation. J Clin Invest 75:1973–1976.

Roche AF (1984): Anthropometric methods: New and old, what they tell us. Int J Obes 8:509–523.

Roche AF, Baumgartner RN (1988): Tracking in fat distribution during growth. In Bouchard C, Johnston F (eds): "Fat Distribution During Growth and Later Health Outcomes." New York: Liss.

Rookus MA, Burema J, van't Hof MA, Duerenberg P, Hautvast JGAJ (1987a): The development of the body mass index in young adults, II: Interrelationships of level, change and fluctuation, a four-year longitudinal study. Hum Biol 59:617–630.

Rookus MA, Burema J, van't Hof MA, Duerenberg P, van der Wiel-Wetzels WAM, Hautvast JGAJ (1987b): The development of the body mass index in young adults, I: Age reference curves based on a four-year mixed longitudinal study. Hum Biol 59:599–615.

Schaie KW (1965): A general model for the study of developmental problems. Psych Bull 64:92–107.

Schmitt LH, Harrison GA (1988): Patterns in within-population variance in stature and weight. Ann Hum Biol 15:353–364.

Seidell JC, Oosterlee A, Thijssen MAO, Burema J, Duerenberg P, Hautvast J, Rujis JHJ (1987): Assessment of intra-abdominal and subcutaneous abdominal fat: Relation between anthropometry and computed tomography. Am J Clin Nutr 45:7–13.

Sheldon WH, Stevens SS, Tucker WB (1940): "The Varieties of Human Physique." New York: Harper.

Sheng HP, Huggins RA (1979): A review of body composition studies with emphasis on total body water and fat. Am J Clin Nutr 32:630–647.

Shively CA, Clarkson TB, Miller LC, Weingand KW (1987): Body fat distribution as a risk factor for coronary artery atherosclerosis in female Cynomolgus monkeys. Arteriosclerosis 7:26–231.

Siegel S (1956): "Nonparametric Statistics." New York: McGraw-Hill.

Siri WE (1956): The gross composition of the body. Adv Biol Med Phy 4:239–254.

Skerlj B, Brozek J, Hunt EE (1953): Subcutaneous fat and age changes in body build and body form in women. Am J Phys Anthropol 11:577–600.

Snedecor GW, Cochran WG (1967): "Statistical Methods." 6th ed Ames, Iowa: Iowa State University Press.

Sparrow D, Borkan GA, Gersof SG, Wisniewski C, Silbert CK (1986): Relationship of fat distribution to glucose tolerance. Diabetes 35:411–415.

Steen B, Bruce A, Isaksson B, Levin T, Ivanborg A (1977): Body composition in 70-year old males and females in Gotnenberg, Sweden, a population study. Acta Medica Scand 611(suppl):87–112.
Stevens SS (1946): On a theory of scales in measurement. Science 103:677–680.
Stokes J, Garrison R, Kannel WB (1985): The independent contribution of various indices of obesity to the 22-year incidence of coronary heart disease: The Framingham Study. In Vague J (ed): "Metabolic Complications of Human Obesity." Amsterdam: Elsevier.
Susanne C (1977): Heritability of anthropological characters. Human Biol 49:573–580.
Szathmary EJE, Holt N (1983): Hyperglycemia in Dogrib indians of the northwest territories, Canada: Association with age and a centripetal distribution of fat. Hum Biol 55:493–515.
Szczotka FA (1981): Canonical decomposition of the process of simultaneous growth of body height, trunk length, biacromial diameter, biiliocristal diameter, and thigh circumference in boys and girls aged 9 to 18 years. Stud Phys Anthropol 7:87–96.
Tanner JM (1951): Some notes on the reporting of growth data. Hum Biol. 23:93–159.
Trotter M, Broman GE Peterson RR (1960): Density of bones of white and negro skeletons. J Bone Jt Surg 42A:50–59.
Vague J (1956): The degree of masculine differentiation of obesities: A factor determining predisposition to diabetes, atherosclerosis, gout, and uric calculous disease. Am J Clin Nutr 4:20–28.
van't Hof MA, Roede MJ, Kowalski CJ (1977): A mixed longitudinal data analysis model. Hum Biol 49:165–179.
Wadden TA, Stunkard AJ, Johnston FE, Wang, J, Pierson RN, Van Itallie TB, Costello E, Pena M (1988): Body fat distribution in adult obese women, II: Changes in fat distribution accompanying weight reduction. Am J Clin Nutr 47:229–234.
Ward GM, Krzywicki HJ, Rahman DP, Quass RI, Nelson RA, Consolazio CF (1975): Relationship of anthropometric measurements to body fat as determined by densitometry, potassium-40, and body water. Am J Clin Nutr 28:162–169.
Wartofsky M (1968): "The Conceptual Foundations of Scientific Theories." London: MacMillan.
Weinsier RL, Norris DJ, Birch R, Bernstein RS, Wang J, Yang M-V, Pierson RN, Van Itallie TB (1985): The selective contribution of body fat and fat pattern to blood pressure levels. Hypertension 7:578–585.
White FMM, Pereira LH, Garner JB (1986): Associations of body mass index and waist:hip ratio with hypertension. Can Med Assoc J 135:313–320.
Woolf CM (1968): Principles of biometry. Princeton, NJ: D Van Nostrand.
Wormersly J, Durnin JVGA (1977): A comparison of the skinfold method with extent of overweight and various weight–height relationships in the assessment of obesity. Br J Nutr 38:281–292.
Young CM, Blondin J, Tensuan R, Fryer JH (1963): Body composition studies of "older" woman, thirty to seventy years of age. Ann NY Acad Sci 110:589–607.
Zerfas AJ (1979): Anthropometric field methods: General. In Jelliffe DB, Jelliffe EF (eds): "Human Nutrition, Vol 2." New York: Plenum Press.

Anthropometric Assessment
of Nutritional Status, pages 83–111

5
Weight–Stature Indices to Measure Underweight, Overweight, and Obesity

T.J. COLE
MRC Dunn Nutrition Unit, Cambridge CB4 1XJ, England

INTRODUCTION

Size and Shape

Body weight is a measure of how heavy a person is, while stature indicates how tall they are. Both these quantities reflect the *size* of the individual. However, they differ in their biological significance, and both contain information other than just the person's size.

Weight is more informative than stature, in that it is more variable—the coefficient of variation (CV) of weight is three to four times the CV of stature. So if weight and stature are to be made equivalent in terms of their size information, stature needs to be scaled up in some way (or equivalently weight scaled down). When this is done appropriately, size can be cancelled out by subtracting scaled stature from weight, and the remaining information indicates the person's *shape* (Colliver et al., 1983).

This then is a general definition of *weight for stature*, a quantity which measures shape largely independently of size. It is widely used in nutritional status assessment because shape is felt to be, in the broadest sense, indicative of body composition (Keys et al., 1972).

Indices of Shape

There are two obvious forms of weight adjusted for stature,

$$W - b.S \quad (1)$$

and

$$W/S^p \quad (2)$$

where W and S represent weight and stature respectively, and the quantities b and p specify how stature is to be scaled. As will be made clear in later sections, *all* the indices of weight for stature that have been proposed over the years can be expressed in one or other of these basic forms.

Equation 2 consists of weight divided by a power function of stature, which does not accord with the general definition arrived at above, of weight less scaled stature. However, it can be put in the required form by using a logarithmic transformation, i.e.,

$$\log (W/S^p) = \log W - p.\log S. \quad (3)$$

This is now the same as equation 1 except that W and S are replaced by log W and log S. On a graph of weight plotted against stature, equation 1 appears as a straight line, while equations 2 and 3 represent a gentle curve. Equally, if weight is plotted against stature on log-log graph paper, then equation 2 is a straight line while 1 is slightly curved. Hence, if b and p, the slopes of the lines, are chosen appropriately, the two shape indices are very similar (Benn, 1971).

The indices in equations 1 and 2 measure absolute rather than relative shape. To be more useful they need to be expressed relative to some reference, and this can be done by incorporating the reference into the equation. Suppose that W_0 and S_0 represent reference weight and stature, obtained either as typical or desirable values. A *typical* value in this context means the average for the population, while a *desirable* value is in some sense optimal for health. If one imagines a hypothetical reference population where obesity or malnutrition is nonexistent, then the desirable value would be the average for this perfect population.

Equations 1 and 2 extend respectively to

$$W - b.S - (W_0 - b.S_0) \quad (4)$$

and

$$W/S^p \; / \; W_0/S_0^p \quad (5)$$

As before, 5 can be put into the same form as 4 by taking logarithms:

$$\log W - p.\log S - (\log W_0 - p.\log S_0) \quad (6)$$

The quantities b, p, W_0 and S_0 are all constants, so that 4 and 5 can be simplified to

$$W - b.S - c \quad (7)$$

and

$$W/S^p/ \; k \quad (8)$$

where c and k are also constants, taking the values $(W_0 - b.S_0)$ and W_0/S_0^p respectively.

The index (5, 8), which can be called *relative* W/S^p, has the useful property that p is independent of the units of measurement. Whether weight and stature are measured in metric or imperial units, the value of index 5 is the same. This property does not hold with index 4, where a change of units requires the scaling factor b to be changed as well.

All the equations (1–8) define an infinite number of different weight-for-stature indices, depending on the precise choices of b and p. Their values should not be negative, as otherwise the index will combine weight and stature positively, which is a measure of size, not shape. Apart from this, b and p can (in principle) lie anywhere between zero and an arbitrarily large positive number. If they are zero, for example, then the index ignores stature entirely and is based only on weight. Conversely if they take a very large value, weight becomes unimportant and the index consists of negative stature. In this case, tall individuals are judged as underweight and the short appear overweight.

Clearly neither of these extremes is particularly useful (!), and the optimal value will lie somewhere in between. However, in order to measure shape optimally, it is necessary to have a precise definition of shape itself.

Criteria for Defining Shape

The precise definition of shape is crucial to the issue of deciding how to construct a weight-for-stature index. Over the years there have been a variety of views on the subject, reflecting the differing backgrounds of the workers involved. Studies involving adults as opposed to children, or concerned with obesity as against malnutrition, or based on low-technology versus high-technology methods, have all used slightly different definitions of shape.

Three conditions commonly identified using weight–stature indices are underweight, overweight, and obesity, and each implicitly defines shape in a different way. They all act as proxies for some underlying state of health or disease, but the disease is different in the three cases. Underweight and overweight are just opposite ends of the same spectrum in the sense that one is a deficit, and the other an excess, of weight relative to some reference weight. However, underweight is also closely linked to malnutrition and is often treated as a proxy for it.

At the other end of the spectrum, overweight and more particularly obesity are proxies for increased risk of several conditions including heart disease and hypertension (Bray, 1987; Weatherall and Shaper, 1988). While overweight is simply an excess of weight, obesity is specifically an excess of body fat.

Both malnutrition and heart disease can result in death, so that the ideal index should be able to predict future mortality accurately. In practice, however, death is a difficult end point to study because of the large sample sizes and long time scales required. Third world studies of malnourished young children (Chen et al., 1980) have provided the most direct evidence of mortality risk related to weight for stature, although large studies of Western world adults have also demonstrated excess mortality at both ends of the weight-for-stature spectrum (Waaler, 1984; Bray, 1987).

Because of the difficulty in linking weight for stature to mortality risk, particularly in the Western world, other criteria for defining weight-for-stature have always been popular. The simplest expresses weight as a fraction of some reference weight based on the subject's stature (and sex and possibly age). The reference weight is obtained from a table, a regression equation, or a chart, and the fraction is often called *relative* weight.

A more recent requirement of weight-for-stature is that it should predict body fat mass, expressed either in absolute terms or as a fraction of body weight. This is not the same as relative weight, which assumes that the amount of body fat is the same irrespective of stature. Expressed in terms of reference populations, relative weight uses as a baseline how people *are*, whereas the prediction of body fat has as its basis how people *ought to be*, i.e., relative to the "perfect" reference population described above.

The two are not the same. For example, if short people tend to be relatively fatter than tall people, then the reference weight for short people will be exaggerated due to the inclusion of their extra body fat. Relative weight then underestimates the level of obesity in short individuals.

Thus the three terms underweight, overweight, and obesity require shape to predict mortality, relative weight, and body fat (Garrow, 1983). In correlation terms this needs high correlations with mortality and body fat, and a zero correlation with stature. An index which is suitable for one of these purposes may not be suitable for the others.

The aim here is to examine the various indices of weight for stature that have been proposed at different times; to show that they are all special cases of the relative W/S^p index, as described in the previous section; to highlight some of their strengths and weaknesses; and to describe the use of one particular index (W/S^2) in more detail.

INDICES OF WEIGHT FOR STATURE IN ADULTS

Weight-for-stature is applied to adults and children in much the same way. Despite this, the two age groups are rarely considered together. Equally, it is unusual to discuss both ends of the nutritional status spectrum, obesity and malnutrition, at the same time. The reasons for this are more historical than physiological, and there are advantages in discussing them together. Nevertheless, while describing the different indices it is helpful to separate adults and children, if only to emphasise the age adjustment that children need, and adults largely do not.

Broca's Index

In 1879 Broca described what is probably the simplest weight-for-stature index, W (measured in kg) $-$ $100.S$ (measured in m). This is a special case of the more general index $W - b.S$.

Relative Weight and Weight–Stature Regression

Relative weight is obtained by expressing the subject's weight as a fraction (or percentage) of some reference weight, based on the subject's stature and sex. At its simplest, the reference weight is obtained from a table (e.g., Montegriffo, 1968). However, Billewicz, Kemsley, and Thomson (1962) showed that in adults weight and stature were linearly related, so that the regression line of weight on stature could be used to provide reference weight for a given stature. Assume the fitted regression line is

$$W = b.S + c + \text{error} \tag{9}$$

where b is the regression coefficient and c is the intercept. Fitting the line by least squares, the error term is minimised by minimising the sum of squares of $W - b.S - c$, so that b is chosen to remove all the stature information from weight. This means that $W - b.S$ contains no stature information, and is an index of shape independent of stature. Broca's index is one particular form of this index.

Using equation 9, the reference weight W_0 for a subject of stature S is defined as

$$W_0 = b.S + c, \tag{10}$$

which corresponds to the average weight for all subjects of stature S: Now, if the subject's weight is W, the relative weight is

$$W / (b.S + c). \tag{11}$$

Hence relative weight based on a regression equation is the same as an index involving just weight, stature, and the two constants b and c which are derived from the reference population.

A modification of relative weight involves not a reference weight but a reference *range* of weights, such as those based on insurance statistics (Metropolitan Life Insurance Co, 1959; Society of Actuaries, 1979). Relative weight in this case is usually calculated using the upper end of the weight range.

W/S^n

The indices W/S, W/S^2, and W/S^3 are all of the general form W/S^n, where n is a whole number. The latter two indices have a long and distinguished history, having first been proposed well over 100 years ago. W/S^3 was discussed by Buffon in the late 18th century, while Quetelet (1869) considered both W/S^3 and W/S^2, preferring the latter. Both have been reinvented since, most notably by Rohrer (1908) (W/S^3) and Kaup (1921) (W/S^2). Keys et al. (1972)

gave W/S^2 the name body mass index, or BMI, although it should more correctly be called Quetelet's index.

The appeal of W/S^3 has always been that mathematically, it is a measure of body density. Density is defined as weight/volume, and on simple dimensional grounds stature^3 is proportional to volume. W/S^3 has also been used in other forms, e.g., $S/W^{1/3}$ or $W^{1/3}/S$, under the general name of ponderal index (Sheldon et al., 1940). The index with stature in the numerator gives larger values in thin subjects, and so measures leanness rather than fatness.

The justification for W/S^2 is more statistical than mechanical, in that (to quote Quetelet, 1869), weight goes as the square of stature (Garrow, 1983). This is discussed further in the next section.

The simplest form of W/S^n, i.e., W/S, is usually called the weight–stature ratio, or more confusingly, relative weight (Killeen et al., 1978). It has not received the detailed attention that W/S^2 and W/S^3 have, but even so it is popular as a simple way of adjusting weight for stature.

Many studies have looked at the correlations of these three indices with stature, preferring the one with the smallest correlation on the grounds that it best approximates relative weight (Khosla and Lowe, 1967; Evans and Prior, 1969; Florey, 1970; Keys et al., 1972). The overwhelming impression from these studies is that in men, W/S^2 is consistently better than W/S and W/S^3, while in women W/S^2 and W/S are equally useful.

High correlation with a proxy for obesity is an alternative criterion for choosing the index, and the obvious proxy here is body fat. Roche et al. (1981) showed that in adults, W/S^2 was the weight–stature index best correlating with both total body fat and body fat expressed as a percentage of weight. The correlations were appreciably higher with total body fat. Norgan and Ferro-Luzzi (1982) and Revicki and Israel (1986) found the same, using estimates of body fat based both on skinfolds and hydrostatic weighing. Garrow and Webster (1985) showed that body fat expressed as F/S^2 was highly correlated with W/S^2, subsequently confirmed by Leonhardt et al. (1987).

Frisancho and Flegel (1982) found that W/S^2 correlated best with triceps and subscapular skinfolds, and Micozzi et al. (1986) found the same for subscapular skinfold in men. However, in women they preferred W/S or $W/S^{1.5}$. Mueller et al. (1985) showed that W/S^2 was well correlated with a clinical rating of obesity based on silhouettes, but this result has to be suspect as the observers did the assessment after doing the anthropometry.

W/S^p

The index W/S^p is different from the indices W/S, W/S^2, or W/S^3 in that the stature power p is estimated from the population being studied. It is commonly called the Benn index, after Benn (1971), who highlighted the link between it and the relative weight regression approach (9) of Billewicz, Kemsley, and Thomson (1962) (see the section on Relative Weight as W/S^p, page 96).

According to Khosla and Lowe (1967) and Benn (1971), the value of p should be chosen to make the index uncorrelated with stature. There are three ways to do this, which all give very similar answers. The simplest is to calculate the correlation between stature and the index for a series of values of p, and to interpolate to find the value that gives a correlation of zero. However, this method does not give a standard error for p, so the precision of the estimate cannot be judged.

The second approach, which Benn (1971) advocated, is to calculate the regression coefficient b of weight on stature (9) for the population, and then to obtain p as follows:

$$p = b.S_0/W_0 \tag{12}$$

where W_0 and S_0 are the population mean weight and stature. Benn also gave a formula for the standard error of p. Note though that the correlation of this index with stature, although very small, is not exactly zero.

The third approach is to take natural logarithms of weight and stature, and to estimate p with its standard error from the regression of log weight on log stature (Khosla and Lowe, 1967):

$$\log W = p.\log S + \log k + \text{error}. \tag{13}$$

This value of p is such that log (W/S^p) has a correlation of precisely zero with log stature.

Many studies, covering thousands of subjects, have calculated the optimal value of p using one or other of these methods (e.g., Lee et al., 1981; Garn and Pesick, 1982). Overall the results confirm the impression from the previous section that p is near to 2 in men, and between 1 and 2 in women.

The philosophy of Benn (1971) is based on relative weight, and so assumes that the reference weight for a given stature should equal the mean weight for that stature in the population. This means that, averaged over the population, relative weight is close to 100%, and this holds at all heights. In other words, relative weight causes the mean level of obesity at different heights to be the same by definition, so that obesity and height are uncorrelated.

This is why p should be chosen to make W/S^p uncorrelated with stature. However, it is important to realise that this is not the only way to choose p. Another obvious criterion is to make it maximise the correlation of W/S^p with a more direct measure of body fat (section on Criteria for Defining Shape, page 85). This general problem of relating W/S^p to another variable is discussed in the next section.

Sjostrom et al. (1986), using a novel estimate of body fat calculated by whole body computed tomography, found that it correlated better with W/S than with W/S^2, although the number of patients was small.

W^q/S^r

Abdel-Malek et al. (1985) showed that percentage body fat in adults was best predicted by an index of the form W^q/S^r, where r and q took the values 3.3

and 1.2, respectively. They estimated the values using a nonlinear regression technique, but it is useful to know that the index can, like the simpler W/S^p (13), be arranged in the form of a linear regression. This greatly simplifies the estimation of r and q, and was used by Abdel-Malek et al. (1985) to obtain the starting values for their iteration.

Suppose that F is some measure of body fat, and W^q/S^r is to be the best index for predicting it. Extending equation 13, the multiple regression of log F on log W and log S

$$\log F = q.\log W - r.\log S + \log k + \text{error} \tag{14}$$

is calculated, where q and $-r$ are the regression coefficients and log k the intercept of the equation. Note that the sign of r is changed. This simplifies to

$$\log F = \log (W^q/S^r) + \log k + \text{error} \tag{15}$$

which confirms that on the log-log scale, W^q/S^r is the index correlating most highly with F. It is likely that the same correlation calculated on the linear scale is also close to optimal.

W^q/S^r appears more general than W/S^p, but in practice it is very similar. It can be rearranged as $(W/S^p)^q$, where p is defined as r/q, so that on the log-log scale the two indices W^q/S^r and $W/S^{r/q}$ are equivalent, i.e., they correlate equally with F. This same point was made by Schey et al. (1984). Thus the index of Abdel-Malek et al. (1985), where r and q were 3.3 and 1.2, is very similar to $W/S^{2.75}$.

Multiple regression is a powerful method for estimating the best value of p when the index is required to predict some third quantity, be it body fat or mortality risk or some other proxy for ill health. The equation 14 is fitted, and p is defined as minus the log S coefficient divided by the log W coefficient.

This method can be used to clarify the correlation of body fat mass with W/S^p. Total body fat can be analysed unadjusted, or adjusted for weight (Womersley and Durnin, 1977; Roche et al., 1981) or adjusted for stature^2 (Garrow and Webster, 1985). There is no obvious reason to prefer any one of these to the others, and it is far simpler to let the regression analysis do the adjustment automatically. This is precisely what the multiple regression equation 14 does, by putting weight and stature on the right side of the equation. Also, by working with logs, the fitted regression treats all the three forms of body fat index equivalently. It also provides the residual error of prediction in proportional rather than absolute terms—the residual standard deviation of log F, multiplied by 100, can be treated as a percentage error.

Multiple regression involving log W and log S is encountered relatively rarely in the literature. However, the same regression using W and S is not uncommon (Hume and Weyers, 1971; Womersley and Durnin, 1977; Watson et al., 1980; Storlien et al., 1987; Boutton et al., 1987). As judged by correlation, W versus log W and more particularly S versus log S are very similar to each other. If the same regression were repeated with W and S logged, then the equivalence of the equation to W/S^p could be found immediately, using the method described above. Again it might or might not provide a better correlation than the original regression, but it would not be very different and would also be informative about p.

INDICES OF WEIGHT FOR STATURE IN CHILDREN

Standards of Weight for Stature and Age

Baldwin (1925) published a set of tables giving mean weight by stature, age, and sex in a large population of U.S. children, covering the range 6–19 years. In theory these tables provide a simple yet satisfactory way of defining weight for stature in children; the appropriate reference weight is obtained from the tables and divided into the child's actual weight, to give a figure for relative weight which is directly analogous to relative weight in adults. The one problem with the Baldwin standards is that due to secular trends in growth they are now very out-of-date.

More recently, Chinn and Morris (1980) produced a weight-for-stature standard in the form of age and sex-specific centile charts, based on 8,000 English children from the National Study of Health and Growth, and covering 5–10 years. This goes one better than the Baldwin tables in that the centile, as well as relative weight, can be assessed. This standard, which is based on regression equations, is discussed in more detail in the section on W/S^p Adjusted for Age (page 94).

Standards of Weight for Stature

Gomez et al. (1956), in order to simplify the assessment of nutritional status in third world children, proposed a classification scheme based on weight and age. Seoane and Latham (1971) suggested splitting it into two parts, weight adjusted for stature and stature adjusted for age. The potential advantages were twofold—not only would the indices be sensitive to both long-term and short-term malnutrition, but weight adjusted for stature would not involve the child's age, an advantage in the developing world where it is often not recorded. Waterlow (1973) subsequently formalised this scheme—stature relative to a reference child of the same age he called *stunting*, and weight relative to a reference child of the same stature was termed *wasting*.

To assess wasting in a population, the reference weight for stature is first obtained from a suitable chart. Like its adult counterpart, this chart takes no account of age, but it differs from the adult chart in two respects. First, it is not a straight line, so it cannot be summarised as a regression line. Second, to take into account the marked skewness of weight during childhood, it is presented not as the mean weight at each stature but as the median, along with other centiles from the 3rd or 5th through to the 97th or 95th. In this form the weight-for-stature chart allows weight to be expressed either as a relative weight, i.e., weight / median reference weight, or else in terms of its centile position according to the standard. Relative weight in this context may be called fraction of the median, or (multiplied by 100) percentage of the median, or most simply, weight for stature.

In the 1960s and 1970s, there was no truly satisfactory child's weight-for-stature standard available. The Harvard standard (Stuart and Stevenson, 1959) and its simplified version (Jelliffe, 1966), although widely used, was inappropriate due to the unrepresentative social mix of the reference population. This changed in 1977 when the American National Center for Health Statistics (NCHS) standard was published (Hamill et al., 1977), based on a large representative sample of U.S. children seen during the 1960s. It was subsequently adopted by the World Health Organisation (WHO) as an international growth reference (Waterlow et al., 1977; Dibley et al., 1987a), and has been used by many countries since to record the nutritional status of their children.

The big disadvantage of the NCHS standard is that the national sample on which it is based did not include suitable data under 2 years of age, and the Fels Research Institute's longitudinal survey was used to make up the deficit. The Fels sample, like the Harvard sample before it, was composed of relatively affluent children, and as a result its growth pattern, and hence the corresponding centiles on the standard, differed from the national sample This has caused problems of interpretation between 2 and 3 years of age, where the two sets of centiles overlap (Cole 1985; Dibley et al., 1987b).

Weight for Stature for Age

Eid (1970) and Shukla et al. (1972) wanted to quantify obesity in young children, but did not find a suitable weight-for-stature standard to use. Instead they obtained the reference weight for each child's stature indirectly, using the weight-and-stature-for-age standards of Tanner, Whitehouse, and Takaishi (1966). Each child's stature was expressed as a stature-age, i.e., the age on the chart where the child's stature matches the median stature. The median *weight* at this stature-age was then used as the reference weight for the child's stature. Cole (1985), working with the NCHS standard, showed that this reference weight is very close to the median on the weight-for-stature standard.

Ehrenberg's Index

Ehrenberg (1968) showed that in many different groups of children, the plot of mean weight against mean stature for ages from 2 to 13 years was closely fitted by the equation

$$\log W = 0.8\,S + 0.4. \qquad (16)$$

This is just a compact way of expressing the weight for stature standard, but it is sometimes used in its own right as the index $\log W - 0.8\,S$. Its advantages and disadvantages are essentially the same as for the weight-for-stature standard.

W/S^n Unadjusted for Age

As with adults, power indices of the form W/S^n have been suggested for use with children (Rao and Singh, 1970; Babu and Chuttani, 1979). W/S, W/S^2, and W/S^3 all change appreciably during childhood, as shown in Figure 1. Their means are shown plotted against age using median stature and weight from the NCHS standard of Hamill et al. (1977). Of the three, W/S^2 changes least during childhood, but even so it shows a sharp increase during the first year of life. Because of the approximate age independence after 1 year, Rao and Singh (1970) and Babu and Chuttani (1979) both suggested that W/S^2 be used.

Two other, noninteger power indices have also been proposed, $W/S^{1.6}$ (Dug-

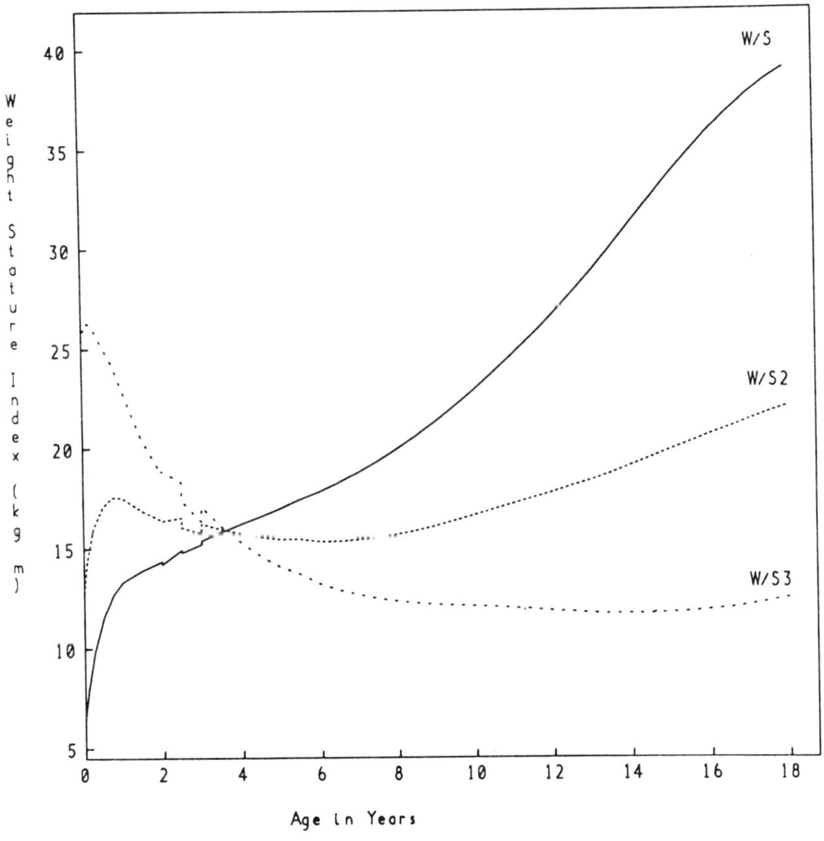

Fig. 1. Values of W/S, W/S^2, and W/S^3 for boys by age during childhood, constructed from the NCHS medians for weight and stature. (Hamill et al., 1977).

dale, 1971) for children from 1 to 5 years of age, and $W/S^{2.4}$ (Dugdale and Lovell, 1981) for ages 5–12 years. The powers 1.6 and 2.4 are chosen to make the index as nearly independent of age as possible. They correspond to the slope of the median weight-for-stature chart over these age ranges.

W/S^n Adjusted for Age

McLaren and Read (1972, 1975) were concerned that the weight-for-stature standard, when used to identify wasting in young children, did not make use of age in the assessment. They proposed instead that the weight–stature ratio W/S should be used, adjusted for age by comparing it with W/S calculated for a reference child of the same age and sex. They published a graph of reference W/S plotted against age to simplify the assessment.

This index can reasonably be called *relative* W/S for age, by analogy with relative weight for stature in adults. However, W/S is only the simplest index of the form W/S^n, and there is no reason *a priori* why it, rather than relative W/S^2 or relative W/S^3, should be considered the best index to use in children. DuRant and Linder (1981) also proposed relative W/S as the best index, but they did not include relative W/S^2 in their analysis. Relative W/S^2 has become popular in recent years as it is almost uncorrelated with stature for much of childhood (Rolland-Cachera et al., 1982). However, there is a short time, early in puberty, when W/S^3 is better than W/S^2 in this respect.

Using the criterion of a high correlation with body fat rather than a low correlation with stature, Michielutte et al. (1984) found W/S^2 to be the best index over the age range 5–12 years for triceps skinfold, with correlations of around 0.8 at the later ages. Storlien et al. (1987) showed that at age 7, W/S^2 was better than three other weight–stature indices for predicting percent body fat (calculated from anthropometry), triceps and subscapular skinfolds, and a visual obesity rating. Killeen et al. (1978) correlated subscapular skinfold with W/S, W/S^2, and W/S^3 in over 6,000 U.S. children age 6–17 years, and found that W/S^2 was consistently the best. They also found that subscapular skinfold was positively correlated ($r = 0.3$) with stature. Himes and Roche (1986) confirmed the association between fat and stature, using radiographic fat thicknesses at two sites.

W/S^p Adjusted for Age

The Benn index W/S^p is used in adults on the grounds that W/S^2 may not be optimal. This applies equally to children, but it is less easy to deal with because the index needs to be adjusted for age. In addition there is the possibility that the optimal p may change with age. This requires the data to be analysed in narrow age groups.

Relative W/S^p adjusts simultaneously for stature and age, and so is equivalent to the standard of weight for stature and age (see section on Standards of Weight for Stature and Age, page 91). It also assumes, like Chinn and Morris (1980), that the plot of weight against stature at each age is linear. The Baldwin

(1925) standard itself is close to linear (see section on Weight for Stature and Age Standards as W/S^p, page 97), so the assumption is reasonable.

As with adults (see section on W/S^p, page 88), the power p in relative W/S^p can be estimated either to provide relative weight or to predict some other measure of obesity. To simplify the age adjustment, Cole (1979) suggested working with relative weight for age (W/W_0) and relative stature for age (S/S_0) rather than weight and stature. The relative weight approach estimates p and its standard error from the regression of log relative weight on log relative stature:

$$\log W/W_0 = p.\log S/S_0 + \log k. \tag{17}$$

This leads to the index

$$W/W_0 \;/\; (S/S_0)^p, \tag{18}$$

which is by definition uncorrelated with relative stature on the log-log scale. So long as the data are analysed in narrow age groups, p can also be estimated from the regression of log W on log S (13).

The appeal of the index (18) is that it can be rearranged as

$$W/S^p \;/\; W_0/S_0^{\,p} \tag{19}$$

which is equivalent to relative W/S^p, as defined in the previous section.

Cole (1979) has shown that for much of childhood, including infancy (Cole et al., 1981), the optimal value for p is slightly greater than 2, providing support for the use of relative W/S^2. However, this does not hold in early puberty, when p is closer to 3 (Chinn and Morris, 1980; Stark et al., 1981; Peckham et al., 1983; Cole, 1986). It confirms the observation of Rolland-Cachera et al. (1982) that W/S^3 is better than W/S^2 during puberty. After puberty the value of p is close to 2, so that W/S^2 is again the most appropriate index, just as it is in adults (see section on W/S^p, page 88).

Chinn and Morris (1980) used their data on 8,000 children to investigate several forms of weight standard for stature and age. The regression of log weight on stature they found fitted slightly better than equation 17, suggesting a more curved weight–stature relationship than W/S^p provides. This is of the same general form as Ehrenberg's equation 16, but there is a fundamental difference between the two. Ehrenberg's curve shows how weight and stature change in children as they grow, whereas the regressions of Chinn and Morris summarise the weight–stature relationship in a group of children *at one particular age.* The two are quite different, as the section on Weight–Stature–Age and Weight–Stature Standards makes clear (page 100).

The case for regressing log weight on stature rather than log stature is not particularly strong, as Cole (1986) showed using other data. Either way the results are likely to be very similar.

Using as their criterion the correlation with triceps skinfold, Schey et al. (1984) obtained values of p ranging between 1.2 and 2.7 for children from 5–12 years. However, the correlations were only trivially better than those obtained using W/S^2. Conversely, Roche et al. (1981) looked at the correlations of total body fat and percent body fat with W/S^2 and W/S^3 in two groups of children aged 5–12 and 13–17 years. Of the eight distinct correlations considered, four were maximised with W/S^2 and four with W/S^3.

RELATIVE W/S^p—A UNIFIED INDEX OF WEIGHT FOR STATURE

The previous sections have shown that many weight-for-stature indices can be expressed either as relative $W - b.S$ or relative W/S^p. This section demonstrates that these two forms themselves are very similar. In addition it shows that the two common types of weight-for-stature standard used with children can both be expressed as relative W/S^p. This unification greatly simplifies the choice of index, as the only important issue to be decided is the value of p (and to a lesser extent the value of k, the reference).

Relative Weight as W/S^p

The adult indices described in the section on Indices of Weight for Stature in Adults consist of two types, the linear form $W - b.S$ (Broca's index, weight-for-stature standard) and the power form W/S^p. Benn (1971), in an important paper, showed that the two were in essence the same, i.e., that the linear (9) and log (13) regression equations predict very similar weights for a given stature.

Rearranging 9 and 13 using 4 and 6 gives the reference weights as

$$W = W_0 + b(S - S_0) \tag{20}$$

and

$$W = W_0.(S/S_0)^p \tag{21}$$

where S is the subject's stature, and W_0 and S_0 are population means. To compare the two, consider U.K. males aged 30–39 years in 1980, where W_0 and S_0 are 75 kg and 175 cm respectively, and the slope b of the regression line is 0.772 kg/cm (Knight, 1984). This makes p, the slope of the log-log regression, 1.80 from equation 12.

The forms of equations 20 and 21 make clear that if S is equal to S_0, then W equals W_0. So it is only when S is somewhat different from S_0 that any differences will show. The 3rd and 97th centiles of adult male stature from the standard of Tanner, Whitehouse, and Takaishi (1966) are 162 cm and 187 cm, for which equation 20 predicts reference weights of 65.0 kg and 84.3 kg. Using 21, the corresponding weights are 65.3 kg and 84.5 kg, which differ from the linear predictions by less than one half of 1%.

This is clearly a trivial difference, and it demonstrates an important principle. Relative weight based on a linear regression equation can be expressed equivalently as W/S^p divided by reference W_0/S_0^p.

Weight-for-Stature-and-Age Standards as W/S^p

The weight–stature–age standard of Baldwin (1925) consists of separate standards of weight for stature by sex and age from 6 to 19 years. Because the age range for each standard is only one year, the corresponding stature range is also relatively small, so that the plot of weight versus stature is very close to a straight line. This line can be fitted by either the regression of weight on stature (Relative Weight and Weight–Stature Regression, page 87) to give $W - b.S$, or the regression of log weight on log stature (W/S^p, page 88; W/S^p Adjusted for Age, page 94) to give W/S^p. The regression of log weight on stature (Chinn and Morris, 1980) is not discussed here.

It is useful to know how straight the two regression lines are, as measured by the correlation coefficient. Table 1 summarises the results, and it is clear that all the correlations are very close to 1 (although those for W/S^p tend to be slightly larger). Thus whichever form of fitted line is used, the plots at each age are all very close to straight lines. This means that the 30-plus tabulated weights at each age can be compactly summarised by the regression line.

Table 1 gives the slope p and constant k for the W/S^p regressions at each age. Thus an individual's weight can be converted immediately to relative weight using W/S^p / k (8). For example, a 16-year-old boy with stature 1.87 m and weight 67 kg, where p is 2.57 and k is 14.5, gives 67 / $1.87^{2.57}$ / 14.5 or 0.925, i.e., 92.5% of the Baldwin reference.

Note that in Table 1 the values for the slope p change steadily with age, starting at about 2, rising to 2.7, and then falling back to 1.7 or 1.8. The constant terms k also change smoothly with age, in the opposite direction. This same pattern of p changing with age was found by Cole (1986) (see section on W/S^p Adjusted for Age, page 94).

The trends in p and k can be summarised as smoothed plots against age, and values for any particular age then read off the graph. In this way the entire Baldwin reference could be summarised in four graphs—p versus age and k versus age for the two sexes. Cole (1986) gives the formula

$$p = 2 + \exp\left[-0.05\,(\text{age} - 11)^2\right] \qquad (22)$$

relating p to age, based on several large data sets including the U.S. health examination surveys HES 2, HES 3, and HANES I. Figure 2 illustrates this curve as a solid line.

It is instructive to repeat the example of the 16-year-old boy (above) using the NCHS standard and equation 22 for p. So p at age 16 is 2.29, while W_0 and S_0 are obtained from the NCHS standard as 62.1 kg and 1.735 m, respectively. This makes W_0/S_0^p 17.58, while W/S^p is 15.98 (67 / $1.87^{2.29}$), so the boy's relative

TABLE 1. Reference Weights for Stature and Age[a]

Age (years)	Number of points	$W - b.S - c$ correlation	$W/S^p / k$ correlation	p	k
Boys					
6	31	0.995	0.997	2.01	15.4
7	30	0.999	0.999	2.21	14.9
8	36	0.999	0.999	2.29	14.7
9	33	0.998	1.000	2.33	14.5
10	33	0.998	1.000	2.44	14.1
11	36	0.998	1.000	2.52	13.8
12	39	0.996	0.999	2.62	13.4
13	38	0.998	1.000	2.63	13.5
14	43	0.999	1.000	2.72	13.1
15	46	0.999	0.998	2.62	13.8
16	39	0.999	0.995	2.57	14.5
17	34	0.998	0.996	2.25	17.7
18	31	0.998	0.998	1.96	21.3
19	29	0.999	0.999	1.87	23.0
Girls					
6	28	0.996	0.997	2.07	15.1
7	33	0.995	0.998	2.20	14.8
8	30	0.998	0.999	2.37	14.4
9	28	0.998	1.000	2.45	14.3
10	36	0.998	0.999	2.50	14.2
11	36	0.996	0.998	2.59	14.0
12	39	0.994	0.998	2.67	13.8
13	38	0.999	0.999	2.64	14.1
14	41	0.996	0.992	2.25	17.1
15	36	0.997	0.995	1.94	20.5
16	33	0.996	0.996	1.76	22.9
17	31	0.997	0.996	1.76	23.1
18	28	0.994	0.994	1.69	24.2

[a]Data from Baldwin (1925) fitted by the regression of 1) weight and 2) log weight on stature by year of age. The first implies an index of the form ($W - b.S - c$), while the second gives the index $W/S^p / k$. The correlation coefficients of weight and log weight with stature are shown, along with the regression coefficients p and constants k from the log regression (equation 13). The standard errors for p lie between 0.01 and 0.05 (median 0.02).

W/S^p is 15.98 / 17.58 = 90.9%. This is very similar to the Baldwin standard figure of 92.5% (above), despite the different values for p and k.

Using equation 21, the reference weight for the boy is 73.7 kg. Extending this calculation to cover other heights and ages, it would be straightforward to construct a modern weight–stature–age standard to replace that of Baldwin (1925).

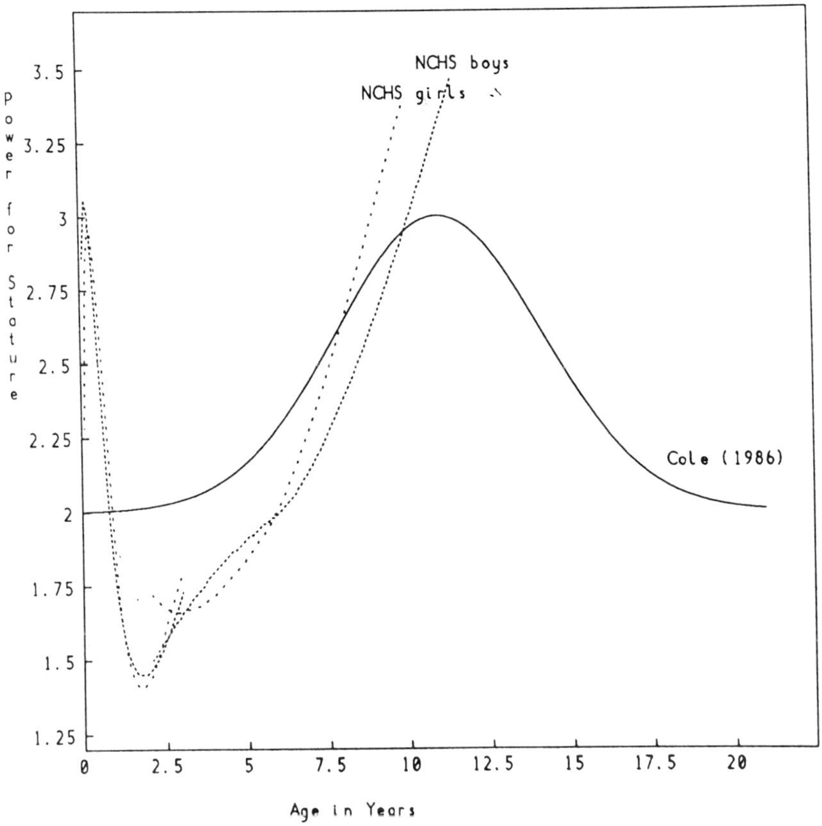

Fig. 2. The power of stature p in the index W/S^p as it changes with age, corresponding to 1) the NCHS weight for stature standard (Hamill et al., 1977) in boys and girls, and 2) the standard of weight for stature and age described by Cole (1986).

Weight-for-Stature Standards as W/S^p

The weight-for-stature standard in children, unlike the equivalent standard in adults, is a curve rather than a straight line. This is because the range in stature covered by the standard is much greater. As a result, the slope of the curve changes from one point on the curve to another. Cole (1985) has shown that each point on the curve corresponds to a particular age, which is the age where that weight and stature are the reference values for age. Put another way, the reference curve of weight versus stature shows weight plotted against stature for the reference child at a series of ages through childhood.

An individual child being assessed on the standard makes use of just two points on the curve—the first corresponds to his chronological age, and the second to his stature-age (i.e., the age where the reference stature is the same as his own). If a straight line is drawn through these two points on the curve, and if the slope of the line on a log-log plot is p with constant k (8), then the child's relative weight for stature is given by $W/S^p/k$ (Cole, 1985).

Figure 2 shows how p changes with age in the NCHS standard for boys (dotted line) and girls (dashed line). Immediately after birth p rises, but it then falls, from 3 to 1.5, in the space of only a few months. Cole (1985) has discussed this issue in some detail, pointing out that this behaviour of the slope in the first 18 months of life is anomalous. It can lead to misleading assessments of weight for stature in very tall or very short children.

THE BEST INDEX FOR CHILDREN

When deciding on a "best" index, it is necessary to specify the criterion that is to be used. For children the alternatives are 1) relative weight for stature and age, 2) relative weight for stature, 3) relative W/S^p chosen to best correlate with body fat, and 4) relative W/S^p chosen to best predict mortality. The previous section has shown that (1) and (2) can, like (3) and (4), be expressed as relative W/S^p. These alternatives are considered in turn, first deciding which of the two relative weight definitions is to be preferred.

Weight–Stature–Age and Weight–Stature Standards

Both the weight–stature–age standard and the weight-for-stature standard can be thought of as sets of age-specific straight lines, with different slopes and constants at each age. The main difference between them is that on the weight-for-stature standard the separate lines join up into a smooth curve, whereas with the weight–stature–age standard the lines are (almost) parallel.

Expressed this way, the differences between the standards can be summarised by the differences in the slope p at each age. (The constant k can be obtained directly from p as W_0/S_0^p, where W_0 and S_0 are the means or references at each age.) Figure 2 shows how p changes with age according to the two standards. Note that the NCHS standard is undefined after age 10 in girls and 11.5 in boys—past this age the slope becomes too steep to be meaningful.

Comparing the two sets of curves, both lie within the range 1.5–3, and between the ages of 3 and 9 years they are very similar. However, in the first 2 years they are materially different, due to sudden changes in the slope of the weight-for-stature standard. This causes problems of assessment because of the way the weight-for-stature standard works—it compares a child's weight with the weight of a reference child of the same stature. If the child is say 15 months old and short (as many third world children are), he or she is compared (say) with a healthy 9-month NCHS child. It is clear that a 9-month baby and a 15-month toddler (even a well-nourished 15-month toddler) are not the same shape—the baby is fatter. However, the standard assumes that the two should be comparable in shape, and so the toddler is rated as underweight.

The weight–stature–age standard avoids this by comparing the short 15-month-old with other children of the same age. This way the child's being short is not equated with his being immature for his age.

At the other end of the age range just prior to puberty, the slope of the weight-for-stature standard is steeper than previously. In particular it is much steeper than the corresponding slope in adults (which is close to 2). Geissler and Miller (1985) and Bray (1987) have both pointed this out, comparing the NCHS standard with adult standards. They interpret it as meaning that something is wrong with the adult standard.

What they forget is that the NCHS standard, because it ignores age and stops before puberty, gives a misleading impression of the relationship between weight and stature in later childhood. It is true that p is near 3 at age 11 as judged by both the standards in Figure 2, but by the age of 16 it has dropped back to 2. Thus if the correct standard is used, there is no discrepancy between childhood and adulthood.

The moral of this comparison is that the weight-for-stature standard, although very convenient, should not be used on children under 2 years. Also it should not be treated as a young version of the adult standard, as it does not extend that far. Thus the only period when it is reliable is during primary school age. Ironically its one advantage, that it can be applied to children whose age is unknown, is no advantage at all in this age range. Even if age is known only very roughly (e.g., to the nearest year or two) this is quite accurate enough to adjust for age as well as stature.

The better alternative is to use the weight–stature–age standard, which is appropriate at all ages throughout childhood. As this is equivalent to relative W/S^p (see section on Weight-for-Stature-and-Age Standards as W/S^p, page 97), it is not difficult to calculate. It is also far more compact than tables or charts.

Correlation With Body Fat

Killeen et al. (1978) and Storlien et al. (1987) both found W/S^2 to be consistently better than other indices, while Schey et al. (1984) concluded that from 5 to 12 years, W/S^2 was effectively as good an index as the more general W/S^p. Roche et al. (1981), with a relatively small sample, found W/S^2 and W/S^3 equally well supported over the age range 5–17 years.

Prediction of Mortality

There have been several studies relating weight for stature to subsequent mortality in children, but none of them have questioned whether the index used was optimal or not. Chen et al. (1980) showed that weight for stature based on the NCHS standard predicted death in the next 24 months, although it was not as effective as weight for age or stature for age. More recently, Bairagi et al. (1985) and Smedman et al. (1987) found that, in contrast to weight for age and stature for age, weight for stature was only weakly related to mortality.

The conclusion is that in this particular context, shape (as measured by weight for stature) is far less relevant than size (i.e., weight for age and stature for age). In turn this suggests that child weight for stature, unlike its adult counterpart, is largely irrelevant as a proxy for mortality.

This hypothesis could be checked by using multiple regression (see section on W^q/S^r, page 89) to predict mortality from both weight for age and stature for age simultaneously. If shape were a useful predictor, then the regression coefficients for weight and stature would be of opposite sign, indicating that weight adjusted for stature was appropriate. Conversely, if the two regression coefficients were of the *same* sign, then weight and stature would be combining to measure the child's *size.*

Relative W/S^2

To summarise, relative weight can be represented by W/S^2 for most of childhood, apart from a period when W/S^3 is better; body fat is best correlated with W/S^2 at all ages; and mortality is only poorly predicted by weight for stature (and so is irrelevant to the discussion). This makes W/S^2 the clear choice.

Using W/S^2, rather than W/S^p as defined by the solid line in Figure 2, ignores the period centred on age 11 years when W/S^3 is preferable to W/S^2. During this time W/S^2 gives a biased measure of relative weight (Chinn and Morris, 1980). The extent of the bias can be seen with an example: an 11-year-old boy 1.544 m tall (i.e., on the Tanner-Whitehouse 97th centile) whose weight is appropriate for stature using slope $p = 3$ (i.e., the correct slope from Fig. 2). W/S^3 at age 11 for a reference Tanner-Whitehouse child is $33.6 / 1.419^3 = 11.76$, so the child's weight, to be appropriate for stature, must be 11.76×1.544^3 or 43.3 kg. If W/S^2 were used to assess this child, the reference value would be $33.6 / 1.419^2$ and the child's value $43.3 / 1.544^2$. This gives a relative W/S^2 of 1.09 (equal to the child's relative stature for age, 1.544 / 1.419). In this case, a very tall child at age 11 (when p is at its maximum in Fig. 2) is assessed by W/S^2 as being 9% overweight. This exaggeration of a tall child's overweight would be reversed in a very short child, where weight for stature would be underestimated to the same extent. Chinn and Morris (1980) tabulate this bias for various combinations of relative stature for age and p.

The bias applies only to relative weight. There is the evidence of Killeen et al. (1978) and Himes and Roche (1986) that tall children at this age tend to be fatter, so that the 9% exaggeration of overweight may well match the likely extra obesity of the tall child. In other words, the stature–fatness correlation may make W/S^2 more appropriate than W/S^3 even at this age, and indeed the evidence is that for body fat correlations, W/S^2 is better than W/S^3 at all ages.

Thus unless there is a very specific interest in relative weight over the age range 9–13 years, when p is elevated, the case for using W/S^2 is incontrovertible. It must be emphasised though that it needs to be adjusted for age, by comparing it with an appropriate age standard.

There are already published centile standards for W/S^2 in childhood from France (Rolland-Cachera et al., 1982) and the United States (Cronk and Roche,

1982). The U.S. standard covers blacks and whites from 6 to 50 years, while the French is from birth to 21 years. However, a more recent version of the French standard extends from birth to 85+ years (Rolland-Cachera, personal communication). Also Cole et al. (1981) describe a child growth slide rule which expresses weight, stature, and W/S^2 as centiles and percentages of the median, using the Tanner-Whitehouse standard as reference.

THE BEST INDEX FOR ADULTS

The two contenders for "best" index in adults are W/S^p (the Benn index) and W/S^2, often called the body mass index, or BMI. As with children, they are considered according to the criteria of relative weight, body fat proxy, and mortality proxy.

Relative Weight

The great strength of the Benn index (Benn, 1971) is that when divided by a suitable reference value, it gives a direct measure of relative weight which is specific to the population under study. The corresponding disadvantage is that p has to be calculated afresh for each population, which in turn means that its value is not known until after the data have been analysed. Also, different studies cannot be compared directly as the basis for adjustment is not the same.

Much play has been made about the importance of calculating p rather than assuming it to be 2, so as to avoid making biased inferences (Lee et al., 1981; Lee et al., 1982; Lee and Kolonel, 1984). However, the examples they cite tend to be rather contrived, and in any case they miss the point. If the populations being compared do differ significantly in their values of p, then it is not permissible to pretend that they are the same, or to use the separate values.

Using W/S^p is equivalent to adjusting weight for stature by covariance analysis, on a log-log scale (equation 13). If this is done for several populations at once, the estimates of p in each population will be different. The correct statistical treatment is to test the p's for significance, and if they are not significantly different a single pooled value for p can be used. Conversely if they *are* significant, then strictly speaking there is no point in comparing the populations for relative weight, as they have already been shown to be different in terms of their p values.

What is not permissible is to compare populations using population-specific p's, as the results of the comparison depend on what stature the populations are standardised to. Take for example two populations, each of mean stature 175 cm and mean weight 75 kg. In population A, p is calculated as 1.7, while in B it is 2.3. Given these values of p and equation 21, adjusted weights can be calculated for each population. If they are adjusted to stature 170 cm, the weights are 71.4 kg for A and 70.2 kg for B, so A is the heavier; conversely if the reference stature is 180 cm, then A's adjusted weight is 78.7 kg and B's 80.0 kg, so B is the heavier. This apparently nonsensical result occurs because the p's for the two populations are different—if they were the same it would not arise. Lee et al. (1982) alluded to this problem, but as quickly dismissed it.

Also, published p values are rarely quoted with their standard errors. Benn (1971) gave a formula to calculate the standard error, and without it the precision of the estimate cannot be judged. For example, in a population of size 2,000 the standard error of p is about 0.1 for men, so the 95% confidence interval is 0.2 on either side of the estimate. For comparison, the range of values across the five ethnic groups quoted by Lee et al. (1981) amounts to 0.44 for the men and 0.41 for the women, hardly wider than the confidence interval. The sample sizes are somewhat larger here, but it is unlikely that the p values are statistically very different.

Correlation With Body Fat

Apart from Abdel-Malek et al. (1985) there has been little attempt to derive W/S^p indices correlating with body fat in adults, although Schey et al. (1984) looked at children. It is well-established that W/S^2 correlates with body fat (Frisancho and Flegel, 1982; Garrow and Webster, 1985; Micozzi et al., 1986; Leonhardt et al., 1987), although there is yet no consensus about how to adjust body fat for body size (see section on W/S^n, page 87). The issue could be clarified using the methods of section W^q/S^r (page 89).

Prediction of Mortality

Several large longitudinal studies have demonstrated a clear U-shaped distribution of mortality according to W/S^2 (Waaler, 1984; Bray, 1987). Mortality is least for W/S^2 in the region around 23 kg/m^2, and it increases steeply outside this range. The rise in mortality is steeper at the lower end than at the higher, although it is the higher end which has had the most attention.

There has been no work investigating whether W/S^p is better than W/S^2 for predicting mortality, although there is a negative correlation between mortality and stature. This suggests that among individuals of the same W/S^2, the taller ones have a lower mortality risk. This in turn implies that the index W/S^p, where p is greater than 2, may predict mortality slightly better than W/S^2. However, Waaler (1984) plots a line of relative mortality by weight and stature, and the slope of this line (converted to a log-log plot) is between 2 and 2.1, so W/S^2 may well be close to optimal.

W/S^2

As with children, W/S^2 in adults is a good index by all three criteria, viz. relative weight, body fat, and mortality. There is thus very little justification for considering any other index.

The potential benefit of this is obvious—W/S^2 can be used throughout life, a single index to cover both childhood and adulthood. However, it is important to know how it changes through the lifetime of individuals, and what its distribution is at different ages, for classification purposes.

NATURAL HISTORY OF W/S^2

Changes Over Life

The pattern of W/S^2 as it changes during childhood is shown in Figure 1—a steep rise during the first year of life, peaking at 9 months, followed by a steady drift down to a minimum at about 6 years. Thereafter it rises again until adulthood.

The changes in the first year of life are dramatic, and they emphasise the need to adjust W/S^2 for age. However, the pattern seen in Figure 1, which is based on Western norms, may be inappropriate in the third world. For example, Raman et al. (1987) have reported that in India W/S^2 stops increasing after 4 months, reaching a maximum value of only 15 kg/m^2.

In adults W/S^2 continues to rise until at least 50 years of age, at the rate of about 1 kg/m^2 per decade (Cronk and Roche, 1982; Waaler, 1984; Millar and Stephens, 1987; Bray, 1987; Rookus et al., 1987). It flattens off earlier in men than in women, which may be because the men who are lighter have an increased chance of surviving.

Several studies have looked at W/S^2 plotted against age in individuals, with a view to predicting W/S^2 later in life. Cronk et al. (1982) split childhood into three periods and looked at polynomial trends in W/S^2 within each period. Most of the variation was explained by the constant and linear terms, and the strongest correlations between periods were mean W/S^2 at 3–9 years versus mean W/S^2 at 10–17 years, and the upward trend in W/S^2 at 3–9 years versus mean W/S^2 at 10–17 years. This shows that W/S^2 in later childhood depends on W/S^2 at about age 6, and also on the increase in W/S^2 from 3 to 9.

Rolland-Cachera et al. (1984, 1987) identified the crucial feature of the W/S^2 curve as being the age when W/S^2 is at a minimum. They called this the age at adiposity rebound, which they found averaged about 6 years (as in Fig. 1). In children with an earlier rebound W/S^2 at 16 and 21 years was increased, whereas in those rebounding later adult W/S^2 tended to be lower than average. Thus one can to some extent predict adult W/S^2 by observing the age in childhood when it starts to rise, after its initial fall.

Classification

Millar and Stephens (1987) recently compared the levels of obesity in the United States, Canada, and Britain by classifying W/S^2 according to age and sex. Their classification, derived from Knight (1984), was 1) up to 20 underweight, 2) 20–25 normal, 3) overweight 25–30, and 4) obese over 30. These ranges are based on the corresponding mortality rates, so that for W/S^2 between 20 and 25, mortality is assumed to be at a minimum.

However, this classification ignores age, when it is known that W/S^2 increases during adulthood. Bray (1987) recommends that the normal range should change with age, increasing by 1 kg/m^2 for each decade of life after 25–34 years, so that for 65+ years, the normal range is 24–29 kg/m^2.

In childhood, there are centile standards for W/S^2 (Cole et al., 1981; Cronk and Roche, 1982; Rolland-Cachera et al., 1982), so that identification of obesity simply involves the child exceeding some specified centile, e.g., the 90th, 95th, or 97th.

For the calculation of new standards it is worthwhile to note that the distribution of W/S^2 in childhood and early adulthood is very skew, in fact more skew than weight (Waaler, 1984; Cole, 1986). To make the distribution less skew, the index can be transformed to either S^2/W or $S/W^{1/2}$. These indices are likely to be fairly close to a normal distribution, allowing the centiles to be calculated from the mean and standard deviation. They can then be back transformed to kg/m^2 units (Cole, 1988).

CONCLUSIONS

W/S^2 is a very simple index to derive, requiring only weight, stature, and a calculator. Not only does it provide a direct measure of over- or underweight, it also acts as a proxy for total body fat and mortality risk, with an overall performance better than for any other weight–stature index. Because of this, W/S^2 has in the last 10 years become the index of choice for adults, while for children it has not yet received due recognition. This ought to change over the next few years.

Against all its advantages, W/S^2 does have several fundamental limitations which reduce its effectiveness as a proxy for body fat (Roche, 1984; Garn et al., 1986; McLaren, 1987). First, there is the problem of frame size, which is addressed elsewhere in this volume (Chapter 8). Second, W/S^2 has been shown to correlate with lean body mass almost as strongly as with body fat, so that subjects with an atypical percent body fat (e.g., athletes) tend to be misclassified by W/S^2. And third, much recent work shows that it is not the totality of body fat, but its distribution within the body into abdominal and subcutaneous fat which determines mortality risk (Vague, 1953; Lapidus et al., 1984; Larsson et al., 1984). The two components correlate equally with W/S^2 (Ashwell et al., 1987), so that it provides no discrimination between them. The ratio of waist circumference to hip circumference is a more useful anthropometric index in this context.

In summary, W/S^2 is a very useful screening tool for identifying obesity or malnutrition in children and adults, but it is probably not accurate enough to make predictions about individuals. However, Quetelet was right—it is the best weight–stature index there is.

The French centile charts for W/S^2 can be obtained from: Section de Nutrition INSERM, 44 chemin de Ronde, 78110 Le Vesinet, France. The Tanner-Whitehouse growth slide rule is obtainable from: Ref 63A, Castlemead Publications, Swains Mill, 4A Crane Mead, Ware, Herts SG12 9PY, England.

REFERENCES

Abdel-Malek AK, Mukherjee D, Roche AF (1985): A method of constructing an index of obesity. Hum Biol 57:415–430.

Ashwell M, Cole TJ, Dixon AK (1985): Obesity: New insight into the anthropometric classification of fat distribution shown by computed tomography. Br Med J 290:1692–1694.

Babu DS, Chuttani CS (1979): Anthropometric indices independent of age for nutritional assessment in schoolchildren. Br J Prev Soc Med 33:177–179.

Bairagi R, Chowdhury MK, Kim YJ, Curlin GT (1985): Alternative anthropometric indicators of mortality. Am J Clin Nutr 42:296–306.

Baldwin BT (1925): Weight-height-age standards in metric units for American-born children. Am J Phys Anthropol 8:1–10.

Benn RT (1971): Some mathematical properties of weight-for-height indices used as measures of adiposity. Br J Prev Soc Med 25:42–50.

Billewicz WZ, Kemsley WFF, Thomson AM (1962): Indices of adiposity. Br J Prev Soc Med 16:183–188.

Boutton TW, Trowbridge FL, Nelson MM, Wills CA, Smith EO, Lopez-de-Romana G, Madrid S, Marks JS, Klein PD (1987): Body composition of Peruvian children with short stature and high weight-for-height, I: Total body-water measurements and their prediction from anthropometric values. Am J Clin Nutr 45:513–525.

Bray GA (1987): Overweight is risking fate. Definition, classification, prevalence, and risks. Ann NY Acad Sci 499:14–28.

Chen LC, Chowdhury A, Huffman SL (1980): Anthropometric assessment of energy-protein malnutrition and subsequent risk of mortality among preschool aged children. Am J Clin Nutr 33:1836–1845.

Chinn S, Morris RW (1980): Standards of weight-for-height for English children from age 5.0 to 11.0 years. Ann Hum Biol 7:457–773.

Cole TJ (1979): A method for assessing age-standardized weight-for-height in children seen cross-sectionally. Ann Hum Biol 6:249–268.

Cole TJ (1985): A critique of the NCHS weight for height standard. Hum Biol 57:183–196.

Cole TJ (1986): Weight/height^p compared to weight/height^2 for assessing adiposity in childhood: Influence of age and bone age on *p* during puberty. Ann Hum Biol 13:433–451.

Cole TJ (1988): Fitting smoothed centile curves to reference data. J R Stat Soc A 151:385–418.

Cole TJ, Donnet ML, Stanfield JP (1981): Weight-for-height indices to assess nutritional status—a new index on a slide-rule. Am J Clin Nutr 34:1935–1943.

Colliver JA, Frank S, Frank A (1983): Similarity of obesity indices in clinical studies of obese adults: A factor analytic study. Am J Clin Nutr 38:640–647.

Cronk CE, Roche AF (1982): Race- and sex-specific reference data for triceps and subscapular skinfolds and weight/stature. Am J Clin Nutr 35:347–354.

Cronk CE, Roche AF, Chumlea WC, Kent R (1982): Longitudinal trends of weight/stature in childhood in relationship to adulthood body fat measures. Hum Biol 54:751–764.

Cronk CE, Roche AF, Kent R, Berkey C, Reed RB, Valadian I, Eichorn D, McCammon R (1982): Longitudinal trends and continuity in weight/stature from 3 months to 18 years. Hum Biol 54:729–749.

Dibley MJ, Goldsby JB, Staehling NW, Trowbridge FL (1987a): Development of normalized curves for the international growth reference: Historical and technical considerations. Am J Clin Nutr 46:736–748.

Dibley MJ, Staehling N, Nieburg P, Trowbridge FL (1987b): Interpretation of Z-score anthropometric indicators derived from the international growth reference. Am J Clin Nutr 46:749–762.
Dugdale AE (1971): An age-independent anthropometric index of nutritional status. Am J Clin Nutr 24:174–176.
Dugdale AE, Lovell S (1981): Measuring childhood obesity. Lancet 2:1224. Letter.
DuRant RH, Linder CW (1981): An evaluation of five indexes of relative body weight for use with children. J Am Diet Assoc 78:35–41.
Ehrenberg ASC (1968): The elements of lawlike relationships. J R Stat Soc A 131:280–302.
Eid EE (1970): Follow-up study of physical growth of children who had excessive weight gain in first six months of life. Br Med J 2:74–76.
Evans JG, Prior IA (1969): Indices of obesity derived from height and weight in two Polynesian populations. Br J Prev Soc Med 23:56–59.
Florey C duV (1970): The use and interpretation of ponderal index and other weight–height ratios in epidemiological studies. J Chronic Dis 23:93–103.
Frisancho AR, Flegel PN (1982): Relative merits of old and new indices of body mass with reference to skinfold thickness. Am J Clin Nutr 36:697–699.
Garn SM, Leonard WR, Hawthorne VM (1986): Three limitations of the body mass index. Am J Clin Nutr 44:996–997.
Garn SM, Pesick SD (1982): Comparison of the Benn index and other body mass indices in nutritional assessment. Am J Clin Nutr 36:573–575.
Garrow JS (1983): Indices of adiposity. Nutr Abstract Editorial. Rev 53:697–708.
Garrow JS, Webster J (1985): Quetelet's index (W/H^2) as a measure of fatness. Int J Obes 9:147–153.
Geissler CA, Miller DS (1985): Problems with the use of "weight for height" tables. J Nutr 115:1546–1549.
Gomez F, Galvan RR, Frenk S, Cravioto JM, Chavez R, Vasquez J (1956): Mortality in second and third degree malnutrition. J Trop Pediatr 2:77–83.
Hamill PVV, Drizd TA, Johnson CL, Reed RB, Roche AF (1977): NCHS growth curves for children birth–18 years. Vital and Health Statistics, Ser. 11, No. 165. Washington, DC: GPO.
Himes JH, Roche AF (1986): Subcutaneous fatness and stature: Relationship from infancy to adulthood. Hum Biol 58:737–750.
Hume R, Weyers E (1971): Relationship between total body water and surface area in normal and obese subjects. J Clin Pathol 24:234–238.
Jelliffe DB (1966). "The Assessment of the Nutritional Status of the Community." WHO Monograph 53. Geneva: WHO.
Kaup J (1921): Ein korperproportionsgesetz zur beurteilung der lange-, gewichts- und index-abweicher populations-altergruppe. Munch Med Wochenschr 68:976–978.
Keys A, Fidanza F, Karvonen MJ, Kimura N, Taylor HL (1972): Indices of relative weight and obesity. J Chronic Dis 25:329–343.
Khosla T, Lowe CR (1967): Indices of obesity derived from body weight and height. Br J Prev Soc Med 21:122–128.
Killeen J, Vanderburg D, Harlan WR (1978): Application of weight–height ratios and body indices to juvenile populations—the National Health Examination Survey Data. J Chronic Dis 31:529–537.
Knight I (1984): "The Heights and Weights of Adults in Great Britain." London: Her Majesty's Stationery Office.

Lapidus L, Bengtsson C, Larsson B, Pennert K, Rybo E, Sjostrom L (1984): Distribution of adipose tissue and risk of cardiovascular disease and death: A 12 year follow up of participants in the population study of women in Gothenburg, Sweden. Br Med J 289:1257–1261.

Larsson B, Svardsudd K, Welin L, Wilhelmsen L, Bjorntorp P, Tibblin G (1984): Abdominal adipose tissue distribution, obesity, and risk of cardiovascular disease and death: 13 year follow up of participants in the study of men born in 1913. Br Med J 288:1401–1404.

Lee J, Kolonel LN (1984): Are body mass indices interchangeable in measuring obesity–disease associations? Am J Public Health 74:376–377.

Lee J, Kolonel LN, Hinds MW (1981): Relative merits of the weight-corrected-for-height indices. Am J Clin Nutr 34:2521–2529.

Lee J, Kolonel LN, Hinds MW (1982): The use of an inappropriate weight–height derived index of obesity can produce misleading results. Int J Obes 6:233–239.

Leonhardt W, Hanefeld M, Julius U, Schulze J, Fischer S, Weck M, Haller H (1987): Predictive value of the index of desirable body weight for total body fat mass as measured by dilution of tritiated water—problems and limitations. Int J Obes 11:221–228.

McLaren DS (1987): Three limitations of the body mass index. Am J Clin Nutr 46:121. Letter.

McLaren DS, Read WW (1972): Classification of nutritional status in early childhood. Lancet 2:146–148.

McLaren DS, Read WW (1975): Weight/length classification of nutritional status. Lancet 2:219–221.

Metropolitan Life Insurance Company (1959): New weight standards for men and women. Stat Bull Metrop Life 40:1–10.

Michielutte R, Diseker RA, Corbett WT, Schey HM, Ureda JR (1984): The relationship between weight–height indices and the triceps skinfold measure among children age 5 to 12. Am J Public Health 74:604–606.

Micozzi MS, Albanes D, Jones DY, Chumlea WC (1986): Correlations of body mass indices with weight, stature, and body composition in men and women in NHANES I and II. Am J Clin Nutr 44:725–731.

Millar WJ, Stephens T (1987): The prevalence of overweight and obesity in Britain, Canada, and United States. Am J Public Health 77:38–41.

Montegriffo VM (1968): Height and weight of a United Kingdom adult population with a review of anthropometric literature. Ann Hum Genet 31:389–399.

Mueller WH, Joos SK, Schull WJ (1985): Alternative measurements of obesity: Accuracy of body silhouettes and reported weights and heights in a Mexican American sample. Int J Obes 9:193–200.

Norgan NG, Ferro-Luzzi A (1982): Weight–height indices as estimators of fatness in men. Hum Nutr Clin Nutr 36:363–72.

Peckham CS, Stark O, Simonite V, Wolff OH (1983): Prevalence of obesity in British children born in 1946 and 1958. Br Med J 286:1237–1242.

Quetelet LAJ (1869). "Physique Sociale. Vol 2." Brussels: C. Muquardt.

Raman L, Vasanthi G, Rao KV (1987): Validity of weight/height in assessing the nutritional status of infants from birth to one year. J Trop Pediatr 33:217–218. Letter.

Rao KV, Singh D (1970): An evaluation of the relationship between nutritional status and anthropometric measurements. Am J Clin Nutr 23:83–93.

Revicki DA, Israel RG (1986): Relationship between body mass indices and measures of body adiposity. Am J Public Health 76:992–994.

Roche AF (1984): Anthropometric methods: New and old, what they tell us. Int J Obes 8:509–523.
Roche AF, Siervogel RM, Chumlea WC, Webb P (1981): Grading body fatness from limited anthropometric data. Am J Clin Nutr 34:2831–2838.
Rohrer F (1908): Ein neue formel zur bestimmung der korperfulle. Korrespondenz-Blatt der Deutschen Gesellschaft fur Anthropologie, Ethnologie und Urgeschichte 39:5–7.
Rolland-Cachera MF, Sempe M, Guilloud-Bataille M, Patois E, Pequignot-Guggenbuhl F, Fautrad V (1982): Adiposity indices in children. Am J Clin Nutr 36:178–184.
Rolland-Cachera MF, Deheeger M, Bellisle F, Sempe M, Guilloud-Bataille M, Patois E (1984): Adiposity rebound in children: A simple indicator for predicting obesity. Am J Clin Nutr 39:129–135.
Rolland-Cachera MF, Deheeger M, Guilloud-Bataille M, Avons P, Patois E, Sempe M (1987): Tracking the development of adiposity from one month of age to adulthood. Ann Hum Biol 14:219–229.
Rookus MA, Burema J, van-t-Hof MA, Deurenberg P, van-der-Wiel-Wetzels WA, Hautvast JG (1987): The development of the body mass index in young adults, I: Age-reference curves based on a four-year mixed-longitudinal study. Hum Biol 59:599–615.
Schey HM, Michielutte R, Corbett WT, Diseker RA, Ureda JR (1984): Weight-for-height indices as measures of adiposity in children. J Chronic Dis 37:397–400.
Seoane N, Latham MC (1971): Nutritional anthropometry in the identification of malnutrition in childhood. J Trop Pediatr Environ Child Health 17:98–104.
Sheldon WH, Stephens SS, Tucker CB (1940): "The Varieties of Human Physique: An Introduction to Constitutional Psychology." New York: Harper.
Shukla A, Forsyth HA, Anderson CM, Marwah SM (1972): Infantile overnutrition in the first year of life: A field study in Dudley, Worcestershire. Br Med J 4:507–515.
Sjostrom L, Kvist H, Cederblad A, Tylen U (1986): Determination of total adipose tissue and body fat in women by computed tomography, 40K, and tritium. Am J Physiol 250:E736–745.
Smedman L, Sterky G, Mellander L, Wall S (1987): Anthropometry and subsequent mortality in groups of children aged 6–59 months in Guinea-Bissau. Am J Clin Nutr 46:369–373.
Society of Actuaries (1979): "The Build Study, 1979." Chicago: Society of Actuaries.
Stark O, Atkins E, Wolff OH, Douglas JW (1981): Longitudinal study of obesity in the National Survey of Health and Development. Br Med J 283:13–17.
Storlien LH, Bird JE, Silva PA (1987): Assessment of obesity in early childhood. Aust Paediatr J 23:131–135.
Stuart HC, Stevenson SS (1959): In Nelson WE (ed): "Textbook of Pediatrics." 8th ed. Philadelphia: WB Saunders.
Tanner JM, Whitehouse RH, Takaishi M (1966): Standards from birth to maturity for height, weight, height velocity, and weight velocity: British children, 1965. Arch Dis Child 41:454–471 613–635.
Vague J (1953): "La Differenciation Sexuelle Humaine: Ses Incidences en Pathologie." Paris: Masson.
Waaler HT (1984): Height, weight and mortality. The Norwegian experience. Acta Med Scand 679 (suppl):1–56.
Waterlow JC (1973): Note on the assessment and classification of protein-energy malnutrition in children. Lancet 2:87–89.
Waterlow JC, Buzina R, Keller W, Lane JM, Nichaman MZ, Turner JM (1977): The presentation and use of height and weight data for comparing the nutritional status of groups of children under the age of 10 years. Bull WHO 55:489–98.

Watson PE, Watson ID, Batt RD (1980): Total body water volumes for adult males and females estimated from simple anthropometric measurements. Am J Clin Nutr 33:27–39.

Weatherall R, Shaper AG (1988): Overweight and obesity in middle-aged British men. Eur J Clin Nutr 42:221–231.

Womersley J, Durnin JVGA (1977): A comparison of the skinfold method with extent of 'overweight' and various weight–height relationships in the assessment of obesity. Br J Nutr 38:271–284.

Anthropometric Assessment
of Nutritional Status, pages 113–122

6
Stature and Weight as Indicators of Undernutrition

W. KELLER
formerly of World Health Organization, Geneva, Switzerland

INTRODUCTION

Stature and weight measure two different effects of undernutrition: inhibition or retardation of linear growth due to deficiency in nutrients or energy, and reduction or reduced increment in body mass, mainly due to energy deficiency.

Measures of growth can be meaningfully applied only to children. A change in stature between successive determinations is a direct measure of linear growth over a period of time. But a single measure of stature provides a relatively insensitive indicator of growth since stature can move only in one direction and does not decrease. This, together with the fact that malnutrition is only one of many causes of growth inhibition, may be the reason why it is seldom used as a measure of the nutritional status of individuals.

A change in weight is by itself not a good measure of growth since weight as a measure of total body mass does not distinguish between body compartments. Weight increases may be due to linear growth, but changes may also be caused by changes in body compartments such as lean body mass, fat, bone, and water. In combination with clinical information weight changes are, however, used in clinical work to assess nutritional status and its changes in adults and children.

Both stature and weight as well as growth in general are very unspecific indicators of nutritional status. To allow a diagnosis of malnutrition in an individual child the finding of reduced weight or height increments must be accompanied by other indications of malnutrition. For nutritional assessments the measurement of stature and weight alone is therefore mostly applied to populations rather than to individuals. In populations epidemiological and probability considerations can be used to arrive at a nutritional diagnosis if nonnutritional factors are excluded as major causes.

In a normal child the measurements of stature and weight increase with age while their velocity of growth decreases with age: It is highest immediately after birth and slows down with increasing age. Measurements are therefore usually related to age. But in many of the poorer developing countries there is no or incomplete birth registration and little formal education, and it is not possible to establish age with certainty. In famine relief it is therefore common to relate weight to stature and to use this as the only indicator of nutritional status. Since in normally nourished child populations boys are on average taller and heavier than girls, measurements are usually also related to sex.

The relationship between weight and stature (or height) has been studied for at least a century, and many indices have been proposed describing in mathematical terms the weight–height relationship. A publication by the League of Nations in 1939 mentioned the following authors of weight–height indices: Quetelet, Pignet, Roehrer, Manouvrier, von Pirquet, Tuxford (Bigwood 1939). The relating of weight to the height of the body provides a measure of the thinness or fullness of the body and can be seen as a rough anthropometric estimate of body composition (Brozek, 1956). The weight–height relation was again proposed in the 1970s (Seoane and Latham, 1971; Waterlow, 1972) expressed as the weight of a child compared to that of a "normal" child of the same height, and in this form it is at present a widely used index of undernutrition and of obesity (Waterlow et al., 1977; WHO Working Group, 1986).

Waterlow (1972) has introduced the terms *wasted* for children with very low weight for their height and *stunted* for those with very low height for their age. By relating weight to height rather than to age, the important distinction can be made between a low body weight that is due to reduced soft tissues (thinness or wasting) and one due to a small skeletal frame. An additional advantage is that weight for height is practically independent of age.

REFERENCE VALUES

In order to go beyond the merely descriptive and to arrive at a judgment or diagnosis, the measurements and indices have to be compared to a norm or reference. Reference populations for children have been established in a number of countries and a reference population has been recommended for international use (Waterlow et al., 1977; WHO, 1981). If reference values are to fulfill their purpose, they should be derived from a generally healthy, well-nourished child population of sufficient size, as suggested by Waterlow (1972; Waterlow et al., 1977). Since in most countries it is difficult to meet these requirements when national reference values are to be established, there is a definite need for international values. The use of an international reference rests upon the assumption that different populations have the same genetic growth potential, which is probably true for most parts of the world (Habicht et al., 1974).

The point is often made that reference values are not standards, norms, or goals, but serve only as value-free reference points for comparisons between populations. If this view were fully accepted it would not be appropriate to use simple anthropometry for the assessment of growth or nutritional status of populations. But nutritional assessments, which are much more common than descriptive comparisons, are of great practical importance, and for them reference populations are by necessity used as standards in spite of their name. In fact, if the reference population is based on data from a generally healthy and well-nourished population, and if there is an equal genetic growth potential in different populations, there seems to be no major reason not to use, with some reservations, a reference population as a norm, representing the growth that could be attained by any child population growing up under similarly favourable conditions. Still, by calling a reference population a reference and not a norm, one makes allowance for the inevitable imperfections and the possibility of still-unknown positive or negative growth factors and avoids the impression that the reference is an established biological standard.

The international reference population which is at present recommended and widely used is based mostly on a population sample of the U.S. population. Its bases and statistical processing have been documented (Hamill et al., 1979; Dibley et al., 1987a) and certain shortcomings described (Dibley et al., 1987b). In the tables published by the World Health Organization (1983), percentile distributions and standard deviations are given for each month of age and each centimeter of height, respectively. The reference population is thus presented as a set of distributions, with a coefficient of variation of approximately 0.9 in the case of weight and 0.95 in the case of height. It is remarkable that very similar coefficients are found in most populations for height and weight distributions, even if the absolute values differ considerably from those of the reference. Guzman (1975) has therefore tentatively ascribed the widths of distributions to a "racial" effect and differences in the absolute values of distributions to environmental influences, which would include nutritional ones.

In order to compare the heights and weights of children to the reference, the measurements from each child can be assigned to percentile ranges or expressed as Z-scores of the reference. Z-scores are formed by subtracting a measured value from the mean or median of the reference for the appropriate age or height (for the weight-for-height index) and dividing the result by the standard deviation: $(M - x)/s$. The resulting percentile or Z-score value is not the diagnosis of "normal" or "pathological" but denotes the probability that the child is not part of the reference population (null hypothesis). For the 5th percentile this probability is 0.05, for a Z-score of -2 it is 0.023. Percentile and Z-score are equally valid, but in many ways the use of Z-scores offers greater flexibility and allows the classification of measurements that are outside the usual range of percentiles.

The Z-scores of a group of children can be arranged as a frequency distribution and, if necessary, weighted for age and sex, compared to the distribution of the reference data. An example is given in Figure 1. Another possibility is the presentation as a cumulative curve (WHO Working Group, 1986). In principle the difference between the found distribution and the reference could be expressed by the difference between the two medians if the two distributions were always of the same width. When this is not the case there is no simple and absolutely correct way to express the differences from the reference in a single figure. The compromise that is usually adopted is the introduction of a cutoff point.

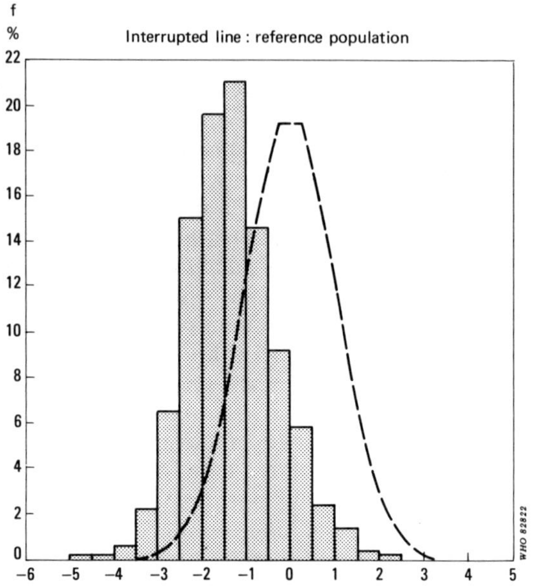

Fig. 1. Distribution of weight-for-height Z-scores in a South Indian child population. Interrupted line: reference population. The distribution is shifted to the left, malnutrition affects all or most individuals. About 26% have Z-scores of less than −2. (Reproduced from Keller, 1983, with permission of the publisher.)

CUTOFF POINTS

A cutoff divides the distribution of values into two: the continuous variable is transformed into a binomial one. The most commonly used cutoffs are points on the frequency distribution of the reference: 80% or 90% of the mean or median(M), the 5th percentile, or two standard deviations below the median. With the cutoff a judgment is introduced: a value below the cutoff is called *stunted* (low height for age), *wasted* (low weight for height), or *underweight* (low weight for age). The anthropometric indices become thus indicators of insufficient growth or undernutrition, and the results of a survey can be expressed in terms of prevalences.

There are differences in the prevalences determined respectively by the cutoffs M − 2sd and 80% or 90% of M which make it difficult to compare results obtained with one or the other of these cutoffs. They are due to the fact that the variance is not a constant proportion of the median over the age or height range of the reference. Depending on the age or height in question, the difference may be between 2 and 12 prevalence % for weight for (standing) height and between 10% and 30% for height for age, depending on the proportion outside the cutoff (calculated for 10 and 50 % prevalence). Results are thus not easily comparable between the two cutoffs.

The division by a cutoff of a continuous distribution into sufficient or insufficient values raises the question of the validity of such a classification. The shift of the distribution to the left as illustrated in Figure 1 means that the population as a whole is affected by whatever causes the reduced weight or height. If a cutoff at -2 standard deviations is introduced, about one-quarter of the population in Figure 1 will be classified as "wasted" and by implication the rest will be considered normal or in any case "not wasted." It is obvious that this is not correct: The right part of the distribution, containing the "fat" children, is as much affected by the shift as the left part. The cutoff, therefore, does not really separate the wasted from the not wasted or the stunted from the not stunted. Instead, as was said before, it identifies those cases for which the probability of belonging to a population like the reference population is less than 0.02275 or 1/44 (for a cutoff at -2 standard deviations). This information is not a direct measure of the prevalence of malnutrition or growth inhibition, but is an indicator of that prevalence, and as such of considerable importance in public health. When the frequencies determined by a cutoff are treated as prevalences, it should be kept in mind that they are only proxies for the unknown true prevalences.

While the anthropometric indicators can serve to assess the degree of malnutrition or growth inhibition in a population, they cannot determine the number of malnourished in it. This is 1) because the manifestations of undernutrition in growth and shape of the body are gradual, and 2) because it is impossible to distinguish in the individual between genetic or other inherent factors and those that act from the environment such as nutrition. For the same reasons the usual epidemiological criteria like specificity, sensitivity, and validity in the narrow sense do not really apply to anthropometric indicators based on cutoffs.

CHOICE OF INDICATORS

Each of the three indicators of undernutrition derived from height, weight, and age is of different biological significance and of different use.

Low weight for height indicates unusually thin or wasted bodies due to a reduction in soft tissue mass. Wasting occurs where there is an imbalance between energy requirements and energy supply to the body. In child populations, this happens mostly due to lack of food in the families or to inadequate feeding habits, but it may also be a result of widespread febrile disease or diarrhea. An epidemic of measles will result in an increase in wasted children. It is not clear to what extent habitually high physical activity of children (child labour) may be responsible for moderate wasting, for instance in rural children of school age. Wasting can develop rapidly in the absence of food or with anorexia, with the clinical pictures of energy-protein malnutrition as the final stage; recovery to normal body proportions may be fast with proper care (Ashworth, 1969). There is indirect evidence that wasting is mainly due to deficiency in energy.

Low height for age is the result of reduced, or stunted, skeletal growth. In laboratory animals any dietary deficiency of an essential nutrient will stunt growth. In child populations there are reports of general stunting in the absence of wasting where energy deficiency cannot be assumed (Keller, 1988). Stunted growth seems to be generally related to poor economic conditions rather than to dietary deficiency, but there is little or no proof of stunting having been caused by a specific deficiency in a population. The continuing secular trend towards increased growth in a number of northern European countries (Tanner, 1976) where widespread nutritional deficiencies are unlikely would speak against such an assumption. Stunted growth is observed in energy-protein malnutrition, but it has also been reported that clinically malnourished children were no more stunted than their healthy siblings (Brock and Hansen, 1965). Little is known about the extent of compensatory growth after a period of growth inhibition, and stunted growth in a child may as well be due to a persisting inhibitory factor as to one in the past. Temporary cessation of growth during diarrhea incidents, followed by periods of accelerated growth, has been reported (Mata, 1983), and since catch-up growth takes longer for length than for weight, repeated infections might produce stunted but not wasted children. While it is thus not certain whether or to what extent stunting indicates undernutrition, there is little doubt that it indicates negative environmental influences on growth.

Low weight for age signifies a low total body mass without indication whether this is due to small size, to thinness, or to a combination of both. As indicator of inhibited growth or of undernutrition, it is less specific than the other two. Weight for age gives no information that is not supplied by weight for height and height for age, more than 95% of its variance being accounted for by the variance of the other two indices (Keller, 1983). Because of its simplicity, it has been suggested to be useful for a rough orientation about trends of change (WHO Working Group, 1986).

Weight-for-age charts for individual children have been used for many years in clinics and maternal and child health services of developing countries. Weights are entered monthly into a chart on which one or several lines indicate the expected weight. In recent years it has been recommended that the weight increment rather than the absolute weight of the child be used as indicator of healthy growth, the reference lines on the chart indicating the desirable slope (WHO, 1986). Today weight charts are used as a tool in child care to monitor a wholesome development in which nutrition is only one of several influences.

The choice of indicators depends to some extent on the purpose for which they are to be used. In addition to individual health care, there are several major areas of application.

Assessment of nutritional status may be part of general socioeconomic, health, or household surveys. A nutritional component is often included in this type of survey in order to obtain an overview of nutritional problems in relation to health or socioeconomic conditions. In the past, faults in sampling design have sometimes prevented a desired geographic or socioeconomic stratification in a national survey.

Monitoring of nutritional status may be part of general health surveillance. Monitoring may be carried out continuously through health centers as in the nutrition surveillance kept by the Centers of Disease Control of the U.S. Public Health Service, where reporting of data is an almost continuous process. Also, it may take the form of a series of surveys at intervals of one or more years of which an example is given in Figure 2. As can be easily seen in the figure, changes are more evident in the whole distribution than in the tail ends outside the 2sd cutoff. However, since distribution curves cannot be expressed in simple numerical terms, more complex monitoring systems prefer reporting the prevalences determined by a cutoff. Usually the indicators are weight for height and height for age; weight for age can easily be added to make historical comparisons with existing data sets that do not include height.

The evaluation of programmes with nutritional objectives is a special case of monitoring. The details of the evaluation must be determined at the planning stage of the programme. Weight for height is a more direct indicator of nutritional effects than height for age, and weight changes due to improved nutrition become measurable before height changes do. For short-term changes weight for height is therefore the better indicator, but if a programme lasts for several years changes in height may occur which make it desirable to monitor the height development as well.

In natural and other emergencies requiring outside relief, the nutritional status of the affected population needs to be determined in order to assess food needs. Children, the most endangered group, are screened by anthropometric indicators. At present, the indicator used by most relief agencies for screening is low weight for height. Although the choice of cutoffs depends to some extent on the available resources and facilities, a cutoff at 80% of the median reference weight for height is usually chosen for participation in supplementary feeding schemes, a cutoff at 70% for admission to special therapeutic feeding, and one at 90% for discharge from the scheme (de Ville et al., 1978). Where ages are not known, a limit of 110 or 115 cm height is often used to identify children below approximately 5 years of age.

In choosing indicators of nutritional status for whatever purpose, the first consideration must be this: What does one want to measure and why? In many cases, but not always, indicators based on weight and on height can give the required answers. The decision on which of these indicators to use depends in the first place on their interpretation. But in practice the consideration of feasibility is equally important, and it may be necessary to compromise between the desired and the feasible.

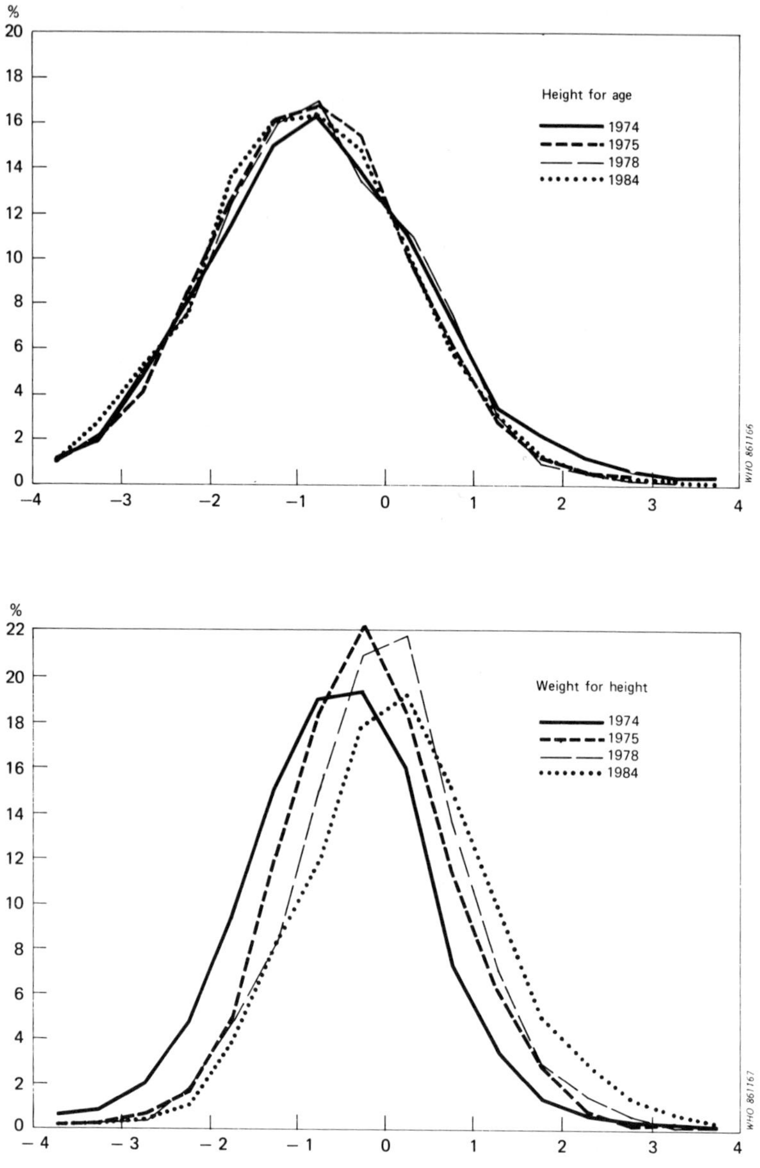

Data from UNRWA

Fig. 2. Changes in distributions of height for age **(top)** and weight for height **(bottom)** in a Middle Eastern child population over a period of 10 years.

INTERPRETATION OF INDICATORS

In summary of what has been said above on the subject, one can state the following:

1. A high proportion of low weights for height in a child population indicates an acute state of undernutrition, sometimes possibly due to widespread infectious disease but usually due to dietary deficiency.
2. A high proportion of low heights for age indicates generally poor living conditions and health which may include poor diets. Specific nutritional deficiencies, for example of trace elements, may play a role, but so far there is little proof.
3. A high proportion of low weights for age may be due to acute undernutrition or poor living condition or both.

These interpretations rest on the validity of the growth reference as representing normal growth (see above). There is evidence that in many populations of varying genetic background so-called elite groups grow to the same heights during childhood as do children in affluent countries (Habicht et al., 1974). It has been argued that elites may be of different ethnic origin from the general population. Although this has sometimes been found to be true, it can hardly be considered a general rule and it probably does not explain the rather consistent findings in the literature. There is less direct evidence supporting the validity of the weight-for-height reference. But if one considers the weight-for-height figures of a large number of different populations (Keller and Fillmore, 1983), there are child populations in all regions of the world where weights for height are similar to the reference, at least at some ages and for the lower parts of the distribution. It seems therefore reasonable to accept the lower percentiles of the reference as representing the weights for height of normally growing healthy children in general. Regarding the upper values of the reference demarcating obesity, there is less certainty, since a problem of obesity is known to exist in the population on which the reference population is based.

Although there exist many problems in the use and interpretation of height and weight indices, heights and weights of children are today the only anthropometric measurements that are used worldwide in assessing the nutritional status and the degree of undernutrition in populations. In the absence of information on other age groups, results are often generalised and extended to the population as a whole. This is most unsatisfactory, and one must hope that a growing interest in the nutritional status of populations and its importance for public health will eventually extend its assessment to other groups.

REFERENCES

Ashworth A (1969): Growth rates in children recovering from protein-calorie malnutrition. Br J Nutr 23:835–845.

Bigwood EJ (1939): "Guiding Principles for Studies on the Nutrition of Populations." Geneva: League of Nations Health Organisation, Technical Commission on Nutrition.

Brock JF, Hansen JDL (1965): Body composition and appraisal of nutriture. In Brozek J (ed): "Human Body Composition." Oxford: Pergamon Press, pp 245–266.
Brozek J (ed) (1956): "Body Measurements and Human Nutrition." Detroit: Wayne University Press.
Dibley MJ, Goldsby JB, Staehling NW, Trowbridge FL (1987a): Development of normalized curves for the international growth reference: Historical and technical considerations. Am J Clin Nutr 46:736–748.
Dibley MJ, Staehling N, Nieburg Ph, Trowbridge FL (1987b): Interpretation of Z-score anthropometric indicators derived from the international growth reference. Am J Clin Nutr 46:749–762.
Guzman MA (1975): Secular trends in height and weight as indicators of the evolution of nutritional status. Proceedings of the Ninth International Congress on Nutrition, Mexico, 1972 4:76–81.
Habicht J-P, Martorell R, Yarbrough C, Malina RM, Klein RE (1974): Height and weight standards for preschool children. How relevant are ethnic differences in growth potential? Lancet 1: 611–615.
Hamill PVV, Drizd TA, Reed RB, Roche AF, Moore WM (1979): Physical growth: National Center for Health Statistics percentiles. Am J Clin Nutr 32:607–629.
Keller W (1983): Choice of indicators of nutritional status. In Schuerch B (ed): "Evaluation of nutrition education in third world communities." Nestle Foundation Publication Series. Bern: Hans Huber Publishers, pp 101–113.
Keller W (1988): The epidemiology of stunting. In Waterlow JC (ed): "Linear Growth Retardation in Less Developed Countries." New York: Raven Press, pp 17–37.
Keller W, Fillmore CM (1983): Prevalence of protein-energy malnutrition. World Health Stat Q 36:129–167.
Mata L (1983): Comments on Black RE, Brown KH, Becker S: Influence of acute diarrhea on the growth parameters of children. In Bellanti JA (ed): "Acute Diarrhea: Its Nutritional Consequences in Children." New York: Raven Press, pp 85–94.
Seoane N, Latham MC (1971): Nutritional anthropometry in the identification of malnutrition in childhood. J Trop Pediatr Environ Child Health 17:98–104.
Tanner JM (1976): Growth as a monitor of nutritional status. Proc Nutr Soc 35:312–322.
de Ville de Goyet C, Seaman J, Geijer U (1978): "The Management of Nutritional Emergencies in Large Populations." Geneva: WHO.
Waterlow JC (1972): Classification and definition of protein-calorie malnutrition. Br Med J 3:566–569.
Waterlow JC, Buzina R, Keller W, Lane JM, Nichaman MZ, Tanner JM (1977): The presentation and use of height and weight data for comparing the nutritional status of groups of children under the age of 10 years. Bull WHO 55:489–498.
WHO (1978): "The Management of Nutritional Emergencies in Large Populations." Geneva: WHO.
WHO (1981): "Development of Indicators for Monitoring Progress Towards Health for All by the Year 2000." ("Health for All" Ser. No. 4) Geneva: WHO.
WHO (1983): "Measuring Change in Nutritional Status." Geneva: WHO.
WHO (1986): "The Growth Chart. A Tool for Use in Infant and Child Health Care." Geneva: WHO.
WHO Working Group (1986): Use and interpretation of WHO anthropometric indicators of nutritional status. Bull WHO 64:929–941.

Anthropometric Assessment
of Nutritional Status, pages 123–140

7
Implications and Applications of Subcutaneous Fat Measurement to Nutritional Assessment and Health Risk Evaluation

STANLEY M. GARN
Center for Human Growth and Development, University of Michigan, Ann Arbor, Michigan 48109-0406

INTRODUCTION

We human beings come ready wrapped in a continuous layer of fat from scalp to sole that waxes and wanes with the weight of fat in general. Even more to the point, the largest proportion of fat in the human body is located just below the skin and is thus accessible to measurement by a variety of noninvasive and nondestructive methods. All of the conventional (and unconventional) measurements employed in nutritional anthropometry are to some extent influenced by the tela subcutanea, and many of the breadth measurements, circumferences, and circumferential ratios are useful primarily because of the subcutaneous fat differences that they reveal.

The good news is that subcutaneous fat serves as a useful measure of caloric status, because it meters calories stored. Moreover, the level of outer fatness relates to size and growth progress throughout the growing period and to lipids, triglycerides, hemoglobin and hematocrit levels, and serum and urinary vitamins throughout the life span. Finally, given the severe limitations of all weight and weight-for-height measures, subcutaneous fat thicknesses are the most practical measures of fatness currently suitable for mass surveys, and nutritional monitoring and assessment in the clinic and in the field.

The bad news is that the subcutaneous fat (whether squeezed or imaged) is more than fat, possibly as much as half lean tissue under some circumstances, and variable in its composition and differently expressed as the result of differences in compressibility. Though easily accessible to measurement by nondestructive and noninvasive techniques and clearly related to fat weight and obesity tissue in general, the tela subcutanea is not just fat but both, more and less.

MEASURING SUBCUTANEOUS FAT

Because of its outer body location and unique density, subcutaneous fat is accessible to imaging and measurement on stored images by a variety of techniques. Because the tela subcutanea is not tightly attached to the deeper tissues on many parts of the body, it can be lifted as folds and measured with simple calipers.

The subcutaneous fat (and other fat stores) absorb less penetrating radiation than most other tissues (Garn, 1957). This makes radiogrammetry possible, using images drawn on a CRO screen or stored as silver granules. While computer-assisted tomographic (CAT) scans can reveal inner fat and outer fat and all between on a single body slice, providing area measurements and volumetric measurements, there are two limitations to its general use. One is expense: many hundreds of dollars for a single scan. The second is the radiation dosage; 1 rad (1,000 millirads) for a typical scan. Filmtype radiogrammetry, once extensively employed, is now grudgingly allowed by human uses committees, even though a typical radiation dose (approximately 3 millirads) is small compared with the normal background exposure. It should be pointed out that a pair of film exposures, say an anteroposterior and lateral leg view, is in effect an elementary scan, far less costly both in dollars and radiation dosage than a CAT scan.

Outer fat can be measured by ultrasonographic means, but the resolution is often inadequate for most outer fat measurements, especially for thinner sections and those with complex tissue masses below (but cf. Borkan et al., 1986). This is a disappointment to those who have seen images of their own bladders projected on a screen or the outlines of their foetuses in utero.

The fact that the subcutaneous fat layer can be pulled up and measured on many parts of the body allows "skinfold" measurement, simply and inexpensively with spring-loaded calipers. In theory what is measured is a double fold of fat plus skin, compressed about 50%. In practice variations in skin thickness are ignored, since they are age dependent, and variations in the degree of compressibility of the skinfold sandwich are also ignored, since the resulting data are ordinarily grouped by age and sex.

Not all outer fat sites are equally good for pinching; at most a half-dozen sites are commonly measured. Only an adult with the elastic-skin syndrome can be caliper pinched at a dozen sites or more. What sites are measured also depends on modesty, on the needs of the measuring program, and on the level of fatness. The triceps and biceps skinfolds are popular, for these sites ordinarily protrude from the usual garb. The subscapular site is popular because it involves rather little disrobing. The abdominal and iliac sites, where the outer fat is thickest in most adults, are less commonly measured—though more useful, and the inner thigh site is but rarely measured—though operationally valuable. A skinfold site at the level of the lowest rib should be added to the list.

In thin and undernourished individuals, skinfold "pinches" can be raised on many parts of the upper and lower leg. In obese men and women, and in superobese children, the truncal skinfolds may exceed the capacity of the skinfold calipers, and are therefore unmeasurable. Besides, there are individuals with an unusually rubbery feel in whom most skinfolds cannot be raised at all. That is why a standard set of skinfolds cannot be employed at all ages, on all subjects, and in pregnant and nonpregnant women alike.

Most skinfolds are not true double folds of fat plus skin, but something less. Compressibility is not the same on all parts of the body, nor in both sexes and over the entire age span (Garn, 1956; Brozek and Mori, 1958; Becque et al., 1986). These technical problems are commonly ignored when using skinfold measurements, since subjects with larger skinfold readings are fatter than those with smaller readings and the rankings reflect fatness in general. Such variables as compressibility must be considered when calculating fat volumes, as in upper arm composition estimates, otherwise the amount of fat is underestimated and the amount of muscle is greatly overestimated (Garn, 1979; Table 2). Compared with well-nourished adults, babies and malnourished individuals are a little more "fat" than may seem to be the case, because skin thickness is less in infants and further diminished in protein-energy malnutrition (cf. Lee and Ng, 1967).

CALIPERS FOR SKINFOLD MEASUREMENT

Skinfold calipers are modifications of fixed-arm calipers, with enlarged contact areas and constant pressure springs added to uniformize the squeeze. The measurements must be taken after a set period of time to uniformize for the squeezing down of the skinfolds (cf. Becque et al., 1986; Katch, 1986).

The Lange (Cambridge) caliper was designed by Dr. K. O. Lange to meet the specifications of the Committee on Nutritional Anthropometry; the Harpenden calipers were similarly designed. They differ in readout (1.0 mm for the Lange and 0.1 mm for the Harpenden): the latter utilizes an industrial micrometer or "mike." They differ also in jaw capacity, so the latest Harpenden is better suited to the obese.

There are now many commercial calipers on the market and some of the throwaway variety, given such names as Fat-O-Meter and the like (cf. Garn, 1983, 1985). The smaller, least expensive calipers are not rugged, often incorrectly calibrated, and may have inadequate jaw capacities. Some of the newer commercial calipers like the Skyndex include such advantages as digital readout and "hold" buttons, and some can be programmed to read both skinfold thickness and estimated fat weight. Digital readout is an advantage, minimizing readout errors, and the "hold" button is a distinct convenience.

Skinfold calipers that employ a dial micrometer can be modified with a multiturn potentiometer for providing a digital display on a digital voltmeter (DVM) or for direct entry of readings on tape or via a computer interface. Digital readout skinfold calipers can also be so adapted. Such technical modifications speed data acquisition and in conjunction with a suitable computer program can challenge the anthropometrist to repeat measurements deemed unlikely for a subject of that age and weight.

REPLICABILITY AND VALIDITY

Assuming care, interest, and motivation, the short-term (i.e., immediate) replicability of skinfold measurements can be slightly in excess of 0.90 in the hands of well-instructed anthropometrists (cf. Garn et al., 1988a). This value of r is comparable to the intercorrelations between the iliac and abdominal skinfolds in older adolescent girls and women and approximates the theoretical maximum for calipers with 1.0 mm readout, a 15 mm (average) skinfold, and an RMS deviation of ±6 mm. Lower replicability can be expected when the skinfolds are smaller, when less care is employed in reading the calipers after a constant time interval, and when the sites are imperfectly located. Moreover there are some subjects who are truly unmeasurable, either because they are so rubbery or because their compressed double folds exceed the useful range of the calipers. In survey work it is common practice to eliminate (censor) improbable skinfold values, though replicability is not much affected by recording errors when the sample sizes are large.

Long-term skinfold replicabilities are of course lower, even for weight stable adult subjects, for the readout errors (±1 mm) may sum or subtract, and it is difficult to remeasure the exact site after a period of time. So the best of the longer-term replicabilities approximate the theoretical value of 0.81, given immediate replicability values of 0.90 and weight stability within ±1 kg. Though 0.81 may be viewed as "good" in serial observations, it is still a limitation when the stability of patterned differences involving pairs of skinfolds is concerned (Garn et al., 1988a).

When compressed double fold skinfolds are compared with radiogrammetric fat shadow measurements, using well-defined and carefully marked sites suitable for both approaches, the results may again be called "good" with correlations exceeding 0.85 (Garn, 1956; Garn and Gorman, 1956; Fig. 1). This is again close to the theoretical value of r, assuming immediate skinfold reliability of 0.90 and radiogrammetric reliability of 0.95 (the latter involving 0.1 mm caliper readout). Such "validity" assumes constant skinfold compressibility, attainable in a narrow age range and for one sex. Spuriously higher skinfold/fat shadow correlations can be attained by selecting fatness extremes (or by pooling age disparate data), but an r of 0.90 is not operationally different from an r of 0.85, and not meaningfully so with Ns of 100 or less.

Comparisons of skinfold measurements with fat-weight estimates obtained from densitometry are limited by the root mean square errors of both techniques and are at best equal to the cross product of their immediate reliabilities. Again an obtained r of 0.81–0.86 is about the maximum that can be expected, ignoring the systematic errors in densitometry introduced by intestinal gases. For obvious reasons the comparisons should involve skinfolds and the weight of fat (FW), not percent fat (%F) as is often done. Subjects of a narrow age range are essential, for the "constants" in the density equations are not that constant (Clarys and Martin, 1986).

Skinfold–fat weight correlations under these conditions and with samples of adequate size do approximate the theoretical maximum, and summed skin-

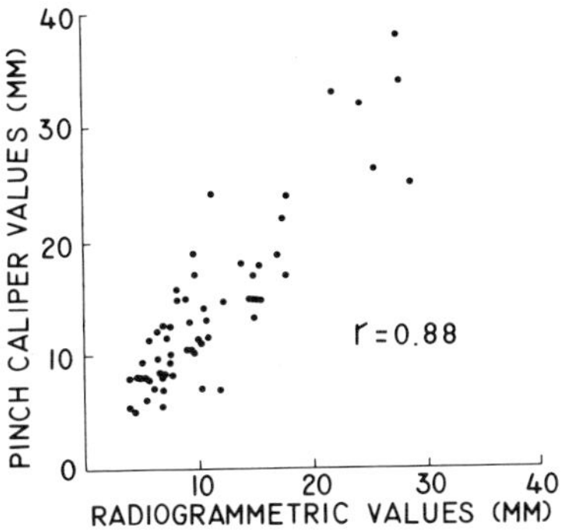

Fig. 1. Relationship between the radiographic fat shadow and the pinch caliper measurement of outer fat at the same site in young adult males (Garn, 1956; Garn and Gorman, 1956). The magnitude of the correlation is dependent upon the site selected, the independent replicabilities of the techniques, and sample size, with a theoretical maximum near 0.85.

folds (Σsf) may exceed individual skinfolds in this respect. While the ideal comparison of skinfolds and fat weight would involve a large sample of a narrow age range then subjected to destructive fat determinations, this (ideal) comparison is unlikely to be made. Fat estimates by underwater weighing have limitations and assume more constancy of the water content of both lean tissue and obesity tissue than is likely.

Obviously, skinfold thicknesses or summed skinfold thicknesses can be converted into an estimated weight of fat either by the regression of weight on skinfold thickness (as we have done) or by the regression of skinfold thickness on fat weight estimated from the densitometric equations. Almost anything can be estimated from regression equations, of course, and their validity is limited by the sample size, the nature of the reference sample, and the techniques used. At best, estimates of fat weight from any regression technique is no better than the raw data, but an estimated FW is useful for survey purposes and is impressive to statistically unsophisticated readers (cf. Katch, 1986).

SKEWNESS AND RELATED PROBLEMS IN OUTER FAT DISTRIBUTIONS

Skinfold and fat shadow distributions, like fat weight distributions, tend to be skewed, with a long tail to the right in well-nourished adults. Since the distributions are skewed and also kurtotic, means and standard deviations and *t*-tests are inappropriate, though most workers use them. Product-moment correlations are also inappropriate for skewed distributions, but most workers use them, even for attenuated or cut-off segments (like the "obese") where the remaining distribution is in consequence saw-toothed in nature.

Many workers, imitating Tanner, employ a $\log_{10}$ transformation of raw skinfold or fat shadow values, unaware that the $\log_{10}$ transformation is not always appropriate and for youngsters and malnourished adults may increase rather than decrease skewness. We have long employed *normalized* *Z*-scores (not simple *Z*-scores), which effectively convert the most skewed skinfold distributions into a closely Gaussian form, and are available on command in many statistical packages, such as MIDAS and SAS.

Though means and sigmas provide inappropriate descriptions for most skinfold distributions, skinfold–skinfold correlations, skinfold–weight correlations, and skinfold–fat weight correlations are not much biased when calculated from the raw (untransformed) values. The skewnesses are of the same nature, and the trend lines often match the calculated regressions closely. In other cases, however, skinfolds or fat shadows are not linearly related to various variables, in which case *r* is less appropriate than a nonlinear measure of relationship. This is especially true when relating skinfolds to age over a long span of years. Age "corrections" in multivariate analyses and residuals from linear age regressions may be incorrect for these reasons.

CORRELATIONS WITH OTHER APPROACHES

Because the subcutaneous fat constitutes the largest part of the total fat stores of the adult human body, some 70%–80% in fact (Martin et al., 1985), it is moderately to highly correlated with "fat" as otherwise measured. A little calculation of the volume of outer fat, using the average midsection thickness and surface area in square meters, will demonstrate why this is so. In truly obese subjects with a 20 cm *uncompressed* outer fat layer at most sites, the tremendous excess of outer fat over inner fat is easily appreciated.

Correlations between subcutaneous fat thickness and "fat" as otherwise measured range from 0.6 to 0.9, depending on sample size and technique and the reliability of each technique. If we assume skinfold reliability of 0.9 and a best-case reliability of 0.95 for another technique, the resulting correlation coefficient of 0.85 represents the maximum possible level of relationship between the two (cf. Borkan et al., 1986).

While underwater weighing (densitometry) has been touted as the "gold standard" for body composition determinations, the limitations must also be considered. The tissue densities used in the simultaneous equations are not that well determined, especially in children and in women. Moreover, the gold standard is more nearly filled gold, i.e., air filled, for intestinal gases may loom large and repeatably in underwater determinations, possibly inflating reliability (though decreasing the validity) of the body composition estimates from weight under water.

The 40_k space, also touted because it is based on the natural radioactivity of the lean body mass (LBM), is similarly limited when it comes to individual determinations. By the 40_k method, the weight of fat is estimated by subtracting the estimated weight of lean from total body weight. A small percentage error in estimating the LBM thus becomes a larger percentage error in estimating FW by subtraction. Whether gold, silver, or platinum by analogy, the 40_K space also yields an approximation to the true fat weight.

The ultimate reference standard for body composition is of course the intact, living body then subjected to total body analysis by dissection. The latter is a tedious procedure, even to an anatomist, and the 40-odd cadavers so far studied are likely to be the last. So we are left with the statement that skinfolds and radiogrammetric fat shadows do correlate to a useful degree with densitometrically derived estimates of body fat.

VALIDATING SKINFOLDS IN NUTRITIONAL ASSESSMENT

It is simple to document the utility of skinfolds in nutritional assessment, for they parallel other measures of nutritional adequacy and they parallel many laboratory measures of blood, serum, and urinary constituents.

During the growing period, and from the end of the first year onward, fatter boys and girls are longer, i.e., taller by as much as 10–12 cm as the adolescent period begins (Garn et al., 1974). They have a more positive energy balance: More energy has been available for growth and more is available for storage as fat. During the growing period in Westernized countries, and throughout life in the Central American countries, fatter individuals are also taller (Garn et al., 1983).

Fatter children, adolescents, and adults have higher hemoglobin and hematocrit levels (Garn and Ryan, 1982, 1983). Exactly why they do is not clear, but it is suggestive of higher food intakes in general. Fatter children and adults in major nutrition surveys (Ten-State, Pre-School, and NHANES) tend to higher serum and urinary vitamins, again suggesting a more ample intake. Indeed the higher serum and urinary vitamin levels and serum albumins of the obese effectively contradict their lower (reported) food intakes, suggesting systematic underreporting on their part.

As skinfolds go up, so does serum cholesterol, age by age and in both sexes (Garn et al., 1975, 1988b). The correlation is not high (0.20–0.30) and the fatness-related range is only 10 mg/dL or so, but the trend is consistent even through the eighth decade. Triglycerides are also fatness dependent, with a slightly higher correlation, while the high-density lipoproteins (HDL) are inversely correlated with skinfolds (see Table 1).

At all ages, systolic and diastolic blood pressures are covariant with the commonly used skinfolds, more so in women than in men. Thus in older adult women aged 50–75, there is a 21 mm increase in systolic blood pressure over the skinfold quintiles, whether the triceps, subscapular, iliac or abdominal skinfolds or the summed skinfolds (Σsf) are used (see Table 2).

There are other independent validations of the validity of skinfolds in nutritional assessment, including the socioeconomic correlates (positive in children and negative in adult women). High skinfold and radiogrammetric fat shadow measurements are predictive of cardiovascular deaths in fifth decade subjects followed for more than a decade (Garn et al., 1987). Of course skin-

TABLE 1. Relationship Between Serum Cholesterol (mg/dL) and Skinfold Quintiles for Four Different Skinfolds and the Summed Skinfold (Σ sf) Value[a]

	Serum cholesterol by skinfold quintile				
Skinfold	1	2	3	4	5
Triceps	129	132	133	136	140
Subscapular	128	132	133	136	142
Iliac	129	133	133	135	141
Abdominal	128	133	134	133	142
Summed skinfolds	129	132	132	134	142

[a]1,589 adult males 20–49, age corrected. Values are for total cholesterol expressed as mg/dL.

folds are far better indicators of fatness than body mass indices that reflect FW, LBW, and leg length as well (Garn et al., 1986b).

WHICH SKINFOLD IS "BEST"

Confronted with a list of skinfold sites indicated for measurement, economy-minded survey directors and minimalist statisticians ask "which one is best?" To this question there are also many answers, *N* times the number of skinfolds, and there is an extensive literature on this subject.

One may, of course, calculate skinfold intercorrelations, deriving from the matrix one skinfold that has the greatest communality with the rest. However, the intercorrelations for the most-used skinfolds are all moderately high, 0.6–0.9 in adults (see Table 3). With most sample sizes it is inadvisable to avow that the triceps or subscapular or iliac or abdominal skinfold holds primacy at a conclusive level of confidence (Garn et al., 1987).

Another approach is to relate skinfold thicknesses to various risk and outcome factors, again with sample size in mind. When this is done by product-

TABLE 2. Systolic Blood Pressure by Summed Skinfold Quintiles From Infancy Through the Eighth Decade[a]

Age		Systolic blood pressure by Σ sf quintile				
group	N	1	2	3	4	5
1–4	320	100	103	103	103	104
5–9	604	111	111	111	115	116
10–14	519	117	118	120	122	127
15–19	389	119	118	120	122	127
12–49	1,793	121	123	125	128	136
50–75	610	140	147	151	154	161

[a]All data refer to female participants in the Tecumseh (Mich) Community Survey, Examination Round 2; age corrected throughout.

TABLE 3. Skinfold Intercorrelation Matrices for Adult Males and Females[a]

Skinfold	Triceps r	Subscapular r	Iliac r	Abdominal r
	1,639 males		1,851 females	
Triceps	—	0.80	0.77	0.75
Subscapular	0.69	—	0.85	0.82
Iliac	0.72	0.75	—	0.91
Abdominal	0.72	0.76	0.87	—

[a]See Garn et al., 1988b.

moment correlations or with nonlinear correlations or using skinfold deciles, no single skinfold emerges as the unchallenged victor in both sexes. There have been efforts to achieve this comparison using the beta coefficients from the regression equations, but differences in relative magnitudes of different skinfolds complicate the decision. A skinfold that is generally thinner will have a higher value of K than one that is generally thicker. So a higher value of K is not to be confused with "better."

Skinfolds also differ in relative thickness over the life cycle, the triceps being thicker than three others in 90% of children and the abdominal skinfold being the thickest in the majority of U.S.A. adults. For technical reasons, the thicker skinfold having greater variance, one might be advocated in the young and in undernourished populations and another in well-nourished older population samples (Garn et al., 1988b).

The obese and the morbidly obese constitute a special problem, for the abdominal and iliac skinfolds may be beyond the jaw capacities of the Lange and other calipers. For pregnant women beyond the first trimester, sites away from the abdomen are indicated. In simple malnutrition and protein-energy malnutrition there are more measurable sites, but they fall in the lowest range of the calipers and have very limited variance.

Summed skinfolds sometimes show slightly higher correlations with specific outcome variables, but summed skinfolds are inevitably weighted by the thicker skinfolds (triceps in the lean and abdominal in the obese). One can also argue that summed skinfolds average out caliper reading and other random measuring errors (Garn et al., 1987). Expediency may dictate one skinfold in survey and monitoring studies, several skinfolds in clinical applications, and a full range of skinfolds for investigative purposes.

LIFE CYCLE CHANGES IN OUTER FAT THICKNESSES

From well before birth through the seventh decade, subcutaneous fat thicknesses at most sites increase through age 50 and then decrease in the later decades. However, the upward course is by no means linear, broken by several periods of decrease in both sexes and a rapid postmenarcheal increase in the female. Life cycle data from 3 major surveys (Ten-State, NHANES I and II, and Tecumseh) are so similar overall and so similar within their inflections as to suggest that this is the "human condition" (see Fig. 2).

Nevertheless, the general trends suggested by such population data are contradicted when the sons of the obese and the daughters of the lean are compared and when skinfold thicknesses are grouped by socioeconomic levels. Sons of obese parents have greater subcutaneous fat thicknesses than the daughters of lean parents. While poor girls are leaner than more affluent girls, low-income women are fatter thereafter than their higher-income age peers (Garn and Ryan, 1981). Such differences in outer fat thickness therefore remind us that samples do differ, and they show the need for caution when using mass data compilations for nutritional standards. Should we define "obesity" in the adult female in terms of the rich, who are less fat, or the poor, who are far fatter (Garn and Clark, 1974; Garn, 1986a)?

Outer fat thicknesses are complicated by developmental status. At 9–12 months, developmentally advanced infants may be leaner than developmen-

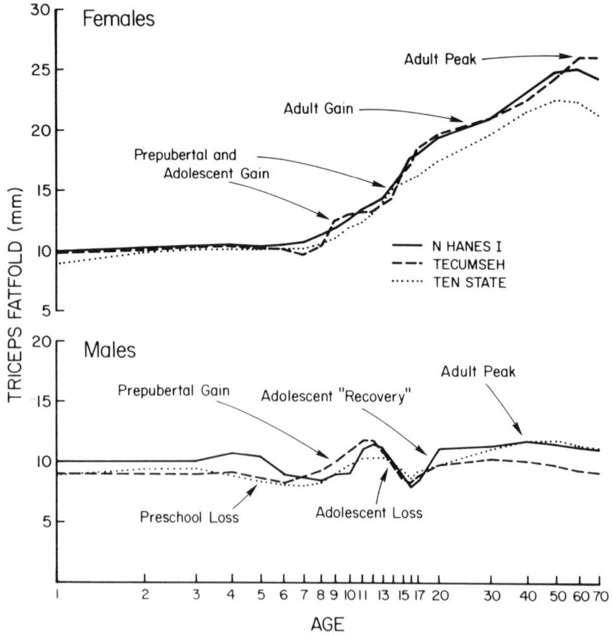

Fig. 2. Changes in the triceps skinfold thickness over the life cycle in females **(above)** and males **(below).** Though the overall trends and points of inflection are remarkably similar in NHANES I, Tecumseh, and the Ten-State Nutrition Survey, the poor and the rich depart from the massed data trend lines (Garn, 1981a) as do early maturers (Garn et al., 1983) and late maturers and nationals of other countries.

tally retarded infants of both sexes. During "adolescence," earlier maturing girls are fatter than their less mature peers (Garn and Haskell, 1960). This problem is further complicated by the fact that earlier maturers remain fatter lifelong (Garn et al., 1986a; Garn and LaVelle, 1985).

Specific fat sites in males and females may change in thickness in directions opposite from the general trend for that sex. Scalp fat is notably thicker in adult males than in females, recalling the cephalic fat pad in anthropoids (Garn et al., 1954). The iliac site is also relatively thicker in adult males than in adult females. Moreover, there is remodeling or redistribution of the fat at adjacent sites on the lower leg even in early adulthood (Garn and Saalberg, 1953). The relative thickness of different skinfolds changes over the life cycle, in part reflecting changes in outer fat thickness and in part reflecting developmental changes (Garn et al., 1988c). So the triceps skinfold is thickest in 90% of children but only a minority of adults (Fig. 3). At and after adolescence the iliac and abdominal sites are generally thicker than the triceps site, except in

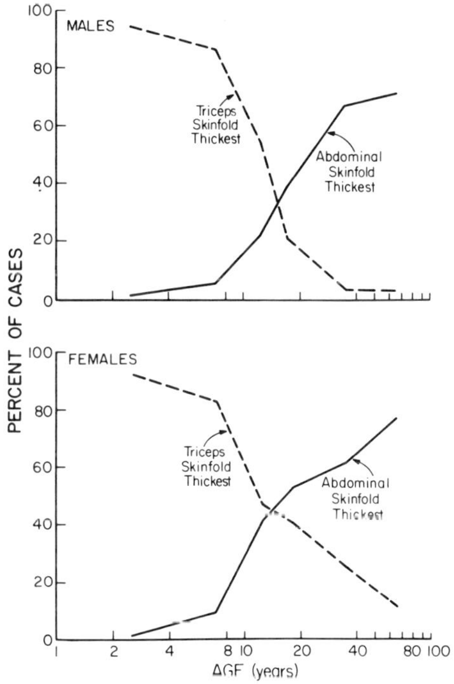

Fig. 3. Lifelong changes in relative skinfold thickness in both sexes. While the triceps skinfold is the thickest of four skinfolds in over 90% of children, this is true only in a minority of adults. The abdominal skinfold is rarely the thickest in children, but it is the thickest of four skinfolds in most adults (cf. Garn et al., 1988c,d).

lean adults. Individual differences and age trends in relative skinfold thickness are not readily discernible from median value, and they raise methodological problems in nutritional assessment.

Lifelong trends in outer fat thicknesses may not be matched exactly in leaner populations, such as the English, and they may be contradicted by trends in third world and marginal populations. In New Guinea, for example, outer fat may decrease after the end of the second decade, and this is true in many Central American populations. Moreover the inverse relationship between socioeconomic status (SES) and outer fat thickness in Westernized women is often different in the third world, where the relationship to SES is positive rather than negative. What we can so fully document in U.S. or U.K. skinfold data is not necessarily the picture for all of humanity, but rather a description of life cycle trends at particular levels of energy balance.

DIFFERENCES IN SUBCUTANEOUS FAT THICKNESS AND GROWTH, AGING, AND MORTALITY

During the growing period, fatter boys and girls grow faster, are advanced in skeletal maturation, and are taller as well. Greater skinfold thicknesses go with a larger lean body mass (LBM), so fatter boys and girls are larger, both inside and out. The implication is that a thicker tela subcutanea is effectively auxogenic, or more correctly, that more energy has been available both for growth and for storage as fat.

Boys and girls with larger fat stores are also higher in the conventional hematological measures (hemoglobin and hematocrit), an important point in nutritional assessment. They also tend to be higher in serum cholesterol and the triglycerides, relevant to the question of "tracking" and to intervention attempts. Obese boys and girls are higher in systolic and diastolic blood pressures than their lean age mates, a point of concern when blood pressure measurements are employed for early identification of potential hypertensives.

In adults, cholesterol and the triglycerides parallel skinfold measurements, regardless of which skinfold is used (Garn et al., 1975a,b, 1988c), though the correlations are low (circa 0.2–0.3). In adults, especially older adults, blood pressure values parallel skinfold values, and over 50% of the truly obese are "hypertensive," even those on antihypertensive drugs (Fig. 4).

It is not surprising, therefore, that the risk of cardiovascular demise rises with skinfold levels. It is more surprising that at the lowest skinfold or outer fat levels, there is also increased risk of demise from all kinds of respiratory disease (Garn et al., 1983c). The relationship between skinfolds and mortality is curvilinear, not linear, so there is no level of outer fatness that is truly ideal or optimal. However, at some level of outer fat thickness, well below the average, mortality is least.

These statements must be modified by noting the age at examination (typically age 40) and the elapsed time of the study. Short-term mortality data reveal an excess risk associated with diminished outer fat; long-term mortality data show an increased risk (primarily cardiovascular) associated with increased outer fat. Moreover, the data are complicated by unrecorded changes

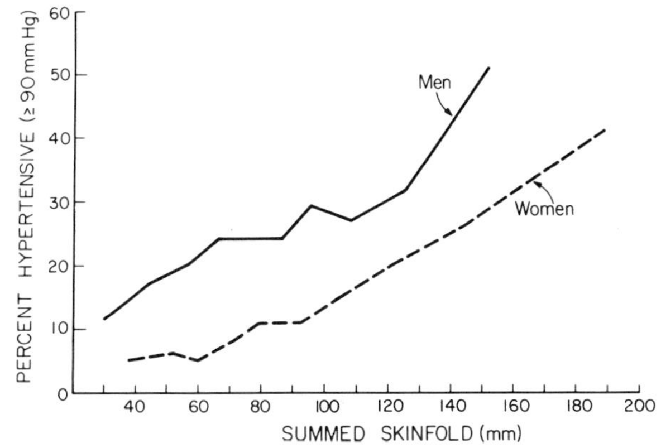

Fig. 4. Percent of hypertensive adults at different levels of fatness in adults aged 20–49. As the summed skinfold thickness increases, as shown here, so does the incidence of hypertension, reaching 40%–50% at the higher levels of fatness. Trends for individual skinfolds (triceps, subscapular, iliac, and abdominal) are closely similar (Garn et al., 1987, 1988c,d).

in fatness between examinations and the time of death, and the mixture of smokers and nonsmokers (Garn, 1986a). Since the smokers are considerably leaner than the nonsmokers, their removal would increase the ideal or "optimal" fatness of the nonsmokers.

FAT PLACEMENT OR FAT PATTERNING AS A POSSIBLE RISK FACTOR

While most students of human body composition have been concerned with the weight of fat or the percent of fat (100 · FW/TBW) and its implications to growth, reproduction, morbidity, and mortality, there has long been an interest in fat placement, fat distribution, or fat "patterning." Vague (1956) is most often mentioned as the pioneer who suggested that the placement or distribution of fat is itself predictive of various diseases. Now we read that upper-body fat, an elevated waist/hip circumference, or a "masculine" fat distribution are separately predictive of diabetes, hypertension, and other ills (Kissebah et al., 1982; Feldman et al., 1969; Bjørntorp., 1986).

It is indeed true that circumferential ratios and skinfold ratios are related to lipid levels and the systolic and diastolic blood pressure levels. Women with a "masculine" fat distribution are more likely to be hypertensive or hyperlipidemic. However, ratios, whether of skinfolds or circumferences, are also highly fatness dependent and so related to various risk factors (Fig. 5). Women with a beer barrel belly are more often hypertensive; they do look like older men, but they are also fat women (Garn et al., 1988b,c).

Correlations between skinfold *ratios* and summed skinfolds (Σsf) are all significant and may approach 0.5–0.6, the relationships being nonlinear as

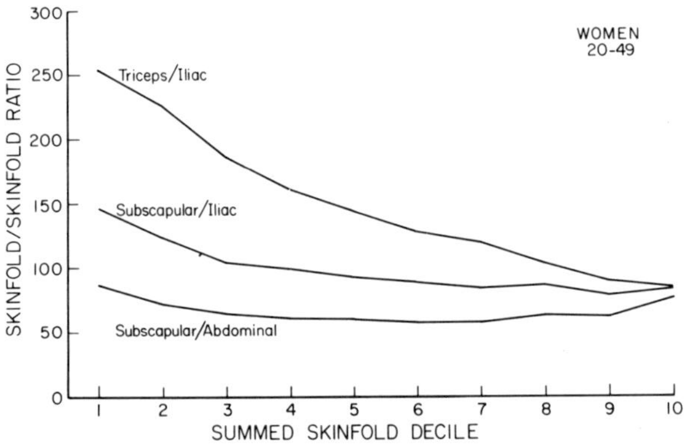

Fig. 5. Relationship between summed skinfold deciles and skinfold ratios in women aged 20–49. All skinfold ratios are fatness dependent in both sexes, to an extent and in a direction dependent upon the construction of the ratios. Circumferential ratios (waist/hip, etc.) are similarly fatness dependent (cf. Garn et al., 1988b,c).

shown by the excess of etas over *r*s. All skinfold ratios involving the triceps, subscapular, iliac, and abdominal skinfolds are fatness dependent, and their independent relationships to various risk factors may stem from this fact (Table 4). With increasing fatness, the abdominal region adds fat faster than the trochanteric region, so differences in waist/hip ratios may simply meter the level of fatness. In very lean individuals, of course, the "waist" is small and constricted, while the bony pelvis places a lower limit on the trochanteric or cristal circumference. There are differences in fat distribution that transcend the level of fatness, but these differences are obscured by simple ratios that are fatness dependent. There are approaches that correct or adjust for fatness (cf. Garn, 1955, 1981b), including the *Z*-scored fatness index of Norgan ($Z_1 - Z_2$), *Z*-score ratios (Z_1/Z_2), and residuals from the regression of one skinfold on the other. The problem is that of adjusting for or "scaling" for fatness, to find methods of expressing differences in placement that are not a product of fatness level per se (Norgan and Ferro-Luzzi, 1986; Garn et al., 1988c).

Given the fact that measuring errors can sum or subtract, it is difficult but not impossible to demonstrate that some of these apparent differences in fat placement persist even after weight gain or weight loss. It is especially difficult to attempt this with ratios, for an apparent lack of difference (zero mean difference) after weight change may be obscured by a large RMS difference, thus questioning the null hypothesis (cf. Ashwell et al., 1986).

SUBCUTANEOUS FAT AND NUTRITIONAL ASSESSMENT

Nutritional anthropometry is only one part of nutritional assessment and measurement of subcutaneous (outer) fat is only part of that part (Garn 1962,

TABLE 4. Magnitude of Fatness Dependence of Skinfold Ratios

	Correlations with summed skinfolds			
	1,639 men		1,851 women	
Skinfold ratio	*r*	η	*r*	η
Triceps/subscapular	−0.10	0.20	−0.50	0.51
Triceps/iliac	−0.45	0.50	−0.57	0.64
Triceps/abdominal	−0.38	0.46	−0.44	0.52
Subscapular/iliac	−0.41	−0.56	−0.35	0.47
Subscapular/abdominal	−0.31	0.55	−0.06	0.32
Iliac/abdominal	0.17	0.20	0.35	0.37

1965, 1966). Measuring subcutaneous fat is no substitute for hematological evaluations, serum and urinary determinations or vitamin levels, serum albumin measurements, lipid determinations, or food frequency data. Yet the amount of fat stored under the skin is a very good indication of the long-term energy balance, and it serves to delineate at-risk individuals and populations at risk for nutritional deficiencies or excesses. Since subcutaneous fat determinations meter the level of fatness, they have unquestioned value in the obesities, for intervention programs, and in explaining morbidity and mortality. In Westernized populations such as ours, skinfold measurements help to define the obese and the superobese, the anorectics, and those at nutritional risk because of inadequate energy intakes relative to their energy expenditures. The effectiveness of therapy for malabsorption states and anorexia can best be followed by serial skinfold measurements.

There is the problem of whether, and to what extent, differences in outer fat placement or patterning are of independent diagnostic value, since skinfold and circumferential ratios are so dependent on the amount of fat. There is the problem of how much of any given skinfold is fat, or at least obesity tissue, and how much is water, and how much is protein. Changes in outer fat thickness versus weight changes, as contrasted with the static comparison of outer fat versus weight, suggests that much more is contained within skinfold changes than just fat alone (cf. Garrow, 1986; Forbes, 1987; Garn et al., 1988b).

There are technical problems, including age changes and sex differences and individual differences in skinfold compressibility at each site and their meaning to skinfold composition. Similar problems haunt all body composition methodologies. Intestinal gases plague those that involve body volume. Variations in body water content affect the measurement of naturally occurring isotopes and NMR determinations as well.

Still, what we measure and label as "subcutaneous fat" is extremely useful and, for many adults, it is the most meaningful aspect of nutritional anthropometry. It can be argued that subcutaneous fat thickness and hemoglobin/hematocrit determinations are, together, the most revealing indications of nutritional adequacy.

ACKNOWLEDGMENTS

I am indebted to Cynthia Housh for her assistance in four versions of the manuscript and to Timothy V. E. Sullivan for data reduction and data analysis. Some of the work described in this paper was supported by the Weight Watchers' Research Foundation and a grant from Gerber Products.

REFERENCES

Ashwell M, McCall SA, Dixon AK (1986): Fat distribution and its metabolism complications: Interpretations. In Norgan NG (ed): "Human Body Composition and Fat Distribution." Euro-Nut (8) The Haag: Koninklijke Bibliotheek, pp 227–245.

Bailey SM, Garn SM, Block WM, Cole P (1977): Definitive estimate of fatness lipid relationships in the normal adult population. Fed Proc 37:593.

Becque MD, Katch VL, Moffatt R (1986): Skinfold compressibility in males and females. Hum Biol 58:33–42.

Bjørntorp P (1986): Fat patterning and disease: A review. In Norgan NG (ed): "Human Body Composition and Fat Distribution." Euro-Nut (8) The Haag: Koninklijke Bibliotheek, pp 201–209.

Borkan GA, Gerzof SG, Robbins AH, Hults DE, Burrows BA (1986): Comparison of computed tomography, skinfolds, and ultrasound assessment of subcutaneous fat thickness. In Norgan NG (ed): "Human Body Composition and Fat Distribution." Eur-Nut (8) The Haag: Koninklijke Bibliotheek, pp 129–141.

Brozek J, Mori H (1958): Some interrelations between somatic, roentgenogrammetric and densiometric criteria of fatness. Hum Biol 30:322–336.

Clarys JP, Martin AD (1986): The concept of the adipose tissue-free mass. In Norgan NG (ed): "Human Body Composition and Fat Distribution." Euro-Nut (8) The Haag: Koninklijke Bibliotheek, pp 49–63.

Feldman R, Sender AJ, Siegelaub AB (1969): Difference in diabetic and nondiabetic fat distribution patterns by skinfold measurements. Diabetes 18:478–486.

Forbes GB (1987): Lean body mass–body fat interrelationships in humans. Nutr Rev 45:225–231.

Garn SM (1955): Relative fat patterning: An individual characteristic. Hum Biol 27:75–89.

Garn SM (1956): Comparison of pinch-caliper and x-ray measurements of skin plus subcutaneous fat. Science 124:178–179.

Garn SM (1957): Roentgenogrammetric determinations of body composition. Hum Biol 29:337–353.

Garn SM (1962): Anthropometry in clinical appraisal of nutritional status. Am J Clin Nutr 11:418–432.

Garn SM (1965): The applicability of North American growth standards in developing countries. Can Med Assoc J 93:914–919.

Garn SM (1966): Malnutrition and skeletal development in the pre-school child. In "Pre-School Child Malnutrition: Primary Deterrent to Human Progress." Washington, DC: National Academy of Sciences—National Research Council, pp 43–62.

Garn SM (1979): Optimal nutritional assessment. In Jeliffe DB, Jeliffe EEP (eds): "Human Nutrition—A Comprehensive Treatise. Vol 2." New York: pp 273–298.

Garn SM (1981a): Socioeconomic aspects of obesity. Contemp Nutr 6:1–2.

Garn SM (1981b): Graphic and numerical analyses of patterned similarities and differences. In Mai LL, Shanklin E, Sussman RW (eds): "The Perception of Evolution:

Essays Honoring Joseph B. Birdsell." Los Angeles: Anthropology UCLA, vol 7, 93–111.
Garn SM (1983): Another inexpensive skinfold caliper. Ecol Food Nutr 13: 197–198.
Garn SM (1985): Still another plastic skinfold caliper. Ecol Food and Nutr 17: 193.
Garn SM (1986a): Smoking and human biology. Hum Biol 57:505–523.
Garn SM (1986b): Family-line and socioeconomic factors in fatness and obesity. Nutr Rev 44:381–386.
Garn SM, Bailey SM, Cole PE (1979b): Synchronous fatness changes in husbands and wives. Am J Clin Nutr 32:2375–2377.
Garn SM, Bailey SM, Cole PE, Higgins ITT (1977): Level of education, level of income and level of fatness in adults. Am J Clin Nutr 30:721–725.
Garn SM, Block WD, Clark DC (1975b): Level of fatness and lipid levels. Ecol Food Nutr 4:235–236.
Garn SM, Clark DC (1974): Economics and fatness. Ecol Food Nutr 3:19–20.
Garn SM, Clark DC, Guire KE (1974): Level of fatness and size attainment. Am J Phys Anthrop 40:447–449.
Garn SM, Clark DC, Guire KE (1975a): Growth, body composition and development of obese and lean children. In Winick M (ed): "Childhood Obesity. Vol 3, Wiley Series on Current Concepts in Nutrition." Wiley-Interscience, pp 23–46.
Garn SM, Cole PE (1980): Do the obese remain obese and the lean remain lean? Am J Public Health 70(4):351–353.
Garn SM, Gorman EL (1956): Comparison of pinch-caliper and teleoroentgenogrammetric measurements of subcutaneous fat. Hum Biol 28:407–413.
Garn SM, Haskell JA (1960): Fat thickness and developmental status in childhood and adolescence. Am J Dis Child 99:746–751.
Garn SM, Hawthorne VM, Pilkington JJ, Pesick SD (1983c): Fatness and mortality in the West of Scotland. Am J Clin Nutr 38:313–319.
Garn SM, Hoff K, McCabe KD (1979a): Maternal fatness and placental size. Am J Clin Nutr 32:277–279.
Garn SM and LaVelle M (1985): Two-decade follow-up of fatness in early childhood. Am J Dis Child 139:181–185.
Garn SM, LaVelle M, Pilkington JJ (1983b): Comparisons of fatness in premenarcheal and postmenarcheal girls of the same age. J Pediatr 103:328–331.
Garn SM, LaVelle M, Rosenberg KR, Hawthorne V (1986a): Maturational timing as a factor in female fatness and obesity. Am J Clin Nutr 43:879–883.
Garn SM, Leonard WR, Hawthorne VM (1986b): Three limitations of the body mass index. Am J Clin Nutr 44:996–997.
Garn SM, Rosenberg KR, Schaefer AE (1983a): Relationship between fatness level and size attainment in Central America. Ecol Food Nutr 13:157–165.
Garn SM, Ryan AS (1981): Replicating the income related reversal of fatness. Ecol Food Nutr 10:237–239.
Garn SM, Ryan AS (1982): The effect of fatness on hemoglobin levels. Am J Clin Nutr 36:189–191.
Garn SM, Ryan AS (1983): Relationship between fatness and hemoglobin levels in the National Health and Nutrition Examination of the U.S.A. Ecol Food Nutr 12:211–215.
Garn SM, Saalberg JH (1953): Sex and age differences in the composition of the adult leg. Hum Biol 25:144–153.
Garn SM, Selby S, Young R (1954): Scalp thickness and the fat-loss theory of balding. Arch Dermatol Syphilol 47:601–608.

Garn SM, Sullivan TV, Hawthorne VM (1987): Does "central" obesity predict coronary artery disease? Lancet 20:1438–1439.
Garn SM, Sullivan TV, Hawthorne VM (1988a): Persistence of relative fatness at different body sites. Hum Biol 60:43–53.
Garn SM, Sullivan TV, Hawthorne VM (1988b): Differential fatness remodelling rates at different body sites. Int J Obes 11:519–525.
Garn SM, Sullivan TV, Hawthorne VM (1988c): Evidence against functional differences between "central" and "peripheral" fat. Am J Clin Nutr 47:836–839.
Garn SM, Sullivan TV, Hawthorne VM (1988d): Fatness dependence of skinfold ratios and its implications to fat patterning. Ecol Food Nutr 21 151–158.
Garrow JS (1986): Methods for measuring changes in body composition. In Norgan NG (ed): "Human Body Composition and Fat Distribution." Euro-Nut (8) The Haag: Koninklijke Bibliotheek, pp 75–80.
Katch V (1986): Assessment of body composition: Comments on prediction. In Norgan NG (ed): "Human Body Composition and Fat Distribution." Euro-Nut (8) The Haag: Koninklijke Bibliotheek, pp 15–30.
Kissebah AH, Vydelingum N, Murray R, Evans DJ, Hartz AJ, Kalkhoff RK, Adams PW (1982): Relation of body fat distribution to metabolic complications of obesity. J Clin Endocr Metab 54:254–260.
Lee MMC, Ng CK (1967): Postmortem studies of skinfold caliper measurement and actual thickness of skin and subcutaneous tissue. Hum Biol 37:91–103.
Martin AD, Ross WD, Drinkwater DT, Clarys JP (1985): Prediction of body fat by skinfold caliper: Assumptions and cadaver evidence. Int J Obes 9:31–39.
Norgan NG, Ferro-Luzzi A (1986): Simple indices of subcutaneous fat patterning. Ecol Food Nutr 18:117–123.
Vague J (1956): The degree of masculine differentiation of obesities: A factor determining predisposition to diabetes, atherosclerosis, gout and uric acid calculous disease. Am J Clin Nutr 4:20–34.

Anthropometric Assessment
of Nutritional Status, pages 141–150

8
Considering Frame Size in Nutritional Assessment

JOHN H. HIMES
Division of Human Development and Nutrition, School of Public Health, University of Minnesota, Minneapolis, Minnesota 55455

INTRODUCTION

The concern for frame size is not new, although the emphases and rationales for considering frame size in nutritional assessment have changed since the early proponents. Throughout, there has been a concern that body build or skeletal robusticity is important for evaluating body size. Frame size usually encompasses bone, joint, and skeletal breadths and depths that are representative of the supportive structure as a whole.

ESTIMATING WEIGHT

As early as 1886, Bornhardt proposed an index based on the product of stature and chest circumference to estimate " ... normal body weight of drafted men as a means of determining fitness for military service." He assumed that one's most appropriate weight was roughly proportional to body surface area, and that chest circumference provided a "volume" measurement in estimating the weight one *ought* to be. Subsequently, investigators devised various indices of appropriate weight, robusticity, and nutritional status that incorporated body breadths, often chest dimensions (Table 1).

The rationale for including what would now be called measures of frame size was that appropriate weight was largely determined by skeletal dimensions. The addition of frame size to the more conventional weight–stature indices introduced by Buffon (1829) and Quetelet (1835) was seen as a major advancement and a recognition of the inadequacy of body length alone to estimate appropriate weight (Gray and Root, 1921). Because of the prevalent nutritional conditions in this early period, the primary emphasis for estimating weight was nutritional sufficiency. Generally, these indices were not viewed as continua of the constructs, but as target levels or optima for weight and nutritional status.

Later, more complicated approaches to determine "normal" body weight of adults utilized a series of standardized and summed ratios of six limb circumferences and body diameters (Willoughby, 1932; Turner, 1943), and multiple

TABLE 1. Selected Early Indices of Nutritional Status Including Measures of Body Frame[a]

Author	Index
Bornhardt (1886)	$\text{Weight} = \dfrac{\text{stature} \times \text{chest circumference}}{240}$
Pignet (1901)	$\text{Robusticity} = \text{stature} - (\text{breast circumference} + \text{weight})$
Oppenheimer (1901)	$\text{Nutrition quotient} = \dfrac{\text{arm girth} \times 100}{\text{chest circumference}}$
Rohrer (1921)	$\text{Nutrition status} = \dfrac{\text{weight} \times 100}{\text{stature} \times \text{shoulder breadth} \times \text{chest depth}}$

[a]For each index, weight is in kg, other dimensions in cm. Bornhardt's formula is converted into metric equivalents from original Russian units.

regression estimates of weight from stature and measures of frame (Boillin, 1930; Ludlum and Powell, 1940). The regression approaches demonstrated that measures of frame contribute significantly to variation in weight beyond that explained by stature.

Associations between weight, stature, and four measures of frame are presented in Table 2 for a sample of college women studied by Boillin (1930). Relative to stature, the frame measures each are more highly correlated with weight than is stature. The partial associations with weight remain strong when stature is held constant (Table 2, second column); and it is clear the frame measures each contribute uniquely to variation in weight (Table 2, third column). These associations between frame and weight are as strong or stronger than those found between subcutaneous fat thicknesses and weight (Himes, 1980).

These early analyses established that selected measures of frame contribute substantially to explaining variation in weight; the investigators then considered the predicted weights as most appropriate or normal. To the degree

TABLE 2. Correlations and Partial Correlations of Stature and Frame Measures With Weight for 815 College Women[a]

Measures	Simple r	Partial r controlling stature	Partial r controlling all other
Stature	0.46	—	0.29
Biacromial width	0.49	0.40	0.16
Chest width	0.63	0.59	0.34
Hip width	0.61	0.54	0.32
Chest depth	0.63	0.61	0.51

[a]Adapted from Boillin, 1930.

that body weight is accepted as a measure of nutritional status, the deviations of individuals from the expected weights constitute a measure of nutrition-related variation in weight. While this regression approach has considerable merit, it was never widely applied because of the complicated presentations, the requirement for multiple measurements, and the need for additional calculations.

For children, similar regression analyses estimating body weight were carried out (Franzen, 1929; Dearborn and Rothney, 1941; McCloy, 1936). These researchers concluded hip width and chest dimensions were the preferred frame measures contributing to variation in children's weight. These regression results were never widely applied to assessing nutritional status of children, although some of the concepts have persisted. A width–length index (100 × hip width/stature) was advocated to capture some of the weight variation explained by frame (Lucas and Pryor, 1931; Pryor and Stolz, 1933). Franzen and Palmer (1934) proposed the ACH index of nutritional status, using two measurements of arm circumference (A), two measurements of chest depth (C), and hip width (H). Width–weight tables for children were published by Pryor (1940, 1966) using categories of hip breadth (biiliac diameter), chest breadth, and stature, although they were so complicated to understand and apply that they were seldom used routinely.

ESTIMATING FAT-FREE MASS

The correlational models of Franzen (1929) and McCloy (1936) expanded emphases from estimating body weight per se to estimating separately indicators of muscle mass and subcutaneous fatness. This work presaged the introduction of theoretical models of total body composition, partitioning body weight into lean and fat compartments. Such a refinement brought significant nutritional and functional specificity to the assessment and meaning of body mass. Measures of frame size were considered important because of their associations with skeletal muscle mass, and because frame measures were approximations of skeletal dimensions, and therefore constituents of the fat-free mass.

Multiple correlation estimates of independently determined fat-free weight and lean body mass from stature and selected frame measures range from 0.89 to 0.98 (Behnke, 1959; von Dobeln, 1959; De Wijn and Zaat, 1968; Wilmore and Behnke, 1969). Clearly, frame is significant in explaining fat-free mass. Moreover, the frame measures contribute substantial information beyond that provided by stature.

Correlations of six frame measures with fat-free mass for a sample of adult men and women are presented in Table 3 (Himes and Bouchard, 1985). Fat-free mass was determined from hydrostatic weighing. Each of the frame measures is significantly correlated with fat-free mass in each sex, and the correlations remain significant after controlling for variation in stature. Multivariate factor analyses of anthropometric dimensions and measures of total body composition confirm the above simple associations by identifying a common

TABLE 3. Correlation of Frame Measures With Fat-Free Mass and Partial Correlations Controlling for Stature[a]

	Men (n = 225)		Women (n = 212)	
Frame measures	*r*	Partial *r*	*r*	Partial *r*
Shoulder	0.54	0.43	0.47	0.35
Elbow	0.45	0.30	0.46	0.38
Wrist	0.47	0.32	0.44	0.30
Hip	0.45	0.36	0.41	0.33
Knee	0.62	0.49	0.52	0.44
Ankle	0.49	0.30	0.48	0.31

[a]Adapted from Himes and Bouchard, 1985; all coefficients are significantly different from zero ($P \leq 0.001$).

factor for lean body mass and body breadths quite independent of stature and other longitudinal body dimensions (Jackson and Pollock, 1976; Skibinska, 1977).

ESTIMATING BODY FAT

The complement of lean body mass, total body fat, is of particular interest in nutritional assessment because of its nutritional specificity for energy and its diagnostic specificity for obesity. Precisely because measures of frame are good estimates of fat-free mass, they provide a means for better identifying that body compartment that is not lean, i.e., body fat. Such a use of frame measures requires that they are minimally correlated with body fat so that variability in frame size only reflects lean tissue variation (Himes and Bouchard, 1985). Further, because fat-free mass is itself positively associated with body fat, estimates of frame size should have minimal associations with body fat beyond that which can be accounted for by associations with fat-free mass. Elbow breadth was selected as an appropriate estimate of frame size over bitrochanteric breadth by Frisancho and Felgel (1983) because of relatively lower correlations with the sum of triceps and subscapular skinfolds.

Table 4 presents first-order correlations of six body frame measures with percentage of total body fat and fat weight determined densitometrically for a sample of adult French Canadians, and corresponding partial correlations controlling for fat-free mass (Himes and Bouchard, 1985). Although none of the correlations with body fat are high, significant proportions of variation in whole body fatness are shared with breadths of shoulder, elbow, hip, and knee. Wrist and ankle breadths have the lowest partial correlations with body fat, in each case approximating zero. Hence, by this criterion, wrist and ankle breadths are preferred estimates of frame size.

There is a paucity of data regarding the usefulness of frame measures in

TABLE 4. Correlations of Frame Measures With Body Fatness and Partial Correlations Controlling Fat-Free Mass[a]

Frame measures	Percent fat First order *r*	Percent fat Partial *r*	Fat weight First order *r*	Fat weight Partial *r*
Men (n = 225)				
Shoulder	0.22	0.26	0.35	0.26
Elbow	0.22	0.25	0.33	0.24
Wrist	−0.01	−0.01	0.11	−0.02
Hip	0.41	0.47	0.53	0.48
Knee	0.23	0.30	0.39	0.30
Ankle	0.07	0.09	0.19	0.08
Women (n = 212)				
Shoulder	0.14	0.26	0.30	0.26
Elbow	0.25	0.38	0.46	0.41
Wrist	−0.08	0.00	0.07	0.00
Hip	0.48	0.62	0.63	0.62
Knee	0.33	0.50	0.53	0.52
Ankle	−0.02	0.08	0.14	0.07

[a]Adapted from Himes and Bouchard (1985); coefficients ≥ 0.14 are significantly different from zero ($P \leq 0.05$).

estimating body fatness in children. Table 5 presents relevant preliminary findings from previously unpublished data (Himes and Bouchard) for a sample of French Canadian youth. Total body fat was determined by hydrostatic weighing (Himes and Bouchard, 1989). Partial correlations of frame measures with percent body fat and fat weight resulted from multiple regressions including stature, weight, and age.

Because body breadths are positively correlated with fat-free mass, it is not surprising that the partial correlations of frame with measures of total body fat are negative. Exceptions to this pattern are the significantly positive partial correlations in girls between biiliac breadth and fat weight, and between knee breadth and both relative and absolute total body fat. These positive associations in girls probably result because the subcutaneous fat included in the measurements of these breadths is sufficient to offset associations with fat-free mass. The stronger associations in boys between total body fatness and breadths of shoulders, wrist, and ankle probably result because, unlike girls, adolescence in boys is associated with large increases in fat-free mass and actual decreases in fatness. Therefore, even with chronological age held constant, the more mature within an age group have relatively more fat-free mass (and larger frames) and less fat than those who are less mature (Tanner, 1962).

TABLE 5. Partial Correlations of Frame Measures with Percent Body Fat (%BF) and Fat Weight (FW) in Youth 8–18 Years of Age[a]

Frame measures	Boys (n = 159) %BF	Boys (n = 159) FW	Girls (n = 157) %BF	Girls (n = 157) FW
Biacromial breadth	−0.26**	−0.25**	−0.15	−0.19*
Elbow breadth	−0.10	−0.11	−0.01	−0.05
Wrist breadth	−0.18*	−0.23**	−0.12	−0.15
Biiliac breadth	−0.12	−0.11	−0.16	−0.20*
Knee breadth	0.05	0.07	0.18*	0.16*
Ankle breadth	−0.16*	−0.16*	−0.02	−0.05

[a]Stature, weight, age, and age^2 were controlled for in the correlations.
*$P \leq 0.05$.
**$P \leq 0.01$.

From Table 5 it is clear that selected measures of frame significantly improve estimates of total body fat in youth beyond those provided by stature, weight, and age.

ESTIMATING HEALTH OUTCOMES

Ideally, one would prefer to validate frame and other anthropometric indicators of nutritional status with important health-related outcomes, such as increased risks of morbidity, dysfunction, or mortality (Himes and Frisancho, 1988). In evaluating nutritional status, there is a lack of studies validating frame measures with health outcomes of purely nutritional etiologies. Frame size has been shown to improve estimation of body fat; and excess body fat, obesity, is known to be a risk factor for morbidity and mortality. To the extent that these relationships hold, indirect associations of frame size with obesity may be considered a partial justification for including measures of frame size when evaluating obesity. Of course, the important question that remains is whether considering frame size per se in defining obesity improves the identification of risks of health-related outcomes. Unfortunately, there are few data to directly address this query.

Early actuarial studies indicated increased risk of mortality among insured men "... in whom the abdominal girth is greater than the chest at full inspiration" (Grant, 1902). More to the point, within categories of weight and stature, relative mortality of insured men increased with categories of chest circumference (Dublin, 1925). Categories of bony chest breadth (BCB) and weight/BCB are positively associated with 16-year cardiovascular mortality in Scots (Garn et al., 1983), but it is unclear whether considering BCB improved identification of those at risk beyond weight alone or weight and stature. Brinkley et al. (1971) have reported smaller biiliac breadths associated with cancers of the cervix, breast, and at other sites compared with controls. Positive associations of elbow breadth with increased risk of breast cancer, within categories of stature, have been reported for a large cohort of U.S. women (Swanson et al., 1988). While it may be questioned whether these health end points are primarily, or even secondarily, of nutritional etiologies, it is apparent that body fatness and frame size are related to nutritional status and that these measures are associated with risks for selected morbidity and mortality.

In 1959, the Metropolitan Life Insurance Company published "ideal" weights for categories of stature and frame size, based on minimum subsequent mortality of insured adults in the United States and Canada. Frame size (small, medium, large) was based on self-appraisal, and no instructions or definitions for its determination were included. Empirical evidence suggests that individuals do poorly at correctly identifying their own frame size (Katch et al., 1982; Horner and Gayton, 1986).

Independently, several measures of frame size were subsequently proposed to be used in conjunction with the 1959 Metropolitan tables: bony chest breadth from radiographs (Garn, 1962; Garn et al., 1983); wrist circumference (Lindner and Lindner, 1973); stature/wrist circumference (Grant, 1980); and elbow breadth (Frisancho and Flegel, 1983). The wrist circumference frame categories of Lindner and Lindner (1973) became widely cited and reproduced in secondary sources and nutrition texts, perhaps because of their simplicity. This popularity is somewhat surprising, because the original privately published source provides no details regarding sample size or characteristics, analyses, or justification. This system provides categories of frame size (small, medium, large) for three categories of stature, irrespective of sex. While the exact category cutoff points in the distributions of wrist circumference and stature were not presented, one can estimate the slope of the wrist–stature relationship from the graphic presentation as approximately 0.25 cm/cm. This slope is almost five times larger than that based on large samples of U.S. military personnel (Churchill et al., 1978).

When Metropolitan Life Insurance Company updated its previous weight-for-stature tables in 1983, elbow breadth (bicondylar breadth of the humerus) was specified as the measure of frame size (Metropolitan Life Insurance Company, 1983). Weights and statures were obtained from approximately 4.2 million insurance policies in the United States and Canada, and elbow reference values were obtained from the 25th and 75th percentiles, within stature categories for U.S. adults participating in the First Health and Nutrition Examination Survey (HANES 1; Johnson et al., 1981). The elbow frame categories were not based on minimum subsequent mortality as were weights for stature.

As noted above (Tables 3 and 4), elbow breadth is a reasonable estimate of fat-free mass, but it has significant positive correlations with absolute and relative total body fat. Consequently, elbow breadth is a biased estimator of frame size. Because of associations with fat, frame size will tend to be underestimated in lean individuals and overestimated in relatively fat individuals, compared with that expected if elbow breadth were unrelated to fatness. For the adults in Tables 3 and 4, the bias amounts to 0.11 mm (± 0.028) of elbow breadth per kg of body fat in men and to 0.21 mm/kg (± 0.032) in women (Himes and Bouchard, 1985).

The 1983 Metropolitan Life Insurance stature–weight tables are frought with concerns besides frame size that are beyond the purview of this report, e.g., self-reported size, representativeness of the sample, length of follow-up. Yet, in the absence of other reference data, one must recommend them for U.S. adults at present, with caveats concerning their limitations. It is likely that fewer and less severe errors will be made using the 1983 Metropolitan tables with elbow as a frame measure, than using them without the frame categories or using other frame-free reference data.

SUMMARY AND CONCLUSIONS

Frame size enhances estimates of body weight, fat-free mass, and total body fat in adults, and probably in children, although there has been relatively little work concerning frame relationships in children. An advantage in considering frame size in nutritional assessment is that deviations from expected status using frame size should be more sensitive and specific to nutritional factors than when frame is not considered. Nevertheless, this statement's strength rests largely on reasoned grounds; much more research is required to validate such an assertion. Specifically, relating frame size to important nutrition-related end points is required. Such studies would hopefully reveal those frame measures, used singly or in combination, that are most closely related to nutritional outcomes.

There has been some research progress since the 1955 recommendations of the Committee on Nutritional Anthropometry of the Food and Nutrition Board (Keys, 1956). At that time, the committee recommended that bicristal diameter (hip breadth) be used in the estimation of the adult individual's standard body weight; this recommendation was based primarily on the work of Brozek (1956). While research in the succeeding three decades has provided more specific details regarding body frame relationships with separate body compartments, frame size has not become a conventional concern in nutritional assessment.

There has been insufficient research to define conventional cutoff points for measures of frame size. Practical and widespread application of frame size in nutritional assessment must await the above validation-related research, and some simplified approaches for graphic or numerical applications. Nevertheless, to the degree that measures of frame size can assist in identifying those at risk for deviations in nutriture and nutrition-related disease, continued effort in these directions is warranted.

ACKNOWLEDGMENTS

Preparation of this chapter was supported in part by Grant HD24684 from the National Institutes of Health, Bethesda, Maryland.

REFERENCES

Behnke AR (1959): The estimation of lean body weight from "skeletal" measurements. Hum Biol 31:295–315.

Boillin ML (1930): Determination of the interrelations, partial and multiple, between various anthropometric measurements of college women. Teacher's College, Columbia University, Contributions to Education, No. 450.

Bornhardt A (1886): Die Körperwägunen der Einberufenen als Mittell zur Bestimmung der Tauglichkeit zum Militardienst. St. Petersburger Medicinische Wochenschrift 3(N.S.):108–109, 196–197.

Brinkley D, Carpenter RG, Haybittle JL (1971): An anthropometric study of women with cancer. B J Prev Soc Med 25:65–75.

Brozek J (1956): Physique and nutritional status of adult men. Hum Biol 28:124–131.

Buffon GLL de (1829–32): Histoire de l'homme. Oeuvres completès. Paris.

Churchill E, Churchill T, Kikta P (1978): "Intercorrelations of Anthropometric Measurements: A Sourcebook for USA Data." AMRL-TR-77-2, Aerospace Medical Research Laboratory, Wright-Patterson Air Force Base, Ohio.

Dearborn WF, Rothney JWM (1941): "Predicting the Child's Development." Cambridge, Mass: Sci-Art Publishers.

De Wijn JG, Zaat JCA (1968): Skeletal frame and body weight. A statistical study for the assessment of appropriate body weight for adolescents and young adults, based on age, height and width measurements of the skeleton. Voeding 29:208–224.

Dublin LI (1925): 1925 report of the committee on Dreyer measurements in relation to life insurance underwriting practice. Proc Assoc Life Ins Med Dir Am 12:204–211.

Franzen R (1929): "Physical Measures of Growth and Nutrition." New York: American Child Health Association.

Franzen R, Palmer GT (1934): "The ACH Index of Nutritional Status." New York: The American Child Health Association.

Frisancho AR, Flegel PN (1983): Elbow breadth as a measure of frame size for US males and females. Am J Clin Nutr 37:311–314.

Garn SM (1962): Anthropometry in clinical appraisal of nutritional status. Am J Clin Nutr 11:418–432.

Garn SM, Pesick SD, Hawthorne VM (1983): The bony chest breadth as a frame size standard in nutritional assessment. Am J Clin Nutr 37:315–318.

Grant FS (1902): Overweights in whom the abdominal girth is greater than the chest at full inspiration. Proc Assoc of Life Ins Med Dir Am 5:323–327.

Grant JP (1980): " Handbook of Total Parenteral Nutrition." Philadelphia: WB Saunders, pp 9–23.

Gray H, Root HF (1921): Weight prediction by the formulae of Bornhardt, of Von Pirquet, and of Dreyer. Boston Med Surg J 1:28–32.

Himes JH (1980): Subcutaneous fat thickness as an indicator of nutritional status. In Greene LS, Johnston FE (eds): "Social and Biological Predictors of Nutritional Status, Physical Growth, and Neurological Development." New York: Academic Press, pp 9–32.

Himes JH, Bouchard C (1985): Do the new Metropolitan Life Insurance weight–height tables correctly assess body frame and body fat relationships? Am J Public Health 75:1076–1079.

Himes JH, Bouchard C (1989): Validity of anthropometry in classifying youths as obese. Int J Obes 13:183–193.

Himes JH, Frisancho RA (1988): Estimating frame size. In Lohman TG, Roche AF, Mart-

orell R (eds): "Anthropometric Standardization Reference Manual." Champaign, Ill: Academic Press, pp 121–124.
Horner C, Gayton WF (1986): Accuracy of body frame-size estimations using the 1983 Metropolitan height and weight tables. Percept Motor Skills 63:26.
Jackson AS, Pollock ML (1976): Factor analysis and multivariate scaling of anthropometric variables for the assessment of body composition. Med Sci Sports 8:196–203.
Johnson CL, Fulwood R, Abraham S, Bryner ID (1981): Basic data on anthropometric measurements and angular measurements of the hip and knee joints for selected groups 1–74 years of age. Vital and Health Statistics, Ser. 2, No. 219 DHHS Publ. No. PHS 81-1669 Washington, DC: GPO.
Katch VL, Freedson PS, Katch FL, Smith L (1982): Body frame size: Validity of self-appraisal. Am J Clin Nutr 36:676–679.
Keys A (1956): Recommendations concerning body measurements for the documentation of nutritional status. Hum Biol 28:111–123.
Lindner P, Lindner D (1973): "How to Assess Degrees of Fatness, A Working Manual." Privately published.
Lucas WP, Pryor HB (1931): Physical measurements and physiologic processes in young children. JAMA 97:1127–1133.
Ludlum FE, Powell E (1940): Chest–height–weight tables for college women. Res Q 11:55–57.
McCloy CH (1936): Appraising physical status: The selection of measurements. University of Iowa Studies in Child Welfare, No. 12.
Metropolitan Life Insurance Company (1983): Metropolitan height and weight tables. Statictical Bull 64:2–9.
Oppenheimer K (1901): Über das Verhältnis des Nahrungsbedarfes zu Körpergewicht und Körperoberfläche bei Säuglingen. Ztschr f Biol 42:147–150.
Pignet (1901): Du coefficient de robusticité. Bull Med: No. 33.
Pryor HB (1940): "Width–Weight Tables for Boys and Girls from 1 to 17 Years—for Men and Women From 18 to 41+ Years." Stanford: Stanford University Press.
Pryor HB (1966): Charts of normal body measurements and revised width–weight tables in graphic form. J Pediatr 68:615–631.
Pryor HB, Stolz HR (1933): Determining appropriate weight for body build. J Pediatr 3:608–622.
Quetelet A (1835): Sur l'homme et le developpement de ses facultes. Paris.
Rohrer F (1921): Der Index der Körperfulle als Mass des Ernährungszustandes. München Med Wchnschr 68:580–589.
Skibinska A (1977): A factor analysis of skeletal measurements in Warsaw students. Ann Hum Biol 4:73–78.
Swanson CA, Jones DY, Schatzkin A, Brinton LA, Ziegler RG (1988): Breast cancer risk assessed by anthropometry in the NHANES I Epidemiological Follow-up Study. Cancer Res 48:5363–5367.
Tanner JM (1962): "Growth at Adolescence." Oxford: Blackwell Scientific.
Turner AH (1943): Body weights optimal for young adult women. Res Q 14:255–276.
von Dobeln W (1959): Anthropometric determination of fat-free body weight. Acta Medica Scand 165:37–40.
Willoughby DP (1932): An anthropometric method for arriving at the optimal proportions of the body in any adult individual. Res Q 3:48–77.
Wilmore JH, Behnke AR (1969): An anthropometric estimation of body density and lean body weight in young men. J Appl Physiol 27:25–31.

Anthropometric Assessment
of Nutritional Status, pages 151–171

9
Ratios and Derived Indicators in the Assessment of Nutritional Status

ROBERT M. MALINA
Department of Kinesiology and Health Education, University of Texas at Austin, Austin, Texas 78712

INTRODUCTION

Ratios of body dimensions have a long history of use in growth studies and in the assessment of nutritional status. The two are related in that the growth status of children is generally accepted as a good indicator of the overall health and nutritional conditions in the community.

Ratios are derived variables which simply express one dimension relative to another in the form of a single number. They can be expressed as a quotient or as a percentage. At times the term *index* is used, but often in the restricted sense of the ratio of one dimension divided by the larger, standard dimension of the same anatomical unit (Simpson et al., 1960; Sokal and Rohlf, 1981). The most commonly used ratio of this type in growth studies is the ratio of sitting height to stature. Measurements of different anatomical elements are also expressed as ratios, for example, the ratio of biacromial breadth to bicristal breadth, or of head circumference to chest circumference. These are ratios of analogous dimensions (Simpson et al., 1960), i.e., breadth versus breadth or circumference versus circumference.

Ratios provide information that is not ordinarily available in the original measurements per se. They are influenced by the relationship between the variables and assume that the two dimensions change in a linear manner during growth. Ratios, however, may not have a normal distribution and do not indicate the form of the relationship between the two dimensions expressed in the ratio (Sokal and Rohlf, 1981). Ratios are affected by the measurement variability associated with each dimension, and have limitations for statistical analysis.

In addition to weight and length/stature per se and ratios of these two indicators of overall body size (which are discussed elsewhere in this volume), two ratios are commonly used in nutritional surveys of children and youth. The first is the ratio of head circumference to chest circumference, and the second is the ratio of sitting height to stature (or crown–rump length to total length). These are used primarily in the context of undernutrition. Though not a ratio, the relationship of arm circumference is stature in the form of the QUAC stick is occasionally used in field surveys of children in areas with a high prevalence of acute and chronic undernutrition. These two ratios and the QUAC stick are the focus of this report.

More recently, several ratios have been used in assessing the relative distribution of subcutaneous fat in children, youth, and adults. Ratios of trunk to extremity skinfolds are used to indicate central versus peripheral patterns of subcutaneous fat distribution. Skinfolds are used either singly, e.g., the ratio of the subscapular to the triceps skinfold, or in combination, e.g., the ratio of the sum of three trunk skinfolds to the sum of three extremity skinfolds (Malina and Bouchard, 1988; Kaplowitz et al., 1987). The ratio of waist to hip circumferences attempts to distinguish "upper body" versus "lower body" fat accumulation in adults (see, for example, Kissebah et al., 1982; Krotkiewski et al., 1983). The validity of these circumferences as indicators of fat distribution in children is not known. Ratios of relative fat distribution will not be considered in this report.

HEAD CIRCUMFERENCE/CHEST CIRCUMFERENCE RATIO

Head circumference is, on average, larger than chest circumference at birth, but by about 9–12 months of age, the two circumferences are approximately equal. Subsequently chest circumference is generally larger than head circumference. This trend reflects the differential growth rates of the two circumferences during infancy and early childhood. In general, head circumference reflects cranial volume and thus growth of the brain, while chest circumference reflects somatic growth of the body.

The age at which chest circumference attains the same size as and eventually is larger than head circumference is commonly used in nutritional surveys. Delayed crossover of chest relative to head circumference is viewed as indicative of stunted somatic growth associated with chronic undernutrition (Dean, 1965; Jelliffe, 1966). Indeed, a disproportionately large head relative to chest circumference is characteristic of severe protein-energy undernutrition early in life.

The relationship between head and chest circumferences in nutritional surveys of preschool children is most often viewed in ratio form:

$$\text{head circumference/chest circumference} \times 100.$$

Data for mean ratios of head circumference to chest circumference derived from measurements of individual children are limited to a longitudinal sample of well-nourished Japanese children (Terada and Hoshi, 1965) and a mixed-longitudinal sample of mild-to-moderately undernourished rural Guatemalan children (Martorell et al., 1975b). The data are shown in Table 1. Standard deviations for the ratios are slightly larger in Guatemalan boys, but generally similar in Guatemalan and Japanese girls. Ratios based on mean head and

TABLE 1. Head Circumference/Chest Circumference Ratios in Infants and Preschool Children

	Japanese[a]				Guatemalan[b]			
Age	n	M	SD	Ratio of means	n	M	SD	Ratio of means
Boys								
Birth					25	108.6	6.1	108.1
15 days					118	105.1	4.8	104.8
1 month	46	103.1	4.4	102.7				
3 months	47	98.1	4.2	98.1	202	101.4	4.7	101.3
6	48	99.0	4.2	98.7	194	101.9	4.5	101.7
9	48	99.9	4.0	99.6	191	103.0	4.4	102.6
12	48	100.1	3.8	100.0	186	101.7	4.5	101.6
15					185	101.1	4.2	100.9
18	48	99.5	3.4	99.4	174	100.6	4.3	100.4
21					162	99.3	4.1	99.1
24	46	98.0	3.6	97.8	180	98.4	4.2	98.3
27	45	97.7	3.3	97.6				
30	45	97.4	3.8	97.3	163	96.5	4.1	96.3
36	39	96.2	3.3	96.2	164	95.0	3.9	94.8
42					166	93.6	4.0	93.4
48					157	92.6	4.1	92.4
60					142	90.7	4.4	90.6
Girls								
Birth					12	108.5	3.4	108.5
15 days					107	105.1	5.7	104.9
1 month	34	103.6	4.5	103.4				
3 months	36	99.6	4.2	99.5	160	102.3	4.5	101.9
6	36	100.6	4.9	100.5	159	100.8	4.5	100.5
9	36	100.8	4.7	100.9	158	101.7	4.3	101.7
12	36	100.9	4.9	100.7	154	101.7	4.6	101.6
15					142	100.9	4.8	100.7
18	36	100.0	4.9	99.8	153	100.2	4.5	100.0
21					136	99.7	4.3	99.5
24	34	98.8	4.8	98.8	141	98.3	4.5	98.3
27	34	98.6	4.8	98.4				
30	33	98.1	4.3	98.0	150	96.6	4.5	96.4
36	33	96.7	4.5	96.6	143	95.0	4.7	94.9
42					146	95.0	3.9	94.8
48					148	93.5	4.2	93.3
60					149	92.1	3.9	92.0

[a]Adapted from Terada and Hoshi (1965), well-nourished children.
[b]Adapted from Martorell et al. (1975b), mild-to-moderately undernourished rural children.

mean chest circumferences are also indicated in the table since many nutritional surveys utilize mean or medians of the two circumferences in calculating the ratios for a sample.

Mean ratios are highest at birth, decline rapidly between birth and 3 months of age, then increase slightly during the first year in Japanese and Guatemalan children. Subsequently, the ratios decline systematically through early childhood. Sex differences in head circumference/chest circumference ratios are not consistently apparent in the Guatemalan children, but the ratios are, on average, higher in Japanese girls than in boys. There is much overlap in the head circumference/chest circumference ratios of the mild-to-moderately undernourished Guatemalan and well-nourished Japanese children, and differences between mean ratios are small (Table 1).

Ratios of mean head and chest circumferences are quite similar to mean ratios based on measurements of individual children (Table 1). This would seem to suggest that ratios based on means may be adequate for population comparisons. However, ratios calculated from median or mean head and chest circumferences indicate different age trends in samples of well-nourished American children (Fig. 1). The ratios decline systematically in Boston children, but tend to remain near 100 in Denver children between 6 and 36 months of age. The latter suggests that the two circumferences are almost the same size in Denver children during infancy and most of early childhood. Further, there are negligible differences in the age- and sex-specific ratios of mild-to-moderately undernourished Guatemalan and well-nourished Denver children (Fig. 2). The latter children were selected as a reference for comparison since the Guatemalan communities are located at a similar altitude as Denver, and altitude may be a factor which influences the growth of both well-nourished and undernourished children (Moore and Regensteiner, 1983; Yip et al., 1988).

The ratio of head to chest circumferences does not, therefore, appear to be a good discriminator between moderately undernourished and well-nourished children. In fact, after two years of age, the ratio is lower in Guatemalan children, which indicates that the former have larger chest circumferences relative to head circumferences than Denver children. This seeming anomaly reflects the fact that head circumference in the mild-to-moderately undernourished Guatemalan children shows greater growth stunting than chest circumference (Malina et al., 1975). Further, Guatemalan children who have head circumference/chest circumference ratios $\leq$ 100 at 4 years of age were no more stunted in growth than the population from which they are drawn (Martorell et al., 1975b).

Measurement variability probably contributes to the differences among samples of well-nourished and undernourished children. Head circumference requires reasonably firm pressure, enough to compress the hair but not the soft tissues, and is a reasonably standardized and accurate measurement in infants and young children. Chest circumference, on the other hand, is more variably measured. It is influenced by the level at which the measurement is taken (e.g., at the xiphoid or breast nipple level), the position of the child (seated or recumbent), the degree of compression of soft tissues (theoreti-

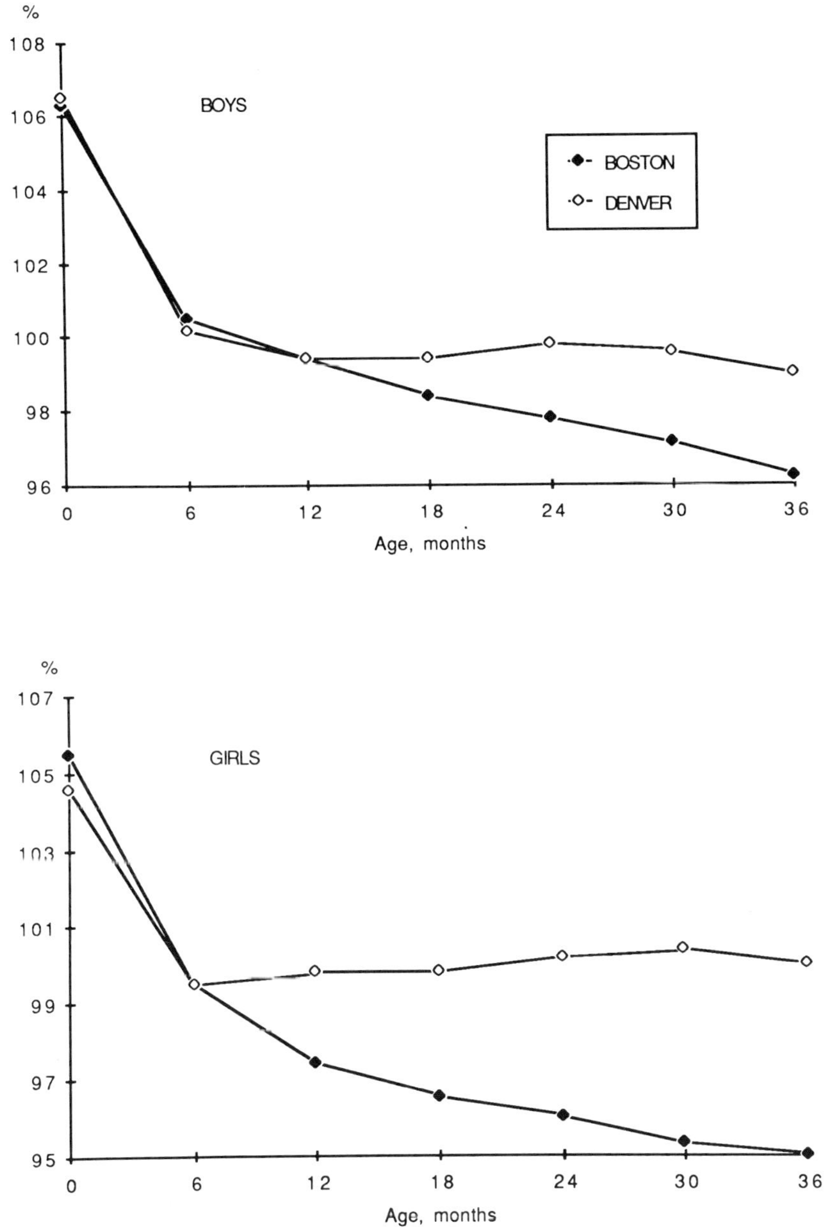

Fig. 1. Ratios of mean/median head and mean/median chest circumferences in well-nourished infants and preschool children from Boston and Denver. (Calculated from data reported by Vaughan, 1969, and McCammon, 1970.)

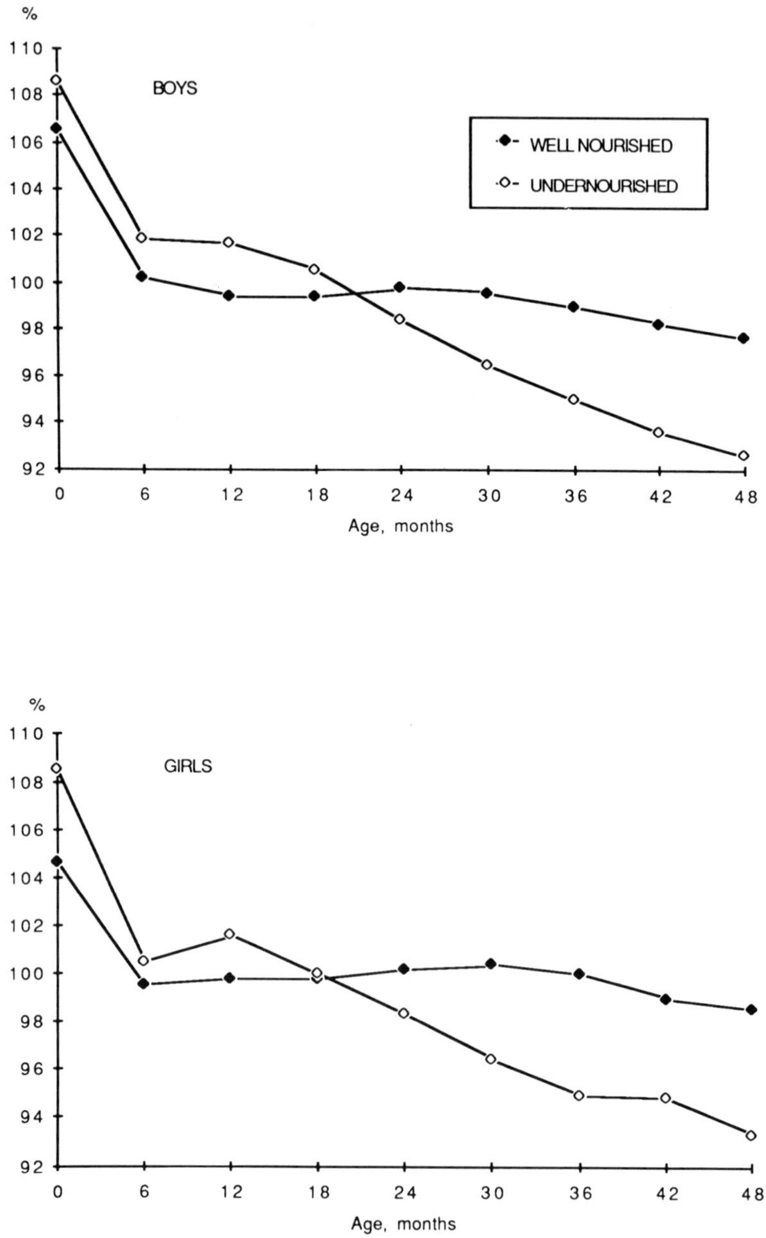

Fig. 2. Ratios of head and chest circumferences in well-nourished infants and preschool children from Denver and mild-to-moderately undernourished infants and preschool children from rural Guatemala. (Drawn from mean ratios reported by Martorell et al., 1975b, and ratios of mean head and mean chest circumferences calculated from data reported by McCammon, 1970.)

cally, skin contact without compression, as well as normal short-term changes in tissue compressibility), and the phase of the respiratory cycle (usually midway between a normal inspiration and expiration). An error of 5 mm in chest circumference can significantly influence the ratio. Assuming that head circumference is measured accurately at 45.7 cm in an 18-month-old child and chest circumference is measured at 45.5 cm or 46.0 cm, the ratio is 100.4 with the former and 99.3 with the latter chest measurement. Measurement variation of 5 mm is not uncommon for chest circumference. For example, among rural Guatemalan children, measurement standard deviations for head and chest circumferences were 1.4 mm and 7.9 mm respectively for immediate remeasurement, and 3.3 mm and 14.6 mm respectively for remeasurement after a one week interval (Malina et al., 1975). Further, the measurement standard deviation of the head circumference/chest circumference ratio was 2.6%, and the ratio of measurement variance to the median population variance was about 38% (Martorell et al., 1975b). Thus, about 38% of the population variance in the ratio is related to variability in measurement, which suggests that the head circumference/chest circumference ratio is a poor indicator of nutritional status in mild-to-moderately undernourished children. It may, however, have utility with severely undernourished children. Among 200 children 1–5 years of age, all of those classified as marasmic (weight for age $<$ 60% of reference data) had head/chest ratios over 100, while only 50% of those classified as marasmic kwashiorkor (weight for age $<$ 60% of reference values + edema) had ratios above 100. Edema is thus a factor which influences circumference measurements. In contrast, only 5% of the children classified as underweight (weight for age 60%–80% of reference data) had a ratio over 100 (Shakir et al., 1972).

SITTING HEIGHT/STATURE RATIO

The ratio of sitting height to stature is expressed as:

$$\text{sitting height/stature} \times 100.$$

The ratio provides an indication of relative trunk or leg length, although the latter is emphasized in nutritional surveys. A child with a ratio of 54% has relatively shorter legs than a child with a ratio of 51%. In the former, sitting height accounts for 54% of stature (and by subtraction, the lower extremities account for 46%), while in the latter, sitting height accounts for 51% of stature (and by subtraction the lower extremities account for 49%).

Changes in the ratio of sitting height to stature during growth are shown in Figure 3. The ratio is highest in infancy and declines during childhood into adolescence as the lower extremities grow at a faster rate than sitting height (head, neck, and trunk). Hence, the lower extremities increase their proportional contribution to stature during growth. The ratio reaches its nadir, on average, in early adolescence when the legs are proportionally long relative to stature. The ratio then gradually rises as late adolescent growth in trunk length occurs. Needless to say, there is considerable variation among individu-

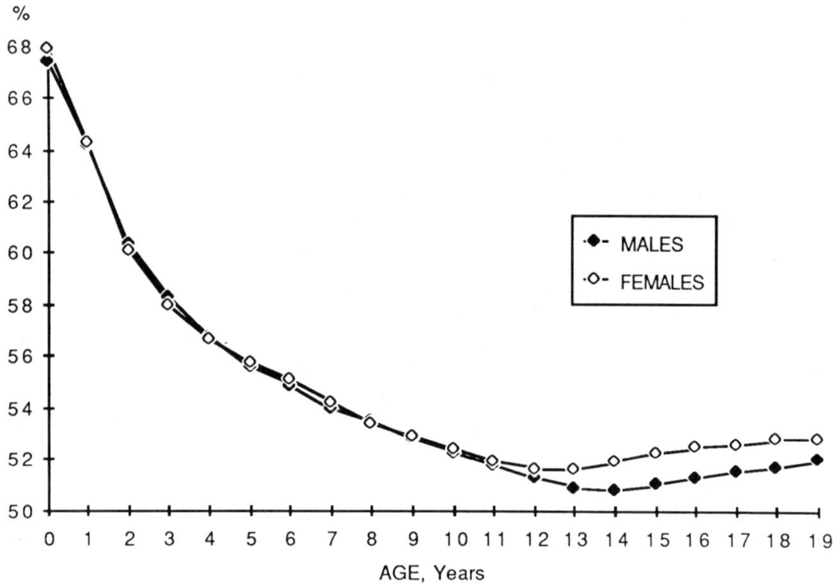

Fig. 3. Median crown–rump length/recumbent length ratios (birth–2 years) and sitting height/stature ratios (3–19 years) in well-nourished Denver children. (Drawn from data reported by McCammon, 1970.)

als in growth rates and in the timing of adolescent growth spurts. The spurt in leg length occurs, on average, earlier than the spurt in sitting height (trunk length).

The utility of the sitting height/stature ratio in nutritional surveys is based on the assumption that the fastest growing body segments are more susceptible to interference by the adverse circumstances associated with chronic undernutrition. Thus, proportional changes in body segments which normally occur during growth might be altered or delayed. On this basis, Thomson and Duncan (1954) suggested that relative leg length may serve as an index of childhood undernutrition.

There is, however, no direct method of measuring lower extremity length in the living. It is usually approximated as subischial length, which is derived by subtracting sitting height from stature (Martin et al., 1988). Hence, for practical purposes, the ratio of sitting height to stature is used primarily as an indicator of relative leg length.

Mean sitting height/stature ratios for a cross-sectional sample of primary school children in the Valley of Oaxaca in southern Mexico are compared to means for a nationally representative sample of well-nourished American children of European ancestry (white) in Figure 4. The Mexican children live under conditions of chronic mild-to-moderate protein-energy undernutrition, and are typical of the primary school age population in this area of Mexico,

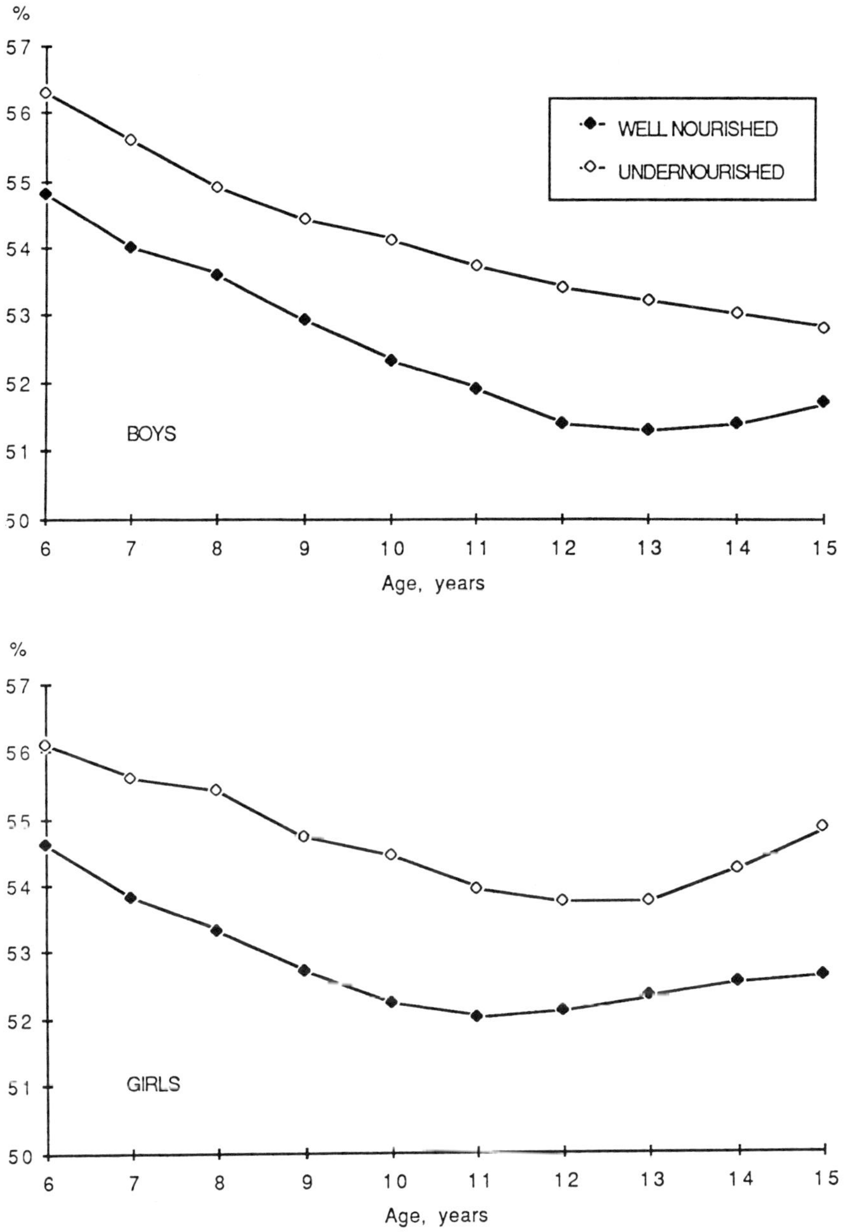

Fig. 4. Mean sitting height/stature ratios in mild-to-moderately undernourished urban and rural Mexican school children compared to well-nourished American white children. (Drawn from unpublished data of Malina and from data reported by Hamill et al., 1973, and Malina et al., 1974, for children in cycles II and III of the U.S. Health Examination Survey.)

which has high infant and childhood mortality rates and no evidence of either short- or long-term secular change in stature (Malina and Himes, 1978; Malina et al., 1980a, 1980b, 1983).

The sitting height/stature ratio is consistently higher in the chronically undernourished Mexican children and is thus indicative of relatively shorter lower extremities. The Mexican children are considerably shorter than the American children, on average approximating only the 5th percentiles of U.S. reference data. The elevated ratios of chronically, mild-to-moderately undernourished Mexican children are due to reduced rates of growth in leg length. For example, mean annual increments for sitting height in a mixed-longitudinal sample of Mexican children 6–12 years of age from a single community in Oaxaca are quite similar to those for well-nourished American children, but mean annual increments for subischial length are consistently lower (Buschang and Malina, 1983; Buschang et al., 1986).

The reduced rate of growth in leg length in undernourished school children presumably represents adverse nutritional conditions during infancy and early childhood, which continue into the school ages. Chavez and colleagues (1977) used the ratio of height of the iliac crest (length from the crest to the soles of the feet) to total length in a comparison of the growth of supplemented and unsupplemented Mexican children from birth to 2 years of age. Mothers of the supplemented children received special rations during pregnancy as did the children postnatally, while mothers of the unsupplemented children and the children themselves received no additional rations. The unsupplemented children had proportionally shorter lower extremities at birth and throughout the first two years of life than did the supplemented children.

Data on the sitting height/stature ratio in undernourished preschool children are not extensive. Means and standard deviations for the crown–rump length/recumbent length ratio in mild-to-moderately undernourished rural Guatemalan children from birth to 7 years of age are summarized in Table 2. Corresponding data for well-nourished children between birth and 2 years are also included in the table. It is of interest that mean ratios are greater in the well-nourished children, which suggests proportionally shorter lower extremities than in the undernourished Guatemalan children. The nutritional significance of the ratio may perhaps be questioned at these young ages.

Measurement variability is an important consideration. Technical errors of measurement[1] based on replicate observations by the same technician in the

[1]The technical error of measurement is defined as the square root of the sum of the squared differences between replicate measurements divided by twice the number of pairs of replicates (Malina et al., 1974):

$$\sigma_e = \sqrt{\Sigma d^2/2N}$$

In the Guatemalan study, measurement standard deviations, the sum of the squared differences between replicate measurements divided by twice the number of pairs of replicates, are reported. The square root of the measurement standard deviation is thus the technical error of measurement.

TABLE 2. Crown–Rump Length/Recumbent Length Ratios in Infants and Preschool Children

	Boys					Girls				
	Guatemala[a]			Denver[b]		Guatemala			Denver	
Age	n	M	SD	n	MD	n	M	SD	n	MD
Birth	32	65.5	3.1	48	67.4	13	65.4	1.4	55	67.9
15 days	116	65.6	2.1			108	65.6	1.9		
3 months	207	65.1	1.8	59	67.0	166	64.9	1.7	67	66.8
6	194	63.9	1.6	64	66.2	159	64.1	1.7	58	66.4
9	190	63.3	1.6	53	65.4	160	63.3	1.4	59	65.4
12	185	62.2	1.6	67	64.2	148	62.4	1.7	65	64.3
15	183	61.7	1.5			147	61.6	1.4		
18	174	61.2	1.3	59	62.0	154	61.2	1.7	58	62.5
21	165	60.8	1.3			137	61.0	1.4		
24	181	60.7	1.2	41	60.8	140	60.8	1.4	43	60.6
30	165	59.8	1.2			150	60.1	1.2		
36	167	59.2	1.2			146	59.5	1.3		
42	163	58.6	1.2			145	59.0	1.4		
48	158	58.0	1.4			148	58.2	1.3		
60	143	56.7	1.4			150	57.0	1.4		

[a]Unpublished data, Institute of Nutrition of Central America and Panama, mild-to-moderately undernourished rural children.
[b]Adapted from McCammon (1970), well-nourished children.

Guatemalan sample were 0.65 cm and 0.77 cm for recumbent length and crown–rump length, respectively (Martorell et al., 1975a). Intraobserver technical errors of measurement for two surveys of school age Mexican children were 0.33 cm and 0.38 cm for stature, and 0.48 cm and 0.77 cm for sitting height, while interobserver technical errors were 0.46 for stature and 0.57 for sitting height (Malina, unpublished data). Corresponding intraobserver technical errors of measurement in the United States Health Examination Survey of children 6–11 years were 0.49 cm and 0.54 cm for stature and sitting height respectively, while interobserver estimates were 0.68 cm and 0.71 cm, respectively, for stature and sitting height (Malina et al., 1974).

Comparative data for well-nourished children older than 2 years are lacking, since sitting height and stature are ordinarily measured at this time. Adjusting either recumbent measurement to approximate sitting or standing values in an attempt to estimate the sitting height/stature ratio from means is hazardous. Recumbent length is greater than standing height by, on average, about 1 cm. However, the difference between the two measurements is not constant. Among preschool children, differences between recumbent and standing measurements can range from 0 to 2.5 cm (Tanner et al., 1966). Measurement variation probably contributes to the differences.

In contrast to the stress of undernutrition, the sitting height/stature ratio can be altered by improved health and nutritional circumstances. Japanese children born and reared in California, for example, have relatively longer legs than children in Japan until adolescence, which suggests an earlier adolescent spurt in the American-born Japanese (Greulich, 1957). Protracted growth of sitting height into late adolescence reduces the proportional differences between American-born and native Japanese young adults. Further, secular increases in the stature of Japanese children between 1957 and 1977 indicate significant increments in leg length compared with sitting height (Tanner et al., 1982; see also Himes, 1979). The secular increase in stature is due almost entirely to an increase in leg length. As a result, sitting height/stature ratios of Japanese children and adolescents have declined substantially (Fig. 5). In contrast, the secular trend towards greater stature has apparently stopped in the United States and several European countries (Malina, 1979; Roche, 1979), and there are negligible differences (in the range of measurement variability) in the mean sitting height/stature ratios of American white and black children 6–17 years in the United States Health Examination Survey (1963–1970) and the second Health and Nutrition Examination Survey (1976–1980).

A major limitation of the sitting height/stature ratio in nutritional surveys relates to racial variation in the proportional contribution of lower extremity length to stature. This is shown in Figure 6 for national samples of American children of European (white), African (black), and Mexican (Mexican-American) ancestry, and of Japanese children. The samples were surveyed between 1976 and 1984, and presumably represent reasonably well-nourished children. Ratios are, on average, lowest in American black children, indicating relatively long lower extremities, and highest in Japanese children, indicating relatively short lower extremities. Ratios for American white children are intermediate. These proportional differences are well documented and reflect genetic rather than environmental differences (Krogman, 1970; Malina, 1973; Eveleth and Tanner, 1976). Mean ratios of Mexican-American children, though generally intermediate between American white and Japanese children, tend to approach those of the former (see also Malina et al., 1987a).

Given population variation in the proportional contribution of leg length to stature, sitting height/stature ratios for undernourished children need to be interpreted with caution. Part of the reduced contribution of leg length to stature in undernourished children may reflect genetic variation. For example, the elevated ratios of undernourished children in southern Mexico (Fig. 4) may reflect, in part, population variation in the proportional contribution of leg length to stature. Thus, the applicability of the sitting height/stature ratio to racially different populations requires the use of race-specific reference data for well-nourished children. In addition, secular changes in the proportional contribution of leg length to stature emphasize the need for current reference data.

QUAC STICK

The QUAC stick relates midarm circumference to stature. The method was initially designed by a Quaker relief services team in Nigeria in 1968–1969 as

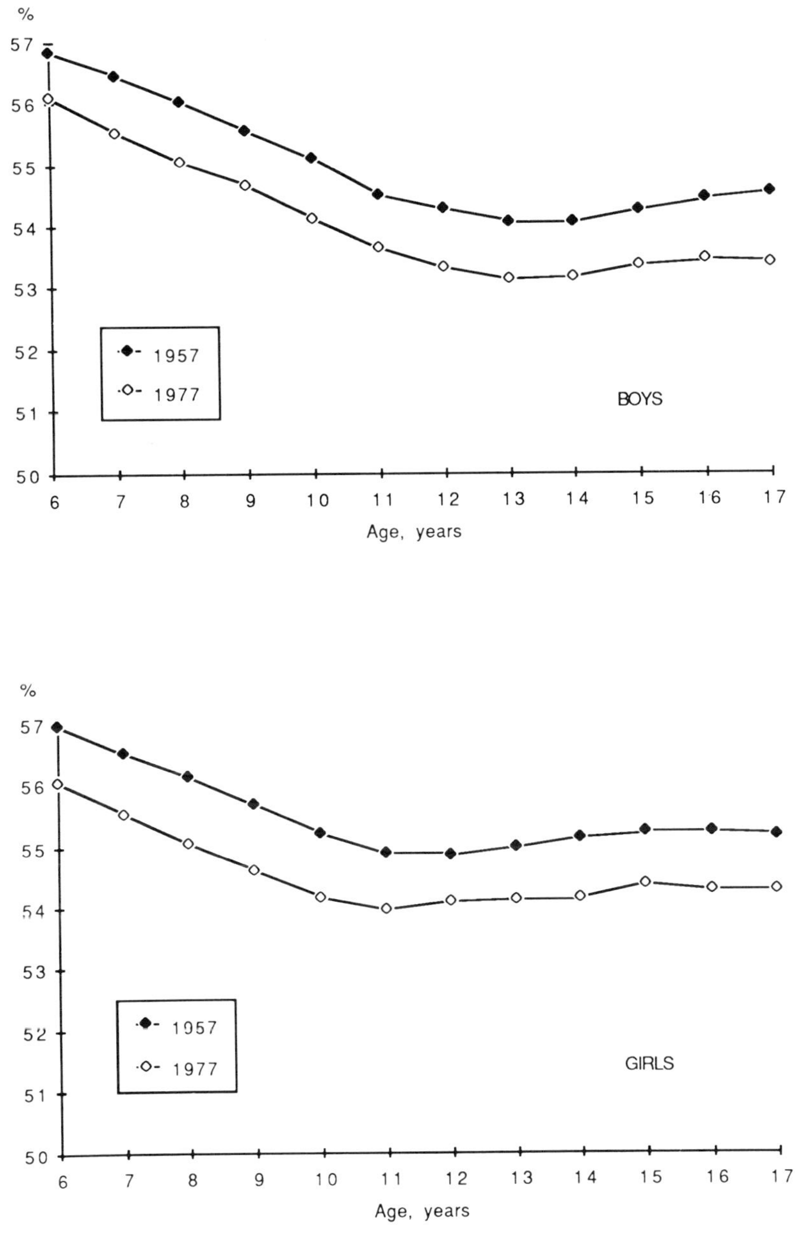

Fig. 5. Sitting height/stature ratios for Japanese children in 1957 and 1977. (Calculated from mean sitting heights and statures reported by Tanner et al., 1982.)

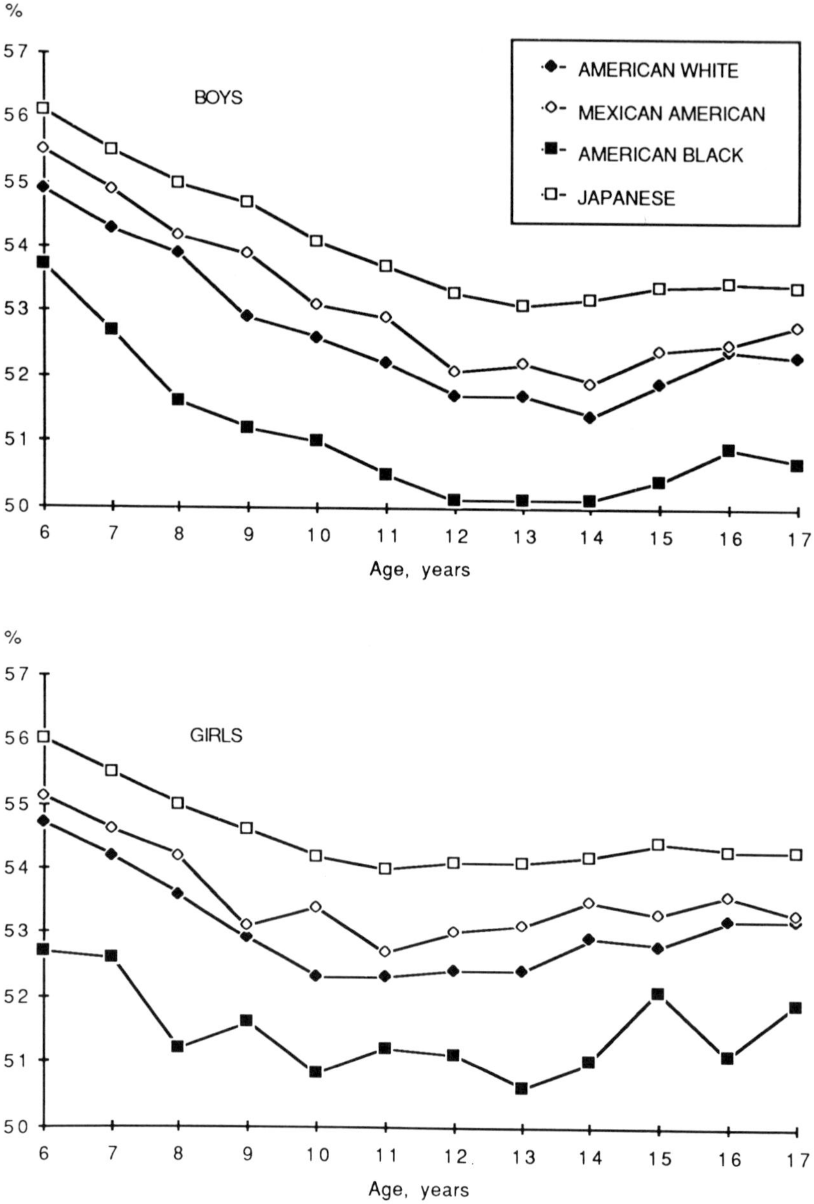

Fig. 6. Racial variation in the ratio of sitting height to stature. (Drawn from mean ratios reported by Martorell et al., 1988, for American black and white children in the second Health and Nutrition Examination Survey [1976–1980] and for Mexican-American children in the Hispanic Health and Nutrition Examination Survey [1982–1984], and from ratios calculated from mean sitting heights and statures reported by Tanner et al., 1982, for Japanese children measured in 1977.)

a nutritional screening device for use during crisis situations. The name QUAC stick is derived from Quaker (QU) and arm circumference (AC) (Arnhold, 1969). A similar device was also described for use in Nigeria by Davis (1971). The QUAC stick attempts to identify which children are most affected by inadequate food supplies associated with emergency or crisis conditions, e.g., the Nigerian civil war (Arnhold, 1969; Davis, 1971) or the East Bengal cyclone (Sommer and Mosley, 1972). Under such conditions, resources are limited and ages of children are ordinarily not precisely known.

The method is designed for rapid assignment of children under 10 years of age into several categories of nutritional status on the basis of midarm circumference relative to stature. Stature reflects the nutritional history of the child, while arm circumference reflects current nutritional status. The primary components of arm circumference are muscle and subcutaneous fat, both of which are affected by acute nutritional insufficiency. Arm circumference is used in lieu of body weight because it does not require a portable scale and it is easily measured.

The QUAC stick is a measuring rod or board upon which values of arm circumference for specific statures are recorded. The 85th, 80th, and/or 75th percentiles of arm circumference for specific statures of well-nourished children are indicated on the stick at the corresponding stature levels (Arnhold, 1969; Davis, 1971; Loewenstein and Phillips, 1973). The three percentile levels are assumed to represent mild, moderate, and severe undernutrition respectively. A child whose stature is above the level on the stick where his/her arm circumference measurement is located, i.e., arm circumference is too thin for his/her stature or is below 85% of that expected for his/her stature, is classified as undernourished. The degree of undernutrition depends on the the percentile levels indicated on the measuring stick. These are often color coded for ease of identification. Conversely, a child whose stature is below the level where his/her arm circumference is located, i.e., arm circumference is above 85% of that expected for stature, is not considered undernourished. Thus, the QUAC stick simply assigns a child to a specific percentile or nutritional status category. It does not permit the computation of means and standard deviations of arm circumference at specific statures.

Arm circumference is measured midway between the acromial and olecranon processes with the arm hanging freely and relaxed at the side. In practice, however, the midpoint may not be located and marked, given the time requirement involved in locating the midpoint and the complexities involved in training nonspecialists who ordinarily carry out such surveys under emergency conditions (Jelliffe and Jelliffe, 1969). Further, published reports generally do not indicate how the midarm level is located and/or whether or not it was marked. Procedures routinely indicate that the measurement was taken at the midarm level or that internationally accepted measurement procedures were used.

Measurement variability of arm circumference is typically not reported, although the measurement has reasonably good reproducibility. Among preschool Jamaican children and with all measurements made by a well-trained observer, maximum and midarm circumferences were compared. Maximum arm circumference was larger than midarm circumference in 36%, smaller than midarm circumference in 36%, and identical with midarm circumference in 28% of the children, and the differences ranged between ±0.3 cm (Jelliffe and Jelliffe, 1969). Among Nigerian children 1–10 years of age, arm circumference measured by two observers differed by less than 0.5 cm in about 87% of the measurements (Merchant, cited by Loewenstein and Phillips, 1973). Technical errors of measurement with the midpoint measured and marked were 0.35 cm and 0.43 cm respectively within and between observers in the United States Health Examination Survey of children 6–11 years of age (Malina et al., 1974). Corresponding values were 0.21 cm and 0.25 cm within observers and 0.26 cm and 0.22 cm between observers in two surveys of mild-to-moderately undernourished Mexican children 6–14 years of age (Malina et al., 1980, unpublished), and 0.49 cm within an observer in preschool Guatemalan children (Martorell et al., 1975a)[2]. Depending upon how the scale is constructed, differences between the 85th, 80th, and 75th percentiles at a given stature are about 0.75–1.0 cm (Arnhold, 1969; Davis, 1971).

The reference data used to establish the 85th, 80th, and 75th percentiles of arm circumference for stature varies among studies. Early studies utilized arm circumference data for healthy Polish children either as reported or smoothed (Jelliffe, 1966; Burgess and Burgess, 1969; El Lozy, 1969). Stature data were derived from samples of healthy local preschool children 1–5 years of age or the extrapolated equivalent percentiles of stature for well-nourished European children, i.e., since mean stature for age of the local preschool children approximates the 10th percentile of British reference data, the 10th percentiles of the British children 5–9 years of age were used in establishing the appropriate arm circumference for stature for children in this age range (Arnhold, 1969; Davis, 1971; Loewenstein and Phillips, 1973). Some have developed local reference data (Sastry, 1972; Sommer and Mosley, 1972), while others have used data from the Ten-State Nutrition Survey in the United States (Trowbridge and Staehling, 1980).

The QUAC stick essentially provides prevalence estimates of the number of children in the respective categories of arm circumference for stature in times of crisis (Arnhold, 1969; Davis, 1971; Sommer and Mosley, 1972; Loewenstein and Phillips, 1973). It appears to be a screening tool for children 1–10 years which apparently identifies the effects of acute undernutrition in contrast to long-term chronic undernutrition.

The efficiency of the QUAC stick to separate mild-to-moderate from severe protein-energy malnutrition (PEM) is related to the criteria used. Weight for age is used most often as the index of nutritional status. A weight for age between 60% and 80% of the reference values for well-nourished children is

[2]See note 1.

accepted as mild-to-moderate PEM, while a weight for age < 60% of the reference values is indicative of severe PEM. Applying these criteria with preschool children in Baghdad, the QUAC stick and weight for age gave similar estimates of overall PEM, but discrepant estimates of severe PEM (Shakir, 1973). The QUAC stick identified more children as having severe PEM than does weight for age. The data for Baghdad children also suggested that arm circumference alone provided estimates of PEM similar to the QUAC stick when precise ages were known (Shakir, 1975).

When mortality is the criterion among Bengali children 1–9 years of age, the relative risk of mortality was 3.4 times greater in children classified as moderate-severe undernutrition by the QUAC stick (< 75% of reference values). When the children were subdivided by age, the relative risk of mortality was much greater in children 1–4 years of age (4.5) than in children 5–9 years (2.0). Further, the risk of death among the younger children was especially greater during the first three months after the QUAC stick assignment and then declined (Sommer and Loewenstein, 1975).

In contrast, the QUAC stick did not appear to be a useful indicator of nutritional status among 6–10-year-old Indian boys from middle and low socioeconomic backgrounds (Sastry, 1972). Among rural, El Salvadoran children 1–4 years of age, the QUAC stick had lower sensitivity (i.e., the ability to correctly identify those with undernutrition, weight for age < 75% or < 65% of reference medians for U.S. children) at given levels of specificity (i.e., the ability to correctly identify those without undernutrition). Compared with arm circumference alone, arm circumference for age, and weight for height, the QUAC stick gave the least satisfactory results (Trowbridge and Staehling, 1980). It should be noted, of course, that the the QUAC stick was used in Nigeria and Bangladesh with children exposed to acute undernutrition, while it was evaluated in El Salvador with children exposed to chronic, probably mild-to-moderate, undernutrition.

The variable results attained with the QUAC stick are probably related to several factors. The reference data per se and the cutoff points for the different categories of nutritional status influence the sensitivity of the device (see Habicht, 1980, for a good discussion of sensitivity and specificity criteria in nutritional screening). Measurement variability is another consideration.

OVERVIEW

The QUAC stick has received more critical evaluation than the ratios of head to chest circumferences and of sitting height to stature. This is related to the purpose of the indicators of nutritional status. The QUAC stick was designed for use in field conditions at times of emergency, i.e., acute undernutrition. The two ratios are more indicative of the nutritional history of the child, i.e., chronic undernutrition. The three have limited utility with mild-to-moderately undernourished children. The QUAC stick and the ratio of head to chest circumferences appear to be useful with the severely undernourished. The application of the sitting heigh/stature ratio as an indicator of nutritional status is limited by racial differences in the ratio and by a lack of data for children varying in degree of undernutrition.

In theory, any two body dimensions can be expressed in the form of a ratio. The ratio or derived indicator should, of course, have biological significance relevant to the problem under study. The two ratios and the QUAC stick described above focus on the growth status of young children, which is presumably affected by the nutritional status among other aspects of the environment. Ratios which indicate functional status may also have utility in nutritional surveys. For example, the ratio of grip strength to body weight may serve as an indicator of functional consequences of chronic undernutrition in school age children. Grip strength is a highly reliable measure which is well suited to field conditions. For example, among school age children in Mexico and Papua New Guinea, grip strength is reduced commensurately with the reduced body size associated with chronic, mild-to-moderate undernutrition (Malina et al., 1987b). Strength per unit body weight is identical with well-nourished children. The utility of a grip strength/weight ratio in more severely undernourished children requires evaluation.

REFERENCES

Arnhold R (1969): The arm circumference as a public health index of protein-calorie malnutrition of early childhood, VXII: The QUAC stick: A field measure used by the Quaker Service Team in Nigeria. J Trop Pediatr 15:243–247.

Burgess HJL, Burgess AP (1969): The arm circumference as a public health index of protein-calorie malnutrition of early childhood, II: A modified standard for mid-upper arm circumference in young children. J Trop Pediatr 15:189–192.

Buschang PH, Malina RM (1983): Growth in height and weight of mild-to-moderately undernourished Zapotec school children. Hum Biol 55:587–597.

Buschang PH, Malina RM, Little BB (1986): Linear growth of Zapotec schoolchildren: Growth status and yearly velocity for leg length and sitting height. Ann Hum Biol 13:225–234.

Chavez A, Martinez C, Ophuis AO, Basta S (1977): Nutrition and development of children from poor rural areas, VI: Effects of mild malnutrition on body morphology during early growth. Nutr Rep Int 15:407–419.

Davis LE (1971): Epidemiology of famine in the Nigerian crisis: Rapid evaluation of malnutrition by height and arm circumference in large populations. Am J Clin Nutr 24:358–364.

Dean RFA (1965): Effects of malnutrition, especially of slight degree, on the growth of young children. Courrier 15:73–83.

El Lozy M (1969): The arm circumference as a public health index of protein-calorie malnutrition of early childhood, III: A modification of Wolanski's standards for the arm circumference. J Trop Pediatr 15:193–194.

Eveleth PB, Tanner JM (1976): "Worldwide Variation in Human Growth." Cambridge: Cambridge University Press.

Greulich WW (1957): A comparison of the physical growth and development of American-born and native Japanese children. Am J Phys Anthropol 15:489–515.

Habicht JP (1980): Some characteristics of indicators of nutritional status for use in screening and surveillance. Am J Clin Nutr 33:531–535.

Hamill PVV, Johnston FE, Lemeshow S (1973): Body weight, stature, and sitting height: White and Negro youths 12–17 years, United States. Vital and Health Statistics, Ser. 11, No. 126.

Himes JH (1979): Secular changes in body proportions and composition. Monogr Soc Res Child Dev 44, Ser. No. 179:28–58.

Jelliffe DB (1966): "The Assessment of the Nutritional Status of the Community." Geneva: WHO.

Jelliffe EF, Jelliffe DB (1969): The arm circumference as a public health index of protein-calorie malnutrition of early childhood, IX: Experience in the Caribbean. J Trop Pediatr 15:209–212.

Kaplowitz HJ, Mueller WH, Selwyn BJ, Malina RM, Bailey DA, Mirwald RL (1987): Sensitivities, specificities, and positive predictive values of simple indices of body fat distribution. Hum Biol 59:809–825.

Kissebah AH, Vydelingum N, Murray R, Evans DJ, Hartz AJ, Kalkhoff RK, Adams PW (1982): Relation of body fat distribution to metabolic complications of obesity. J Clin Endocrinol Metab 54:254–260.

Krogman WM (1970): Growth of head, face, trunk, and limbs in Philadelphia White and Negro children of elementary and high school age. Monogr Soc Res Child Develop 35, Ser. No. 136.

Krotkiewski M, Bjorntorp P, Sjostrom L, Smith U (1983): Impact of obesity on metabolism in men and women: Importance of regional adipose distribution. J Clin Invest 72:1150–1162.

Loewenstein MS, Phillips JF (1973): Evaluation of arm circumference measurement for determining nutritional status of children and its use in an acute epidemic of malnutrition: Owerri, Nigeria, following the Nigerian Civil War. Am J Clin Nutr 26:226–233.

McCammon RW (1970): "Human Growth and Development." Springfield, Il: CC Thomas.

Malina RM (1973): Biological substrata. In Miller KS, Dreger RM (eds): "Comparative Studies of Blacks and Whites in the United States." New York: Seminar Press, pp 53–123.

Malina RM (1979): Secular changes in growth, maturation, and physical performance. Exer Sports Sci Rev 6:203–255.

Malina RM, Bouchard C (1988): Subcutaneous fat distribution during growth. In Bouchard C, Johnston FE (eds): "Fat Distribution During Growth and Later Health Outcomes." New York: Liss, pp 63–84.

Malina RM, Brown KH, Zavaleta AN (1987a): Relative lower extremity length in Mexican American and in American Black and White youth. Am J Phys Anthropol 72: 89–94.

Malina RM, Habicht JP, Martorell R, Lechtig A., Yarbrough C, Klein RE (1975): Head and chest circumferences in rural Guatemalan Ladino children, birth to seven years of age. Am J Clin Nutr 28:1061–1070.

Malina RM, Hamill PVV, Lemeshow S (1974): Body dimensions and proportions, White and Negro children 6–11 years, United States. Vital and Health Statistics, Ser. 11, No 143.

Malina RM, Himes JH (1978): Patterns of childhood mortality and growth status in a rural Zapotec community. Ann Hum Biol 5:517–531.

Malina RM, Himes JH, Stepick CD, Gutierez Lopez F, Buschang PH (1980a): Growth of rural and urban children in the Valley of Oaxaca, Mexico. Am J Phys Anthropol 55:269–280.

Malina RM, Little BB, Shoup RF, Buschang PH (1987b): Adaptive significance of small body size: Strength and motor performance of school children in Mexico and Papua New Guinea. Am J Phys Anthropol 73:489–499.

Malina RM, Selby HA, Buschang PH, Aronson WL (1980b): Growth status of school children in a rural Zapotec community in the Valley of Oaxaca, Mexico, in 1968 and 1978. Ann Hum Biol 7:367–374.

Malina RM, Selby HA, Buschang PH, Aronson WL, Wilkinson RG (1983): Adult stature and age at menarche in Zapotec-speaking communities in the Valley of Oaxaca, Mexico, in a secular perspective. Am J Phys Anthropol 60:437–449.

Martin AD, Carter JEL, Hendy KC, Malina RM (1988): Segment lengths. In Lohman TG, Roche AF, Martorell E (eds): "Anthropometric Standardization Manual." Champaign, Il: Human Kinetics, pp 9–26.

Martorell R, Habicht JP, Yarbrough C, Guzman G, Klein KE (1975a): The identification and evaluation of measurement variability in the anthropometry of preschool children. Am J Phys Anthropol 43:347–352.

Martorell R, Malina RM, Castillo RO, Mendoza FS, Pawson IG (1988): Body proportions in three ethnic groups: Children and youths 2–17 years in NHANES II and HHANES. Hum Biol 60:205–222.

Martorell R, Yarbrough C, Malina RM, Habicht JP, Lechtig A, Klein RE (1975b): The head circumference/chest circumference ratio in mild-to-moderate protein-calorie malnutrition. Environ Child Health 21:203–207.

Moore LG, Regensteiner JG (1983): Adaptation to high altitude. Annu Rev Anthropol 12:285–304.

Roche AF (1979): Secular trends in stature, weight, and maturation. Monogr Soc Res Child Dev 44, Ser. No. 179:3–27.

Sastry JG (1972): Evaluation of QUAC-stick for growth assessment in children. Indian J Med Res 60:747–751.

Shakir A (1973): QUAC stick in the assessment of protein-calorie malnutrition in Baghdad. Lancet 1:762–764.

Shakir A (1975): Arm circumference in the surveillance of protein-calorie malnutrition in Baghdad. Am J Clin Nutr 28:661–665.

Shakir A, Demarchi M, El-Milli N (1972): Pattern of protein-calorie malnutrition in young children attending an outpatient clinic in Bagdhad. Lancet 2:143–146.

Simpson GG, Roe A, Lewontin RC (1960): "Quantitative Zoology." Rev ed. New York: Harcourt, Brace & World.

Sokal RR, Rohlf FJ (1981): "Biometry: The Principles and Practice of Statistics in Biological Research." 2nd ed. San Francisco: Freeman.

Sommer A, Loewenstein MA (1975): Nutritional status and mortality: A prospective validation of the QUAC stick. Am J Clin Nutr 28:287–292.

Sommer A, Mosley WH (1972): East Bengal cyclone of November, 1970: Epidemiological approach to disaster assessment. Lancet 1:1029–1036.

Tanner JM, Hayashi T, Preece MA, Cameron N (1982): Increase in length of leg relative to trunk in Japanese children and adults from 1957 to 1977: Comparison with British and with Japanese Americans. Ann Hum Biol 9:411–423.

Tanner JM, Whitehouse RH, Takaishi M (1966): Standards from birth to maturity for height, weight, height velocity, and weight velocity: British children, 1965, I. Arch Dis Child 41:454–471.

Terada H, Hoshi H (1965): Longitudinal study on the physical growth in Japanese, 3: Growth in chest and head circumferences during the first three years of life. Acta Anat Nippon 40:368–380.

Thomson AM, Duncan DL (1954): The diagnosis of malnutrition in Man. Nutr Abstr Rev 24:1–18.

Trowbridge FL, Staehling N (1980): Sensitivity and specificity of arm circumference indicators in identifying malnourished children. Am J Clin Nutr 33:687–696.

Vaughan VC (1969): Growth and development. In Nelson WE (ed): "Textbook of Pediatrics." 9th ed. Philadelphia: WB Saunders, pp 15–57.

Yip R, Binkin NJ, Trowbridge FL (1988): Altitude and childhood growth. J Pediatr 113:486–489.

Anthropometric Assessment
of Nutritional Status, pages 173–183

10
Anthropometric Assessment of Fat-Free Body Mass

T.G. LOHMAN
Department of Exercise and Sport Sciences, University of Arizona, Tucson, Arizona 85721

INTRODUCTION

The fat-free body mass (FFB) includes all body components including fat-free adipose tissue and excluding all body fat (lipid). It contains muscle, bone, and all organs and both intra- and extracellular substances. The fat-free body has been estimated to have a density of 1.100 g/cm^3 and a water content of 73.8% in reference man (Brozek et al., 1963). Behnke (1959) has added a small amount of fat in the fat-free body mass and defined the lean body mass (LBM) as the fat-free body plus a small amount of essential lipid. This lipid remains during fasting and starvation and is believed to be essential for life. It is found in bone marrow, the central nervous system, and cell membranes throughout the body. Lean body mass has a density of 1.095 in young adult males, and the estimation of excess fat and lean body mass can be derived from the following equation (Behnke, 1959):

$$\text{Excess} f = \frac{5.053}{D} - 4.614 \qquad (1)$$

Body cell mass excludes all extracellular materials of the fat-free body as proposed by Moore et al. (1963) and is considerably smaller than the FFB and LBM. The focus of this paper is in the prediction of FFB from anthropometric dimensions including height and weight. Emphasis is given to approaches which use various combinations of skeletal breadths, circumferences, and skinfolds in the young adult population. Applications of various approaches to children and the elderly, obese, and athletic population are discussed. Studies which employed body density as the criterion method for evaluation of anthropometric assessments were selected for this review.

ASSUMPTIONS AND LIMITATIONS OF BODY DENSITY AS A CRITERION METHOD FOR FAT-FREE BODY

Most research evaluating anthropometry as an index of fat-free body mass have used body density as the criterion method. Fat-free body is calculated from body density, assuming the density of the fat-free body is 1.100 g/cm^3

and that the density of fat is 0.900 g/cm^3. Siri (1956) has shown that the relation of the fat content of the body can be estimated from the above constants using the equation:

$$\%\ \text{fat} = \frac{495}{D} - 450 \qquad (2)$$

and estimated an error of ±4% fat in the general population if this approach were used. Bakker and Struinkenkamp (1977) in a review of literature confirmed the results of Siri (1956), and Lohman (1981) extended these results to an error of 2.5% fat for prediction from body density in a more homogenous population, e.g., young adult males, or female young adult athletes. FFB is derived from body fat content using the following equation:

$$\text{FFB, kg} = \text{body wt, kg} - \frac{\%\ \text{fat}}{100}(\text{body wt, kg}) \qquad (3)$$

A 2.5% fat error results in an FFB of 1.9 kg for young adult males with a mean FFB of 65 kg and an error of 1.5 kg for young female adults with a mean FFB of 45 kg (Table 1).

The primary reasons for this error in body fat estimates from body density come about because of variation in the water and bone mineral content of the fat-free body from individual to individual. An increase in the water content of FFB from 0.738 to 0.745 and a decrease in bone mineral content from 0.068 to 0.060 result in a decrease in the fat-free body density from 1.100 to 1.0930. This change in FFB density results in a 2.5% overestimation of body fat content from use of the constant 1.100 and the Siri equation (2).

Because fat-free body mass has errors of 1.9 kg in young adult men and 1.5 kg in young adult females, an anthropometric method is expected to have larger errors than those theoretically possible because of the imperfect relation between anthropometry and body composition. Using this analysis, we can set a scale of how well anthropometric dimensions predict FFB using

TABLE 1. Estimated Error for FFB From Body Density in Young Adult Males and Females[a]

Variable	Men	Women
Wt (kg)	76.5	60.0
% Fat	15.0	25.0
FFB (kg)	65.0	45.0
% Fat error	2.5	2.5
FFB error (kg)	1.9	1.5

[a]Estimated from Lohman (1981).

density as a criterion, and assign a subjective descriptor to the results, e.g., excellent, good, etc. (Table 2). If, for example, the majority of research showed that a particular anthropometric approach estimated FFB with standard errors of 2.5 kg in men and 1.8 kg in women, then we would conclude that the error due to anthropometry for men was 1.8 kg ($\sqrt{(2.5)^2 - (1.9)^2}$) and for women was 1.7 kg ($\sqrt{(1.8)^2 - (1.5)^2}$).

For another method that yielded a standard error of estimate of 4.0 kg for males and 3.2 kg for females from most studies in the literature, we would conclude that this approach was less satisfactory and could be classified as fair. Using this approach we will see that height and weight yield the least satisfactory approach, skeletal dimensions next, and skinfolds and circumferences yield the best approach.

HEIGHT AND WEIGHT

The prediction of fat-free body from height, weight, and the combination of height and weight has not received a great deal of attention. The popular equations of Hume and Weyers (1971) have been used most often when height and weight only were available. The work of Wilmore and Behnke (1968), Pollock et al. (1976), Katch and McArdle (1973) and Durnin and Womersly (1974) all do not report the prediction accuracy for estimation of FFB from height and weight. This overlooked relationship is important because of the number of epidemiological studies using height and weight to estimate obesity and body composition in relation to health and diseases. Also, if an anthropometric approach is not better than height and weight in predicting FFB, then there is no need to supplement height and weight measures with additional anthropometric dimensions if only FFB estimates are needed.

TABLE 2. Errors for Predicting FFB From Anthropometric Dimensions and Subjective Evaluation

Standard errors of estimate (kg)[a]		Actual error of anthropometric approach[b]		
Men	Women	Men	Women	Subjective rating
2.0–2.5	1.5–1.8	0–1.8	0–1.8	Ideal
2.5	1.8	1.8	1.0	Excellent
3.0	2.3	2.3	1.7	Very good
3.5	2.8	2.9	2.4	Good
4.0	3.2	3.5	2.8	Fairly good
4.5	3.6	4.0	3.3	Fair
>4.5	>4.0	—	—	Not recommended

[a]Prediction errors from anthropometric dimensions estimating FFB including error in body density.
[b]Actual error in FFB after density error in FFB is removed.

In the work of Womersley and Durnin (1977) various indices and height and weight were used to estimate %fat from body density. The SEE (standard error of estimate) for the best index (W/Ht^2) was 4.98% fat for men (20–29-year-olds) and 6.08% fat for women (20–29-year-olds). Corresponding errors on FFB in these samples would be 3.6 kg (men) and 3.8 kg (women). The work of Hume and Weyers (1971) estimating total body water from weight and height in a more heterogeneous sample of men (N = 30) and women (N = 30) yielded a SEE of 2.1 l (men) and 1.8 l (women). This would be increased to 2.9 kg and 2.5 kg in men and women if body water was used to estimate FFB. No other investigator using height and weight to predict FFB has found such low SEE values. Weight alone has been shown to predict %fat almost as closely as body mass index (Womersley and Durnin, 1977) in both young men and women, while height alone has been less effective in estimating FFB in young adult men with an SEE of 6.3 kg and more effective in women with a SEE of 3.5 kg several investigators have found (Slaughter and Lohman, 1980). In summary, height by itself is less closely associated with FFB than body weight. Prediction errors from height and weight together are between 3.5 kg and 4.0 kg for FFB. In future studies with anthropometric dimensions, height and weight equations also need to be developed and compared with additional anthropometric dimensions under study.

SKELETAL DIMENSIONS

The primary questions in using skeletal dimensions to estimate fat-free body mass are as follows: 1) how many skeletal dimensions are needed for estimating fat-free body mass, 2) are various skeletal dimensions more effective than height and weight in estimating fat-free body, 3) which skeletal sites are the best predictors of fat-free body, and 4) what is the typical standard error of estimates for equations based on skeletal dimensions.

To answer questions 1 and 2 we must first look to see if one skeletal dimension is effective in estimating fat-free body or if a combination of such dimensions is needed. How equations using one or more skeletal dimensions compare with fat-free body estimates based on height and weight can then be considered. The use of skeletal dimensions and its relation to fat-free body mass is illustrated in the research of Wilmore and Behnke (1969, 1970) in the young adult nonathletic population and has been extended to the college athletic population by Sinning et al. (1984, 1985).

The correlations between any single skeletal dimension and fat-free body mass range from .14 for head breadth to .76 for bideltoid breadth for men. The standard error of estimate for the latter correlation is 5.2 kg. For females, the correlations ranged from .03 to .64 with the bideltoid and elbow breadth yielding the highest correlation and a SEE of 3.6 kg (Wilmore and Behnke, 1970). Wilmore and Behnke then evaluated several equations which employed four to eight skeletal dimensions along with height using the approach developed by Behnke (1959, 1961) and explained in detail by Behnke and Wilmore (1974). They found in young adult men that four to eight dimensions increased the correlation up to .82 (SEE = 4.7 kg). The chest, bitrochanteric, ankle, and wrist gave the highest correlation with various other combinations of biocromial, biiliac, knee, and elbow yielding slightly lower predictions. In females various combinations of skeletal breadths were not evaluated without circumferences. When considered on the basis of correlations of each skeletal dimension with fat-free body, biocromial, bitrochanter, ankle, and wrist all show similar relationships with FFB (r = .60). Himes and Bouchard (1985) found correlations between .41 and .62 between skeletal dimensions and FFB in a large sample of men and women between the ages of 18 and 59 years. The association of FFB and height was partialled out, and the relation of skeletal dimensions to FFB decreased to between .30 and .49 (partial correlation) showing that a significant but not large amount of variation in FFB can be accounted for in these dimensions over that of height.

In summary, up to four skeletal dimensions appear more adequate in estimating fat-free body than one dimension does; however, standard errors of estimate are only fair, and this approach is only somewhat of an improvement over height and weight in most samples investigated. The one exception to these results not predicting FFB with low SEE values was found by Wilmore and Behnke (1968) in a sample of 54 young adult males where a standard error of estimate for predicted fat-free body from skeletal dimensions was 2.5 kg using biacromial, bitrochametric, wrist, and ankle diameters. In a larger sample this low a prediction error was not found, and no other investigators have found standard errors much below 4 kg.

CIRCUMFERENCES AND SKELETAL DIMENSIONS

The primary question to be answered in this section is the use of circumferences in addition to skeletal widths to estimate fat-free body mass. Secondly, which circumferences are usually used. Again, we turn to the large sample size and large number of circumferences measured by Wilmore and Behnke (1969, 1970). In this sample we find that when weight, circumferences, and skeletal widths are used together (one to four skeletal widths and circumferences), the standard error of estimate in men is 2.5 kg and in women 1.9 kg. The circumferences and skeletal widths yielding the lowest SEE values for men were biiliac breadth, abdomen 1, abdomen 2, and knee circumferences. Biiliac breadth and abdomen 1 were particularly related to FFB, while abdomen 2 and knee circumferences were negatively related in the multiple regression equation. For women, weight, wrist breadth, and abdomen 2, hip, and forearm circumference all contributed to the prediction of FFB from 19 circumferences and 10 skeletal breadth dimensions. Hip circumference was negatively related to FFB while the other four dimensions were all positive. No equations were presented without body weight. Katch and McArdle (1975) cross-validated Wilmore and Behnke's equations on 69 women and found SEE of 3.0 kg on their sample.

In summary, SEE values for circumferences and skeletal dimensions are found to predict FFB when under 3.0 kg and to be of advantage over use of height and weight and skeletal dimensions alone. Few cross-validation studies have been done on these and other equations using FFB as the dependent variable.

SKINFOLDS AND BODY WEIGHT

Skinfolds by themselves cannot be used to predict FFB; however, when used with body weight, they can be successful in achieving a good prediction. Lohman (1981) recommended triceps, subscapular, abdomen, and thigh skinfolds as most often contributing to the prediction of body density. More recently Lohman (1988) recommended the following four skinfolds to be used in any future battery of skinfold sites: triceps, subscapular, paraumbilicus (abdomen), and calf (medial) where an optimal set of sites is being developed for estimation of body composition. Most investigators have used skinfolds to estimate body density rather than FFB, and the equations of Jackson and Pollock (1985) are now in general used for the young adult population.

For estimation of FFB, Wilmore and Behnke (1969) studied seven skinfolds in a large sample of young adults and found that abdomen, thigh, and knee skinfolds in combination with height and weight best predicted FFB with a SEE of 2.8 kg. Using only abdomen skinfolds and body weight an SEE of 3.0 kg was found. For young adult women (Wilmore and Behnke, 1970) the triceps, subscapular, and thigh skinfold along with body weight predicted FFB with a SEE of 1.9 kg. Cross-validation by Katch and McCardle (1975) of the Wilmore and Behnke (1970) equations in another sample of young adult women yielded an SEE of 2.9 kg.

One of the lowest SEE values in prediction of FFB from skinfolds, and skinfolds in combination with circumferences and skeletal breadth, was found in a sample of 68 young adult men. Unique to this study, the criterion method of estimating FFB was from the mean of estimates using both body density and whole body potassium 40. In addition, FFB from body density was based on the mean of two days of measurement, and that from potassium was based on the mean of three days. The standard errors of estimate were as low as 1.6 kg for selected equations using skinfolds and body weight or skinfolds and circumferences along with skeletal dimensions and height and weight (Lohman et al., 1978).

In summary, skinfolds and body weight yield an SEE below 3.0 kg in the young adult population for prediction of FFB. Few of these equations have been cross-validated using the method of Lohman (1981), and only a limited number of studies have used skinfolds together with body mass to predict FFB, though this approach appears to be a useful one.

LIMITATIONS OF EQUATIONS USING SKINFOLDS AND CIRCUMFERENCES

While skinfold and circumference equations offer more accurate prediction of fat-free body mass compared with use of height, weight, and skeletal dimensions, their use is not without limitations (Lohman, 1982). Two major categories of limitations have been described by Lohman (1988) as population- and investigator-specific factors. If an equation derived from one population is applied to another population, a systematic overestimation or underestimation of FFB may result because of biological factors affecting the relation of anthropometry to FFB. For example, if the amount of muscle mass in relationship to height differ between two populations and the fat content is not different, then the relationship of circumferences to estimated FFB will yield different equations in the two populations. Similarly, if the skinfold distribution is different in two populations, then the relation of skinfolds and body weight to FFB will differ.

In addition to biological factors affecting the skinfold and circumference equations, investigator-specific equations have been developed because of the use of nonrandom samples, small sample sizes, a limited set of anthropometric dimensions analyzed in a given study, and unstandardized anthropometric procedures. These effects were illustrated in a methodological study of skinfolds using four different calipers and four different investigators taking the measurements (Lohman et al., 1984). Mean fat content for the sample varied 7% depending on caliper and investigator combinations. Thus, unless the measurement procedures are carefully standardized and carried out by experienced anthropometrists using the techniques employed by the original investigator from which the equations were derived, systematic errors will be present and will add to the prediction errors presented in the previous sections. For this reason, future investigators who wish to develop improved prediction equations for FFB in various populations should use a set of standardized anthropometric dimensions such as those recently developed at a national conference (Lohman et al., 1988).

PREDICTION EQUATIONS FOR SPECIFIC POPULATIONS

The development of FFB prediction equations for specific populations is important to improve the usefulness of anthropometric estimations of FFB. Since most of the research has been done on the young and middle-aged adult population, cross-validated equations for children and the obese, athletic, and aging populations are greatly needed. In these populations, however, the assumption that the density of the fat-free body is 1.100 g/cm^3 is in question and specifically, in children and the aging population, research has shown the fat-free body to have a density of less than 1.100 g/cm^3 (Haschke, 1983; Lohman et al., 1984; Boileau et al., 1985). It is likely that in the obese and athletic samples the density of fat-free body also deviates from the reference mean value, and thus use of equations based on this assumption may lead to systematic errors in predicted FFB. A second important point in the development of equations for a specific group is the use of skinfolds in certain populations and circumferences in other populations. In the obese, for example, Bray and Gray (1988) have shown that circumferences have a smaller interinvestigator reliability than skinfolds do and may be measured with a smaller technical error. Tran and Weltman (1988) have developed circumference equations on a larger sample of obese men and found that use of two abdomen circumferences and an abdomen to hip circumference ratio along with body weight predicted the FFB mass with an SEE of 3.1 kg in the original sample and 4.1 kg in a cross-validation sample. Additional studies comparing circumferences, skinfolds, and body mass index in obese samples are needed for general use of this approach in the obese.

For the athletic young adult population Sinning et al. (1984, 1985) have cross-validated many published anthropometric equations using body density as the criterion method. Because all equations evaluated predicted body density rather than FFB, these results are not directly applicable to the scope of this paper. From any of these equations, however, FFB can be calculated given body weight and predicted percentage fat using the following formula:

$$\text{FFB, kg} = \text{Weight, kg} - \frac{\%\,\text{Fat (Weight, kg)}}{100} \qquad (4)$$

In his review of skinfold equations Lohman (1981) has shown that one can predict body composition just as accurately whether one uses %fat or FFB equations and illustrated these results using the published data of Sloan (1967). Though the correlations are higher when FFB is predicted from anthropometry and body weight, the standard errors of estimate when converted into comparable errors for percentage fat are similar to those obtained from body density equations. Because all anthropometric equations derived from the athletic population use body density as the criterion variable, %fat and FFB may be overestimated and underestimated where athletic groups differ from reference man in their bone mineral content. Since these deviations were not taken into account and the density of the fat-free body was assumed at 1.100 g/cm^3, the equations would overestimate %fat and underestimate FFB when bone mineral content was below reference man (less than 6.8% FFB), and underestimate %fat and overestimate FFB where the bone mineral content was greater than reference man. These differences in the bone mineral content and density of the fat-free body among athletic groups need to be estimated in future research.

In children, the problems of applying anthropometric equations from adults to the younger population have been reviewed by Lohman (1986). In 1975, Lohman et al. presented skinfold equations for estimating FFB in children 8–12 years of age. The authors found that the triceps plus subscapular sites with body weight yielded the best fit for predicting FFB (derived from whole body potassium 40 assuming a potassium content of FFB of 2.68 g/kg) with an SEE of 1.8 kg. Since it has been shown that young males have a potassium content of 2.4 g/kg (Haschke, 1983; Lohman, 1986), these equations will slightly underestimate the FFB mass in children. Boileau et al. (1981) found that two skinfolds and two circumferences at one skeletal width estimated body density satisfactorily in two independent samples of male children. Many other authors have developed skinfold equations from body density and body potassium criterion methods. All these equations overestimate the fat content of the body and underestimate the FFB (Lohman, 1986).

Equations which may minimize this systematic error arising from lower FFB densities in children have been proposed by Lohman (1986) and Slaughter et al. (1988). These equations are based on body density, body water, and bone mineral measurements to enable more accurate determination of %fat and FFB in this population. For the elderly, the most widely used anthropometric equations have been developed by Durnin and Womersley (1974); however, because these equations do not account for the increase in FFB density–associated bone mineral content loss with age, their use will overestimate the fat content and underestimate the FFB mass. New equations are now being developed by several investigators to alleviate this problem.

FUTURE CROSS-VALIDATION STUDIES

The development of anthropometric equations to estimate FFB has been carried out mainly in young adult athletic and nonathletic populations, and general equations are available for use in these populations. Better equations need to be developed in the obese and in the general population for children and for the elderly. The proper cross-validation of equations has been outlined by Lohman (1981), and this procedure has been applied to the young adult female (Sinning et al., 1984) and male (Sinning et al., 1985) athletic populations. For an equation to be successfully cross-validated it should 1) produce only slightly higher SEE values in the new sample than in the original sample, 2) produce a small error for the mean of the predicted value versus the mean measured value, and 3) produce a similar standard deviation of predicted values as the measured values using the criterion method (Lohman, 1981). Results can be compared with the equations given in Table 3, which have been developed in the young adult populations.

TABLE 3. Equations Predicting FFB From Skinfolds and Body Weight

Population	Regression equation
Males	
Wilmore et al. (1968)	FFB, kg = .79 body weight − .37 waist S + 10.3
Sloan (1967)	FFB, kg = 9.6 body weight, kg − .40 thigh S − .46 subscapular S + 4.2
Lohman et al. (1978)	FFB, kg = .90 body weight, kg −3.5 triceps S −.52 suprailiac S +5.6
Females	
Wilmore et al. (1970)	FFB, kg = .68 body weight, kg − .16 subscapular S − .10 triceps S −.054 thigh S

SUMMARY

Various anthropometric approaches to the estimator of fat-free body mass have been discussed. In general, larger prediction errors are found for use of height and weight and skeletal breadth dimensions than for skinfolds and circumferences. The standard errors of estimate for skinfolds or circumferences are between 2 kg and 3 kg as compared to SEE values larger than 4 kg when skeletal dimensions or height and weight are used. Cross-validation studies of anthropometric equations estimating FFB are few in number, and, thus it is recommended for future research that both %fat and FFB equations be reported. Optimal equations in many populations have yet to be developed. Future research must use standardized anthropometric procedures and multicomponent models to estimate FFB and %fat if improved prediction equations are to be developed in many populations other than young adults.

REFERENCES

Bakker HK, Struinkenkamp RS (1977): Biological variability and lean body mass estimates. Hum Biol 49:187–202.

Behnke AR (1959): The estimation of lean body weight from skeletal measurement. Hum Biol 31:295–315.

Behnke AR (1961): Quantification assessment of body build. J Appl Physiol 16:960–968.

Behnke AR, Wilmore JH (1974): "Evaluation and Regulation of body build and Composition." Englewood Cliffs, NJ: Prentice-Hall.

Boileau RA, Lohman TG, Slaughter MH (1985): Exercise and body composition in children and youth. Scand J Sports Sci 7:17–27.

Boileau RA, Wilmore JH, Lohman TG, Slaughter MH, Riner WF (1981): Estimation of body density from skinfold thicknesses, body circumferences and skeletal widths in boys aged 8 to 11 years: Comparison of two samples. Hum Biol 53:575–592.

Bray GA, Gray DS (1988): Anthropometric measurements in the obese. In Lohman TG, Roche AF, Martorell R (eds): "Anthropometric Standardization Reference Manual." Champaign, Ill: Human Kinetics, pp 131–136.

Brozek J, Grande F, Anderson JT, Keys A (1963): Densitometric analysis of body composition: Revisions of some quantitative assumptions. Ann NY Acad Sci 110:113–140.

Durnin JVGA, Womersley J (1974): Body fat assessment from total body density and its estimation from skinfold thickness measurements on 481 men and women aged 16 to 72 years. Br J Nutr 32:77–97.

Haschke F (1983): Body composition of adolescent males, Part II: Body composition of the male reference adolescent. Acta Paediatr Scand Suppl 307:11–23.

Himes JH, Bouchard C (1985): Do the new Metropolitan Life Insurance Weight-Height Tables correctly assess body frame and body fat relationships. Am J Public Health 75:1076–1079.

Hume R, Weyers E (1971): Relationship between total body water and surface area in normal and obese subjects. J Clin Pathol 24:234–238.

Jackson AS, Pollock ML (1985): Practical assessment of body composition. Phys Sports Med 13:76–90.

Katch FI, McArdle WD (1973): Prediction of body density from single anthropometric measurements in college-age men and women. Hum Biol 45:445–454d.

Katch FI, McArdle WD (1975): Validity of body composition prediction equations for college men and women. Am J Clin Nutr 28:105–109.

Lohman TG (1981): Skinfolds and body density and their relation to body fatness: A review. Hum Biol 53:181–225.
Lohman TG (1982): Use of body composition methodology in sports medicine. Phys Sports Med 10:46–58.
Lohman TG (1986): Applicability of body composition techniques and constants for children and youth. In Pandolf K (ed): Exerc Sport Sci Rev 14:325–357, New York: MacMillan.
Lohman TG (1988): Anthropometry and body composition. In Lohman TG, Roche AF, Martorell R (eds): "Anthropometric Standardization Reference Manual." Champaign, Ill: Human Kinetics, pp 125–129.
Lohman TG, Boileau RA, Massey BH (1975): Prediction of lean body mass in young boys from skinfold thickness and body weight. Hum Biol 47:245–262.
Lohman TG, Pollock ML, Slaughter MH, Brandon LJ, Boileau RA (1984): Methodological factors and the prediction of body fat in female athletes. Med Sci Sport Exerc 16:92–96.
Lohman TG, Roche AF, Martorell R (1988): "Anthropometric Standardization Reference Manual." Champaign, Ill: Human Kinetics.
Lohman TG, Slaughter MH, Selinger A, Boileau RA (1978): Relationships of somatotype to body composition in college-aged men. Ann Hum Biol 5:174–180.
Moore FD, Oleson KM, McMurrey JD, Parker HV, Ball MR, Boyden CM (1963): "The Body Cell Mass and Its Supporting Environment." Philadelphia: WB Saunders.
Pollock ML, Hickman T, Kendrick I, Jackson A, Linnerud AC, Dawson G (1976): Prediction of body density in young and middle-aged men. J Appl Physiol 40:300–304.
Sinning WE, Dolney DG, Little KD, Cunningham LN, Racaniello A, Siconolfi SF (1985): Validity of "generalized" equations for body composition analysis in male athletes. Med Sci Sport Exerc 17:124–130.
Sinning WE, Wilson JR (1984): Validity of "generalized" equations for body composition analysis in women athletes. Res Q Sport Exerc 55:153–160.
Siri WE (1956): The gross composition of the body. Adv Biol Med Physiol 4:239–280.
Slaughter MH, Lohman TG (1980): An objective method for measurement of muscle-skeletal size to characterize body physique with application to the athletic population. Med Sci Sport Exerc 12:170–174.
Slaughter MH, Lohman TG, Boileau RA, Horswill CA, Stillman JR, Van Loan MD, Bemben DA (1988): Skinfold equations for estimation of body fatness in children and youth. Hum Biol 60:709–723.
Sloan AW (1967): Estimation of body fat in young men. J Appl Physiol 23:311–315.
Tran ZV, Wettman A (1988): Predicting body composition of men from girth measurements. Human Biol 60:167–175.
Wilmore JH, Behnke AR (1968): Predictability of lean body weight through anthropometric assessment in college men. J Appl Physiol 25:349–355.
Wilmore JH, Behnke AR (1969): An anthropometric estimation of body density and lean body weight in young men. J Appl Physiol 27:25–31.
Wilmore JH, Behnke AR (1970): An anthropometric estimation of body density and lean body weight in young women. Am J Clin Nutr 23:267–274.
Womersley J, Durnin JVGA (1977): A comparison of the skinfold method with extent of "overweight" and various weight–height relationships in the assessment of obesity. Br J Nutr 38:271–284.

Anthropometric Assessment
of Nutritional Status, pages 185–196

11
Anthropometric Assessment of Bone Mineral

ALAN D. MARTIN
Sport and Exercise Sciences Research Institute, University of Manitoba, Winnipeg, Manitoba R3T 2N2, Canada

INTRODUCTION

Interest in bone mineral has increased dramatically in recent years with the expanding public realization that bone is not simply an inert tissue. Bone is constantly being broken down and re-formed. As well as this remodeling process, the amount and architecture of the skeleton undergo many changes throughout the life span. The skeleton increases steadily in size and level of mineralization throughout the growing period with several years of rapid growth during puberty (Gilsanz et al., 1988). By about the end of the second decade bone lengths reach their maximum. Following this is a variable period of some 10 years in which skeletal mass is consolidated. Bone mass reaches a peak in the third or fourth decade and declines gradually for the rest of the life span (Mazess, 1982). This age-related loss, observed in all populations that have been examined, is accelerated sharply in women for the 10 to 15 years following menopause. There are large individual differences in the rate of bone loss, both within populations and between different ethnic groups (Ahuja, 1969).

Progress in our understanding of the skeleton has been limited by the inability to accurately measure bone mass. Traditional radiography cannot detect bone loss until more than 20% of bone mass has been lost. Recent advances in quantitative computed tomography (QCT) and dual energy x-ray absorptiometry (DEXA) have made these the methods of choice for bone density assessment (Mazess, 1983). However, they involve radiation exposure, which limits applicability, particularly in children and young women, though the radiation dose from DEXA is considerably less than with QCT (Hangartner, 1986). Both require expensive, nonportable equipment. Ultrasound technology, though promising, is still in the preliminary stages of development. While anthropometry has served as a valuable, noninvasive, inexpensive, and portable approach to the estimation of body fat, attempts to use it to predict bone mass have been sparse. There are several clear problems. Anthropometry measures bone dimensions. How are these related to skeletal volume and skeletal mass? Knowing skeletal mass, is it possible to estimate the amount of bone mineral? These are the questions that will be addressed in this chapter, but first it is necessary to look more closely at the nature of bone itself.

THE STRUCTURE OF BONE

Bone is a dynamic tissue, consisting of a fibrous, collagenous protein or osteoid, stiffened by an extremely dense filling of calcium phosphate (Currey, 1984). Unmineralized collagen has little stiffness, as is readily seen in its roles in skin, ligaments, and blood vessels, where elasticity is of primary importance. The mineral to osteoid ratio in bone is an important determinant of stiffness, and pathological reduction in this ratio, i.e., osteomalacia, results in bones that are easily deformed under normal loads. It is important to distinguish this from the more common situation of osteoporosis, in which substantial loss of both mineral and osteoid occurs with little change in their ratio, leading to brittleness and the characteristic low-trauma fractures (Martin and McCulloch, 1987).

There are two types of bony tissue, cortical and trabecular, and every bone in the body is made up of these two types. Cortical or compact bone is dense and forms the outer shell of all bones and predominates in the shafts of long bones. Trabecular bone provides the filling for small bones and is found also in the ends of long bones. Its large surface area, due to a honeycomb configuration, makes it more metabolically active than cortical bone, and thus more sensitive to the influence of factors such as mechanical loading. Cortical bone makes up about 80% by weight of the total skeleton (Mazess, 1982). Surprisingly, little is known about the weight of the skeleton. The literature reveals that there have been few direct assessments of total skeletal mass using cadavers.

DIRECT MEASUREMENT OF THE MASS OF THE SKELETON

We have recently completed a series of 25 cadaver dissections, the Brussels Cadaver Study, aimed in part at supplementing the available data on skeletal mass (Martin, 1984; Drinkwater, 1984). These have been summarized along with the limited data available prior to the Brussels study (Clarys et al., 1984) yielding a total of 42 subjects. Typically, bone constitutes about 10%–20% of body weight, but this value will, of course, depend on the fatness of the subjects. After all dissectible adipose tissue is removed, the skeleton makes up about 20%–21% of the remainder, i.e., the adipose tissue-free mass (ATFM), with a standard deviation of about 2.5% of the ATFM (Fig. 1). Absolute skeletal mass ranged from 6.7 kg to 11.7 kg with a mean of 9.3 kg for the men (SD = 1.4 kg) and 7.7 kg (SD = 1.3 kg) for the women (Clarys et al., 1984). The relationship between skeletal mass and anthropometry in the cadavers of the Brussels study will be described later.

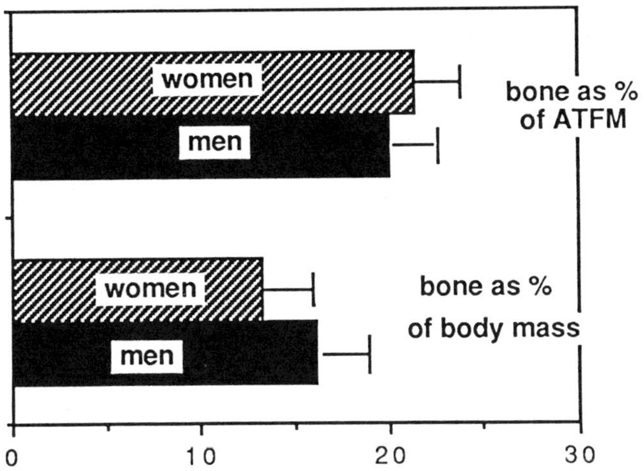

Fig. 1. Skeletal mass as a percentage of body mass and adipose tissue-free mass. Data are means and standard deviations for 42 cadavers (Martin, 1984).

AGING BONE LOSS

The rapid loss of bone in women immediately following menopause is clearly related to the reduction in circulating estrogen. However, the slower, more prolonged loss observed in both men and women remains unexplained and may be due to a combination of the following factors: declining levels of physical activity (Martin and Houston, 1987); inadequate nutrition (Parfitt, 1983); age-related impairment of metabolism (Orwoll and Meier, 1986); or a variety of drugs including nicotine and alcohol (Lees et al., 1987). While this bone loss is not associated with any symptoms, a time is reached when insufficient bone remains at certain sites to withstand even very mild physical trauma, and osteoporotic fractures result. Those are now at epidemic proportions in North America, with an estimated 1.3 million fractures and treatment costs of $3.8 billion annually (Peck, 1984). In 1980 there were an estimated 267,000 hip fractures, the most serious manifestation of osteoporosis, with direct costs alone exceeding $1.3 billion (Lindsay et al., 1984). A 50-year-old Canadian woman has a 15% probability of a future hip fracture (Martin et al., 1987), and with the aging trend of most Western populations, incidence and costs of osteoporosis will continue to rise steadily.

The ages at which fractures occur reflect different rates of loss for the two types of bone. Trabecular bone loss begins earlier in life and is greater through menopause than cortical loss. Those sites with a higher trabecular to cortical ratio will therefore reach the fracture threshold sooner. This explains the early occurrence of vertebral and wrist fractures (type I or postmenopausal osteoporosis), while the predominantly cortical bone of the proximal end of the femur typically is not subject to fracture until after age 70 (type II or senile osteoporosis) (Riggs and Melton, 1983).

THE PREDICTION OF SKELETAL MASS

Attempts to predict skeletal mass date back to Matiegka (1921). He made the observation that the "osseous parts of the extremities give us a good idea of the skeleton as a whole," and thus based his prediction equation on the breadths of wrist, ankle, humerus, and femur. Specifically, he used the mean of four measurements: the bicondylar femur, biepicondylar humerus, radioulnar breadth, and bimalleolar breadth. This quantity he termed "*O*" (for osseous) and multiplied its square by stature, *S*, and a constant to get skeletal mass, i.e.,

$$\text{skeletal mass} = O^2 \times S \times k$$

With the breadth in cm, he used the constant $k = 1.2$ g/mL. This equation can be rewritten as:

$$\text{skeletal mass} = 0.75 \times 10^{-4} \times S \times (\Sigma b_i)^2$$

where b_i are the four breadths in cm and the mass is in kg. Matiegka clearly acknowledged the tentative nature of his choice of constant, and expressed his hope that subsequent cadaver dissections would provide a more accurate value. Alexander (1964) used essentially the same prediction equation but chose a constant that yielded a 43% higher prediction. In the same year von Dobeln devised an equation based on four bone dimensions: right and left radioulnar breadths and right and left bicondylar femur breadths:

$$\text{skeletal mass} = 1.614 \times 10^{-4} (S^2FR)^{0.712}$$

where *S* is stature, *F* is the sum of the two femur breadths, and *R* is the sum of the radioulnar breadths (all in cm), giving skeletal mass in kg (von Dobeln, 1964).

The fundamental difficulty with these predictions is the same as that faced when attempting to predict any body constituent from anthropometry: The lack of validation data. When these prediction formulae were devised there was not a single subject for which both anthropometric bone breadths and skeletal mass were known. This situation was corrected after the completion of the Brussels Cadaver Study. Data from this study included extensive anthropometry as well as the masses and densities of the skeletons and all major bones of 25 older Belgian cadavers (Martin, 1984). This has enabled, for the first time, a check on the validity of the available equations for predicting skeletal mass. More important, it permits a closer examination of the relationships between bone dimensions and bone mass than has up to now been possible, leading to improved prediction equations.

ASSUMPTIONS UNDERLYING SKELETAL MASS PREDICTION

The problem is analogous to that of the anthropometric prediction of fat or muscle masses. An indirect measurement is made on one or more of the skeletal components with the assumption that these are representative of the whole skeleton. Since bone is less accessible than adipose tissue, the possibilities are fewer, but problems of compressibility of the tissue to be measured are minimal. Those regions where subcutaneous soft tissues are negligible are the best choices—hence the selection of extremities and limb joints. In addition, potentially useful indicators are head girth, trunk breadths such as biacromial and biiliac, and various lengths including stature. Inherent in the use of these anthropometric indicators are several assumptions.

First, it is assumed that the anthropometric measurement accurately reflects the actual bone dimension; second, that the mass of an individual bone is directly related to its dimensions, and third, that the mass of a given bone reflects the total skeletal mass. This sequence of assumptions is outlined in Figure 2. The validity of these assumptions can be assessed using data from the Brussels Cadaver Study, which also included osteometry of selected bones, i.e., measurements made directly on the separated bones.

The first assumption is that anthropometry reflects osteometry. Osteometry on the Brussels cadavers included biepicondylar breadth of the humerus and bicondylar breadth of the femur. Scatter plots of the anthropometric mea-

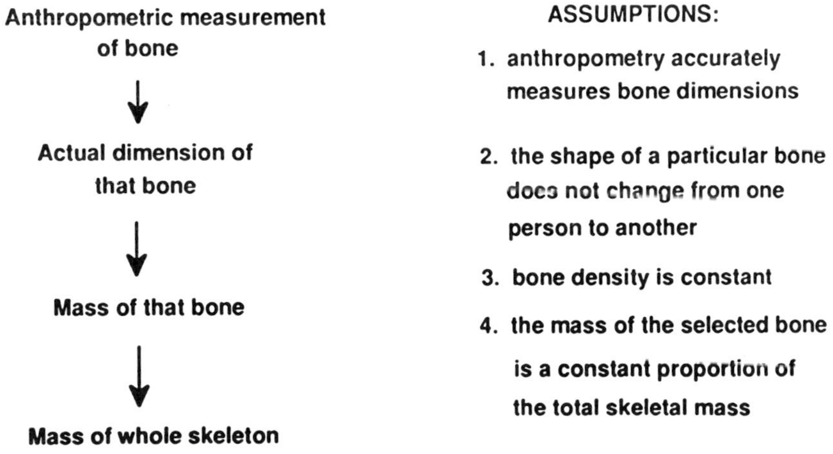

Fig. 2. Assumptions underlying the anthropometric prediction of skeletal mass.

surements are shown in Figures 3 and 4. As expected, in every case the anthropometric value exceeded the osteometric value, the deviation from the line of identity ($y = x$) being less for the men than for the women. The regression equations predicting osteometric values are:

Humerus breadth		
men and women	$y = .757x + 0.899$	$r = .86$ SEE $= .26$ cm
men	$y = .665x + 1.715$	$r = .93$ SEE $= .20$ cm
women	$y = .596x + 1.828$	$r = .72$ SEE $= .21$ cm
Femur breadth		
men and women	$y = .794x + .408$	$r = .65$ SEE $= .52$ cm
men	$y = .832x + 0.370$	$r = .84$ SEE $= .34$ cm
women	not significant at .05 level	

These data suggest that in the Brussels sample the humerus is more amenable to accurate anthropometric measurement than the femur. This may result, in part, from the greater overlay of soft tissue found in an older population, and may be less true in a younger sample.

The second assumption concerns the transformation from a given bone dimension to the mass of that bone. This requires that both shape and density of a particular bone do not change from one person to another.

Constancy of Bone Shape

Using the Brussels data, the relationship between bone dimensions and bone volumes has been investigated for humerus, femur, and ulna. If bone shape were constant from one person to another, then any one dimension of the bone should predict bone volume as well as any other dimension. However, the breadths of the humerus, femur, and ulna all showed greater correlations with bone volume than did the lengths of these bones, suggesting that bone shape is a function of size. Hence, the combination of a length and a breadth should predict bone mass better than either one of these alone.

Femur volume can be predicted accurately by osteometry; the square of bicondylar breadth multiplied by femur length gives a correlation coefficient of 0.92 with measured femur volume and a standard error of 38 mL (7%) for all 25 cadavers. This confirms that skeletal mass predictions should include a measure of length, rather than just bone breadths. The length need not necessarily be the length of a specific bone; rather it might be stature, which gives an overall reflection of bone length.

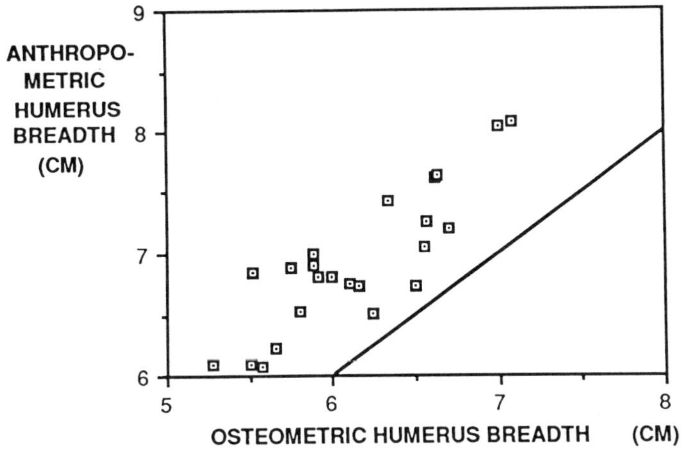

Fig. 3. The relationship between anthropometric and osteometric humerus breadths for 23 cadavers.

Bone Density

Since it is a decrease in bone density that increases susceptibility to osteoporotic fractures, it appears that variations in bone density may be great enough to render skeletal mass prediction by anthropometry highly inaccurate. The problem is that two humeri, for example, may have the same size, i.e., biepicondylar breadth, but due to different densities, will have different

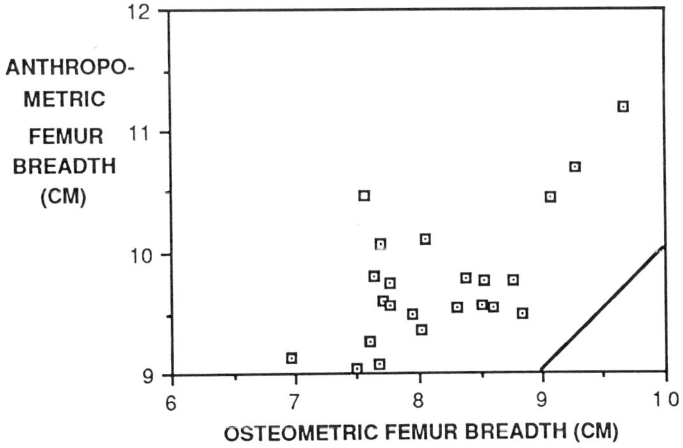

Fig. 4. The relationship between anthropometric and osteometric femur breadths for 23 cadavers.

masses. Unaided anthropometry cannot detect this and will yield the same predicted mass for each of these two bones. The Brussels data include bone densities determined by hydrostatic weighing of each bone. This is the straightforward mass per unit volume meaning of density and should not be confused with the term bone density as it is used in connection with indirect techniques such as photon absorptiometry.

Fresh bone densities for selected bones are shown in Table 1, which also gives the mean values for 25 cadavers. These range from 1.164 g/mL for the pelvis to 1.403 g/mL for the cranium. Of particular interest is the variability in density; for the whole skeleton the observed standard deviation was 0.039 g/mL. Thus, for the Brussels sample, with an anthropometric prediction equation that is accurate at the mean skeletal density of 1.24 g/mL, the two extreme subjects, with skeletal densities of 1.15 and 1.33 g/mL, will have predicted skeletal masses with errors due to density of about 7%. Most differences will be smaller than this, so this error, while not insignificant, may not be a major one. If there were a relationship between bone size and bone density, e.g., if larger bones were denser than smaller ones, then it might be possible to offset this error. However, a correlation analysis showed no significant relationship (at the 5% level) between the following pairs of variables:

humerus osteometric breadth and humerus density ($r = .13, p > .25$)
femur osteometric breadth and femur density ($r = .15, p > .25$)
stature and overall skeletal density ($r = .16, p > .25$)
skeletal mass and overall skeletal density ($r = .21, p > .25$)

Thus, this error appears to be inherent in the use of unaided anthropometry to predict skeletal mass. While skeletal density and size appear to be unrelated, density and age are related ($r = -.49, p < .01$ for males and females combined). The regression equation: skeletal density (g/mL) = 1.392 − .00206

TABLE 1. Fresh Bone Densities: Means for 25 Cadavers

Bone	Density (g/mL)	SD
Pelvis	1.164	0.037
Tibia	1.242	0.055
Humerus	1.262	0.054
Femur	1.267	0.053
Clavicle	1.315	0.058
Radius	1.353	0.070
Ulna	1.395	0.078
Cranium	1.403	0.061
Whole skeleton	1.236	0.039

× age (years) suggests a .02 g/mL decline in skeletal density per decade. A separate analysis demonstrated that this loss was distributed over almost all the individual bones, though not the cranium. Thus it may be advisable to incorporate age into any anthropometric equation for the prediction of skeletal mass, to help offset the error due to density variation.

The third general assumption (Fig. 2) is that the mass of a selected bone is a constant proportion of total skeletal mass. That is, if an anthropometric measure can accurately predict the mass of a given bone, does that necessarily reflect the rest of the skeleton? Table 2 shows the correlation coefficients for the masses of humerus, ulna, femur, and pelvis with segmental and total skeletal mass.

As expected, the mass of a bone is most highly correlated with the bone mass of its own body segment, e.g., humerus and upper limb. Humerus mass shows the highest correlation with skeletal mass, r = .92; the femur value is r = .83. Trotter (1954), who studied the 24 male skeletons of the Terry collection, found the correlation between femur mass and skeletal mass to be .96 (she did not report a correlation for the mass of any other bone with skeletal mass). The high value can be attributed to the fact that her material was defatted and dehydrated, thus eliminating some sources of variability.

The mass of the skull is not significantly related to the masses of individual limb bones. This may have important implications for the prediction of skeletal mass, since the bone mass of the adult head contributes some 10% to the body's total bone mass. This contribution takes on far greater importance when infants and children are being assessed. Thus, for improved predictive accuracy, it may be that an anthropometric measurement of the head is required, a tactic not previously used by workers in this area.

CHOICE OF VARIABLES FOR SKELETAL MASS PREDICTION

The validity of the assumptions discussed in the previous section will be clearly reflected in the correlation coefficients between the anthropometric variables and actual skeletal mass. Values for nine selected variables are shown in Table 3. The three best predictors are upper limb breadths with wrist breadth having the highest correlation (r = .85) with skeletal mass.

TABLE 2. Correlation Coefficients Between the Masses of Individual Bones and the Masses of Bone in the Various Body Segments

Segment	Humerus mass	Ulna mass	Femur mass	Pelvis mass
Head	n.s.	n.s.	.354	.545
Right arm	.989	.978	.712	.788
Right leg	.839	.785	.984	.794
Trunk	.882	.880	.744	.889
Whole skeleton	.924	.911	.827	.908

TABLE 3. Correlation Coefficients Between Skeletal Mass and Selected Anthropometric Variables

Dimension	*r*
Wrist breadth	.85
Hand breadth	.83
Humerus breadth	.78
Foot breadth	.76
Stature	.76
Head girth	.70
Ankle breadth	.61
Femur breadth	.60
Bi-acromial breadth	.55

This is remarkable for several reasons. First, wrist breadth is rarely measured in common anthropometric assessments, perhaps because it spans two separate bones. Second, it is included in the prediction equations of both von Dobeln and Matiegka, neither of whom had the advantage of comprehensive dissection data. The common choices for indicators of frame size or skeletal mass are the humerus and femur breadths. However, femur breadth, while significantly correlated with skeletal mass (r = .60), appears to be a poor predictor (unexplained variance 64%), unless used in conjunction with other variables. Hand and foot breadth, though infrequently measured, are also highly related to skeletal mass.

EVALUATION OF THE PREDICTIONS OF MATEIGKA AND VON DOBELN

Skeletal masses were estimated for all the Brussels cadavers using the prediction formulae of von Dobeln and Matiegka. Matiegka overpredicted, on average, by 2.07 kg, slightly better than von Dobeln (2.17 kg). Matiegka's constant, 0.75, was then corrected to bring his mean for prediction to the actual mean for the cadavers. The new value was found to be 0.60. Thus his revised equation is: Skeletal mass (kg) $= 0.60 \times 10^{-4} \times S \times (\Sigma b_i)^2$ (where S is stature in cm and Σb_i is the sum of four breadths: femur, humerus, wrist, and ankle, all in cm).

The choice of revised constant gave a mean error of prediction of zero. The absolute deviations expressed as percentages of the actual skeletal masses had a mean value of 6.5% and a standard error of 0.95%. The equation appears to be a useful predictor of skeletal mass and in the absence of further data, particularly in younger adults, must be considered to be the best available.

RELATIONSHIPS OF BONE MINERAL TO SKELETAL MASS

Having estimated skeletal mass, is it then possible to predict total body bone mineral? Clearly this is only possible if bone mineral is a reliably fixed fraction of skeletal mass. Though data are limited, Trotter's work suggests that in her skeletal sample the mineral to osteoid ratio was surprisingly constant (Trotter and Peterson, 1955). However, anthropometry will be unable to detect variations in this ratio. Thus, at best, the anthropometric estimation of bone mineral will be reliable only in the presence of a normal mineral to osteoid ratio since it is the matrix that constitutes the bulk of bone. This rules out its application to skeletons suffering from nutritional deficiencies leading to osteomalacia.

It may be possible to combine anthropometry with techniques such as photon absorptiometry, which can provide a measure of bone mineral density at a few selected sites. In this way a selection of skeletal breadths complemented by bone mineral density measurements at the distal forearm, lumbar spine, and hip could prove useful. However, just as a single bony breadth may not be a good indicator of total skeletal mass, so one or two bone mineral density measurements may not give enough information on overall skeletal density. It is well established that appendicular density is not a good predictor of axial density (Mazess, 1983).

SUMMARY

There are some important obstacles to the anthropometric assessment of bone mineral. Variability in bone density, not detectable with anthropometry, could cause moderate errors in skeletal mass prediction. Strategies for circumventing this could be adopted. Since some of the variability in bone density is associated with age, it may be possible to incorporate age as a variable into any prediction equation. An alternative is to make a direct estimation of bone density using DEXA or QCT and use this to improve prediction accuracy. This would appear to be a fruitful direction for future research. Though it is clear that anthropometric estimation of skeletal mass has its limitations, Matiegka's equation modified in light of cadaver validation as presented in this chapter should prove a useful first approximation in the absence of other cadaver-validated approaches. Improvements in the future can only come from more dissections, ideally incorporating a noninvasive measure of bone density, and carried out with a cadaver sample that is both large and with a wide range of ages.

REFERENCES

Ahuja M (1969): Normal variation in the density of selected human bones in north India. J Bone Jt Surg 51B:719–735.

Alexander ML (1964): The post-mortem estimation of total body fat, muscle and bone. Clin Sci 26:193–202.

Clarys JP, Martin AD, Drinkwater DT (1984): Gross tissue masses in the human cadaver. Hum Biol 56:459–573.

Currey J (1984): "The Mechanical Adaptations of Bones." Princeton, NJ: Princeton.

Drinkwater DT (1984): "An Anatomically Derived Method for the Anthropometric Estimation of Human Body Composition." Burnaby, B.C., Canada: PhD thesis. Simon Fraser University.

Gilsanz V, Gibbens DT, Roe TF, Carlson M, Senac MO, Boechat MI, Huang HK, Schultz EE, Libanati CR, Cann CE (1988): Vertebral bone density in children: Effect of puberty. Radiology 166:847–850.

Hangartner TN (1986): The radiologic measurement of bone. J Can Assoc Radiol 37:143–152.

Lees B, Devenport M, Simpson R, Stevenson JC (1987): Relation of physical and lifestyle factors to vertebral and femoral neck bone density in premenopausal women. In Christiansen C, Johansen JS, Riis BJ (eds): "Osteoporosis 1987." Copenhagen: Osteopress, pp 111–112.

Lindsay R, Dempster DW, Clemens T et al. (1984): Incidence, cost and risk factors of fracture of the proximal femur in the U.S.A. In Christiansen C, Arnaud CD, Nordin BEC et al. (eds): "Osteoporosis. Denmark: Glostrup pp 311–316.

Martin AD (1984): "An Anatomical Basis for Assessing Human Body Composition: Evidence From 25 Dissections." Burnaby, B.C., Canada: Simon Fraser University. PhD thesis.

Martin AD, Houston CS (1987): Osteoporosis, calcium and physical activity. Can Med Assoc J 136:587–593.

Martin AD, McCulloch RG (1987): Bone dynamics: Stress, strain and fracture. J Sports Sci 5:155–163.

Martin AD, Silverthorn KG, Houston (CS) (1987): Age-specific increases in hip fracture in Canada. In Christiansen C, Johansen JS, Riis BJ (eds): "Osteoporosis 1987." Copenhagen: Osteopress, pp 111–112.

Matiegka J (1921): The testing of physical efficiency. Am J Phys Anthropol 4:223–230.

Mazess RB (1982): On aging bone loss. Clin Orthop 165:239–252.

Mazess RB (1983): The non-invasive measurement of skeletal mass. In Peck WA (ed): "Bone and Mineral Research Annual 1." Amsterdam: Excerpta Medica, pp 223–279.

Orwoll ES, Meier DE (1986): Alterations in calcium, vitamin D and parathyroid hormone physiology in normal men with aging: Relationship to the development of senile osteopenia. J Clin Endocrinal Metab 63:1262–1269.

Parfitt AM (1983): Dietary risk factors for age-related bone loss and fractures. Lancet 2:1181–1184.

Peck W (1984): Consensus conference: Osteoporosis. JAMA 252:799–802.

Riggs BL, Melton LJ (1983): Evidence for two distinct syndromes of involutional osteoporosis. Am J Med 75:899–901.

Trotter M (1954): A preliminary study of the weight of the skeleton. Am J Phys Anthropol 12:537–551.

Trotter M, Peterson RR (1955): Ash weight of human skeletons in percent of their dry, fat-free weight. Anat Rec 123:341–358.

von Dobeln W (1964): Determination of body constituents. In Blix G (ed): "Occurrences, causes and prevention of overnutrition." Upsala: Almquist and Wiksell, pp 103–106.

Anthropometric Assessment
of Nutritional Status, pages 197–212

12
Anthropometric Assessment of Body Fat and Fatness

N.G. NORGAN
Department of Human Sciences, University of Technology, Loughborough, Leics. LE11 3TU, United Kingdom

INTRODUCTION

Disorders of energy nutrition are the primary nutritional problem in the world today. In the developed countries there is much concern about fatness, but for most, the concern is not overnutrition but the familiar, pervasive condition of chronic energy deficiency. Energy is stored in the body as fat, so a measure of body fat content is a measure of energy stores and of energy nutritional status. There is then a need for simple, valid, safe, and inexpensive measurements of body fat. Anthropometry is a family of related techniques that goes some way to meeting these requirements. It is becoming apparent that in addition to the amount of fat in the body, the location of the fat deposits may be a separate and additive risk to health and well-being. Thus, an assessment of body fat in the context of nutritional status should attempt to assess both the amount of fat and its location. This information should then be compared with reference data and, if necessary, remedial treatment instituted.

DESCRIPTIONS OF BODY FAT AND FATNESS

Fat is stored as triglyceride (tri-acylglycerol) in adipose tissue. The total body adipose tissue mass (TBAT) may be conveniently subdivided into the subcutaneous adipose tissue mass (SCAT) and the internal adipose tissue mass (IAT). SCAT is not uniformly distributed. It appears as discrete pads on the abdomen, over the iliac crest and sacrum, between the scapulae, on the inner thigh, and over the trochanter. Its distribution varies in the sexes, with men having greater proportions on the trunk and women greater proportions on the limbs. Several patterns of distribution of SCAT and of TBAT have been described, but interest is focussing on the internal:external distribution in the abdominal region.

Anthropometry is a dimensional approach which, in the first instance, describes adipose tissue mass. However, adipose tissue mass is not synonymous with fat mass as fat is a chemical entity, not an anatomical component. Fat has become the variable most often studied. It is important to distinguish between *body fat*, an amount of fat, and *body fatness*, a compositional description. The numerical and statistical properties of amounts (kg) differ from those of composition (proportion or percentage). Although the two are intercorrelated, $r = 0.7–0.8$, they each have some unique variation. As they may pose separate risks to health, it is important to distinguish between them. Here, body fat refers to fat mass (FM) and body fatness to percentage of the body weight as fat (%Fat). Some fat, the so-called essential fat, is located in muscle, the nervous system, bone marrow, and cell membranes, and women have sex-specific fat in the reproductive organs and breasts. However, these are not important as long-term energy stores and are not considered here.

PRINCIPLES OF THE ANTHROPOMETRIC ASSESSMENT OF BODY FAT AND FATNESS

The anthropometric assessment of body fat and fatness is based on the measurement of skinfold thicknesses, weight, stature, circumferences, and diameters. Anthropometry has only an indirect relationship with fat and fatness and these relationships must be established and validated. As there is no direct in vivo method for fat and fatness, a criterion method has to be identified. In the case of fatness, this is usually taken to be densitometry. The rationale of the method should be established. There should be a theoretical and not solely a random basis to the relationship. This should include the form of the relationship and the number and type of independent variables. In practice, the selection of the anthropometric variables has been left to statistical procedures such as stepwise multiple regression. The problems of replacing biological theory with statistical edict have been described by Jackson (1984). Newer methods of maximum R^2 improvement or ridge regressions are thought to provide more effective models (Mukherjee and Roche, 1984). Large sample sizes (>50–75) should be used with at least 30 subjects for each independent variable because small numbers render the selection to be based more on chance. Ideally, random sampling should be performed but this has yet to occur. Instead selection is made on criteria thought to be unrelated to body composition.

To assess the derived relationships several principles of cross-validation have been enunciated (Katch and Katch, 1980; Lohman, 1981; Jackson, 1984). The usual approach has been to examine the correlation between the criterion variable (F^c) and the anthropometric method (F^a). However, without random sampling the standard error of estimate (SEE) is a better statistic for comparing relationships. Nowadays, it is recommended to cross-validate the established relationships on a second independent sample. The measured and estimated fat indices are compared using the following statistics.

(1) The constant error = $(\bar{F}^c - \bar{F}^a)$, the mean difference between the two methods. (2) The correlation coefficient. (3) The standard deviations of the measured and estimated scores: These should be of a similar size; lower SD of F^a indicates that fatness is being underestimated in fat subjects and/or over-

estimated in the lean. (4) The standard error of estimate $= \sqrt[SD]{1 - r^2}$. (5) The total error $= \sqrt{\Sigma[(F^a - F^c)^2]/N}$ which combines the constant error and the SEE.

There is usually a fall in the estimation performance, lower r, higher SEE, of a relationship in cross-validation because of the inclusion of variables by capitalisation on chance. Ideally, the relationship should be validated on more than one group to establish its applicability, by careful cross-validation studies such as those of Thorland et al. (1984); Sinning and Wilson (1984); Sinning et al. (1985). A further test would be to use the method on the same group of subjects in different laboratories to establish the sources of technical or methodological variation and error.

ANTHROPOMETRIC ASSESSMENT OF BODY FAT AND FATNESS

Human beings differ from each other and vary throughout their life span so that the nature of the indirect relationships between anthropometry and fat and fatness also vary. The most appropriate method for assessing the fat content of an individual or group will depend on who is being measured and when. The measurement techniques of the anthropometric variables are not given here because full descriptions are available (Lohman et al., 1988). Techniques vary and the actual procedure used should always be described.

Assessment of Body Fat and Fatness Using Skinfold Thicknesses

A skinfold is a direct measure of SCAT and dermis thickness, and a series of representative skinfold measurements would characterise the average SCAT thickness and represent an estimate of SCAT mass. If the proportion of adipose tissue as fat and the proportion of fat situated subcutaneously are constant, then skinfold thicknesses should be good estimators of body fat.

Matiegka (1921) first proposed that body fat be calculated from the product of skinfolds, surface area, and derived constants in this way. The method has been neglected but was recently validated by cadaver dissections (Drinkwater et al., 1986). The problem is in establishing the constants and the error involved in the estimation of surface area. Katch et al. (1970) found that the approach provided estimates that agreed well with those from densitometry and other anthropometric approaches. Earlier, Chien et al. (1975) estimated SCAT and IAT mass from 10 skinfolds, surface area, and body density and showed that skinfolds were linearly related to FM. Our attempts, involving considerable refinement of previous methods, suggest this approach is unfruitful (Davies et al., 1986).

The dimensional approach has been less popular than the compositional approach. Skinfolds are most commonly used to estimate body density from which body fatness (%Fat) then fat content (FM) can be derived. The preference for compositional measures is because the relationship between the criterion variable and skinfold thicknesses can be established and tested. Before describing these, the assumptions involved should be examined more closely.

The assumptions. First, skinfold thicknesses are usually measured as a compressed double fold. Compression varies according to the site, sex, age, nutritional status, and even within groups homogeneous for these variables. Martin et al. (1985) regard compressibility as presenting the major problem since it is both large and difficult to predict. However, its true significance is not clear. Using ultrasound or radiographs to measure uncompressed SCAT has not been found to be superior to caliper measurements in the estimation of density (Sloan, 1967; Jones et al., 1986a) except in the obese (Kuczmarski et al., 1987). Second, a skinfold includes the dermis, and dermis thickness is neither negligible nor a constant fraction of the skinfold. This is not the major violation although its significance is unknown. Correcting readings for dermis thickness does not markedly increase the correlation with SCAT mass (Martin et al., 1985). Third, the sites selected for measurement may not represent the average SCAT thickness. However, skinfolds are highly intercorrelated and tend to behave as a single variable, measurements at one site providing a good estimator of thickness at others (Himes, 1980). Principal component analysis suggests most of the variation in multiple skinfolds can be accounted for by one component (Jackson and Pollock, 1976; Mueller and Reid, 1979). Fourth, the fat content of adipose tissue varies at different skinfold sites, according to weight and fat status and probably age and sex. Fifth, the ratio of internal to external fat varies, but without valid methods data is scarce and estimates show wide differences (Brown and Jones, 1977).

The effect of these variations will be to decrease the reliability, accuracy, and validity of skinfold thicknesses as estimators of body fat and fatness.

The relationships. Body density has been estimated from one to ten skinfolds. The SEE is not lowered to any marked extent by using three or more skinfolds, but to reduce the risk and effect of individual difference in fat patterning three to five are recommended. The skinfolds most often selected are the triceps and subscapular, and an abdominal site. The best combination has been suggested as triceps and thigh with chest and abdomen in young men and with suprailiac and subscapular in young women (Lohman, 1981). Data for other groups are lacking. The sum of the several skinfolds is a better estimator than the individual sites. Multico-linearity of skinfolds contributes to the specificity of equations as individual regression coefficients have large SEE and are unstable. Summing skinfolds reduces these effects.

The relationship between skinfolds and fat is, in theory, linear, but that with fatness is curvilinear; therefore logarithmic or quadratic transformation of the data is required. There is no real difference in the effects of these transformations on the correlation with density (Jackson and Pollock, 1978; Norgan and Ferro-Luzzi, 1985), but the quadratic form may perform better at the ends of the range (Jackson and Pollock, 1978).

The first equation to estimate fatness from skinfold thicknesses was that of Brozek and Keys (1951) using six skinfold thicknesses. A similar equation from Sloan (1967) using thigh and subscapular skinfolds has had some popularity. The most commonly used equations are however the logarithmic equations of Durnin and Womersley (1974) and the quadratic equations of Jackson, Pollock, and colleagues (Jackson and Pollock, 1978; Jackson et al., 1980).

Durnin and Womersley's equations were based on a sample of 481 British 16–72-year-olds, of a wide range of fatness, 5%–50% in males and 10%–61% in females. They take the form of body density = $c + b$.log (sum of skinfolds) and represent the first attempt to derive equations of general applicability. Separate equations are available for the sexes and the different age groups. The skinfolds used are biceps, triceps, subscapular, and suprailiac or some combination of these. The pooled SEE were 8.4 in men and 10.5 kg·m^{-3} in women, which are equivalent to ±3.5%Fat and ±5%Fat in two-thirds of the cases.

The equations of Jackson, Pollock, and colleagues were based on a large sample of 557 adults aged 18–61 years and with fatness ranging from 1%–33% for men, 4%–44% for women. They take the form

$$\text{body density} = c + b_1.(\text{sum of skinfolds}) + b_2.(\text{sum of skinfolds})^2 - b_3.(\text{age}).$$

The sum may be chest, axilla, triceps, subscapular, abdomen, suprailiac, and thigh or three of these: in men, chest, abdomen, and thigh; in women, triceps, suprailiac, and thigh. SEE were 7.7 and 8.3 kg·m^{-3} for men and women but were reduced if circumferences were added, 7.3 and 8.0 kg·m^{-3}. The equations were carefully cross-validated on 177 other subjects.

How accurate are the estimates? Lohman (1981) reviewed the literature and concluded that the pooled SEE of density from 35 samples was 7 kg·m^{-3} in young men and 9 kg·m^{-3} in other groups. An SEE of 7 kg·m^{-3} is equivalent to 3.1%Fat, or 2.2 kg FM. These SEE of density are close to the value expected (9.8 kg·m^{-3}) arising from biological and technical sources such as the measurement error of the skinfolds (0.5%), the variation in the relationship of a finite number of skinfolds to subcutaneous fat (1.8%), and the known variation in subcutaneous to total body fat (2.5%).

The error of the estimate is often expressed as %Fat, as above. This is a major source of confusion as the SEE of density is not the same as the total SEE of %Fat. The estimation of %Fat from density has an error arising from the variability in the composition of the fat-free mass, particularly the mineral and water content. Siri (1961) suggested this to be equivalent to less than 3.5%Fat in two-thirds of cases. Lohman (1981) suggested a figure of 2.7% in white college-aged men. Such variation is not well quantified in other groups such as women, children, the elderly, and patients. The total error, due to estimating density from skinfolds and %Fat from density, may be 4.6%Fat, assuming the errors to be independent and additive. Thus, biological variation in fat-free mass makes a significant contribution to the inaccuracy of assessing fatness.

Some of the error of estimate of density comes from the measurement of density itself. The precision of density measurement is probably 1.5–2.0

$kg \cdot m^{-3}$ (Lukaski, 1987a), but if residual volume is not measured directly it may be 3 $kg \cdot m^{-3}$. Jackson (1984) states that half of the inaccuracy of the estimation of density may be due to the original measurements of density.

These SEE may be low enough, and compare favourably with other methods, to be of practical value if the results can be applied to other samples. Jackson and Pollock's equations were carefully cross-validated, but usually equations have proved to be specific to the populations on which they were drawn up. There is a tendency for %Fat to be underestimated in the fat and overestimated in the lean. Specificity has technical and biological factors. The validity of anthropometric estimates of fat and fatness will be reduced if the measurement procedure differs from that in the original research. The methodological problems in skinfold measurement have been discussed (Himes, 1980; Lohman, 1981; Pollock and Jackson, 1984; Lohman et al., 1988). Variations in measurement techniques can be an important factor, but a major influence has been poor statistical criteria (Jackson, 1984). Much of the variability in the biological factors are associated with age, gender, fitness, and fatness.

A further difficulty is that there has been disquiet about "gold standard" criterion methods for some time (Wilmore, 1983; Ross et al., 1986). There is a move away from two-compartment models of body composition to multicompartment models using density, body water, and mineral (Lohman, 1984). Equations relating anthropometry to %Fat determined from several measures of body composition may have lower SEE as well as increased general validity.

In general, Jackson and Pollock's equations seem to perform well enough in groups of similar characteristics, although this is not always so (Norgan and Ferro-Luzzi, 1985). For groups such as athletes, the equations may require adjustment or population-specific equations be used. There are in the literature equations with lower SEE, but low SEE should not be the sole basis for selecting an equation. Many equations have not been cross-validated and fail to perform well in other groups. Equations should only be applied to groups of similar age, gender, fatness, and probably nutritional status too and, if possible, only after validation on a sample using the principles described earlier.

Using Skinfold Thicknesses Themselves as Proxies for Fatness

In view of the errors and limitations of the assessment of fat and fatness, several authors propose that accurate estimates of body composition of an individual are not possible and that the skinfold thicknesses themselves be used (Johnston, 1982; Martin et al., 1985). There is considerable merit in this suggestion, particularly for children, women, and the elderly. Skinfolds may be compared with reference centiles cross-sectionally or longitudinally, in the same way as height or weight. The O-scale system of Ross and Ward (1984) derives an adiposity rating from six skinfolds and centile data. In its short form, it includes a rating of proportional weight as fatness and leanness which may change to different degrees.

Skinfolds do not increase progressively with age during growth. They show gains and losses at times when FM may be increasing progressively. It might be expected that SCAT areas would provide a better estimate of fatness than skinfolds, but this has not proved to be the case (Himes et al., 1980; Norgan and Ferro-Luzzi, 1985). Fat areas explain 13% more of the variance in FM than skinfolds, but no more of %Fat.

The validity of skinfolds alone as indicators of nutritional status is considered in Chapter 7 this volume.

Circumferences

The theoretical and empirical validity of circumferences as estimators of body composition have been considered by Wilmore and Behnke (1974) and cross-validation has been investigated (Sinning and Hackney, 1985). Problems with the repeatability of skinfold thickness measurements, the training required, and the assumptions made in interpreting them have led to the suggestion that circumferences, being more repeatable, may be better for estimating body fat and fatness.

Circumferences do indeed seem to be more repeatable (Mueller and Malina, 1987), but there is little difference in SEE from skinfolds alone or several circumferences alone (Katch and McArdle, 1973; Lohman, 1988). Jackson and Pollock (1976) suggest a circumference may be less useful as it represents both fatness and leanness. One way over this may be to use two girths, one limb girth as a suppressor variable to eliminate the lean weight from the other (Jackson, 1984).

The effect of the addition of frame size (skeletal breadth) is variable. They do not appear in the equations for children but do for women, and less frequently for men (Roche, 1984).

The place of circumferences is in combination with skinfolds and breadths. Equations with all three types of measurement show a decrease in SEE, especially in women and middle-aged men (Pollock and Jackson, 1984; Lohman, 1988), in some studies but not in others (Womersley and Durnin, 1977; Norgan and Ferro-Luzzi, 1985). It is not yet possible to state the ideal set of measurements. The successfully validated equations of Jackson and Pollock have waist and forearm girth in men and gluteal circumference in women.

Weight and Stature

Weight and stature were the earliest and simplest anthropometric measurements used in the assessment of nutritional status and body fatness. Relative weight or weight for stature have in the past been keystones. Nowadays, weight and stature are most commonly used as indicators of fatness in the form of indices of W/S^n where n is usually taken as 2. The exponent chosen is that with the highest correlation with a measure of fatness and the lowest correlation with stature. The advantage of W/S^n over the computationally simpler W/S^2 is small. The index explains about half the variation in %Fat of population groups but is more highly correlated with FM (r = 0.88) than %Fat (r = 0.75) (Norgan and Ferro-Luzzi, 1982). It estimates %Fat less well than skinfolds although this is not always the case (Roche et al., 1981) particularly in the elderly (Womersley and Durnin, 1977). Its performance can be improved by allowing for age (Norgan and Ferro-Luzzi, 1982) and gender, but not for frame size (Roche, 1984). W/S^2 or body mass index has become the measurement of overweight and obesity of the epidemiologist and in the clinical context. It is simpler and thought to be more objective than skinfolds, particularly in the obese. However, it does not separate the moderately obese from the muscular individual, nor does it take into account the changing composition with age. It does, however, have the advantage of having been related to morbidity and mortality data, while measurements of fatness have not.

Comparison of Methods

The correlations of anthropometric variables with density are of the order of -0.6 for weight, -0.7 for W/S^2, -0.8 for skinfolds, and some -0.85 for skinfolds, circumferences, and diameters (Himes, 1980; Garrow, 1983; Pollock and Jackson, 1984). The associated SEE might be 12–14, 11–13, 9–10, and 8–9 $kg{\cdot}m^{-3}$. Thus the extent of the improvement by the more comprehensive or sophisticated measurements is not marked. In children and groups other than young adult men and women, the SEE may be higher. These cases should be considered.

Assessment of Body Fat and Fatness in Other Groups

The methods described above rest on assumptions about the relationship between the anthropometric method and a criterion variable, its relationship with fat or fatness, and a constancy in these relationships. In children, the elderly, and patients, or with changing nutritional states, where assessments are most often made, the relationships vary.

Children and growth. It has been appreciated for many years that the model of body composition of two compartments of fixed composition did not hold in children. During growth there is a fall in the proportion of water and an increase in the proportion of the other constituents, particularly minerals. With higher water and lower mineral contents the density of the FFM (fat-free mass) is lower with the result that adult equations overestimate fatness. Lohman (1986) has suggested values for density of FFM in boys and girls of different ages from which equations to estimate fatness and fat content can be derived from densitometry or other body composition techniques. Until recently, problems arose because equations were drawn up on heterogeneous groups of prepubescent, pubescent, and postpubescent subjects and few were cross-validated. Boileau et al. (1985) published quadratic equations for estimating %Fat from sum of triceps and subscapular skinfolds based on %Fat calculated from density, water, and forearm bone mineral measurements. These have been applied successfully to other groups (Lohman, 1986) and hence represent the best available method. Johnston et al. (1982) published equations for 12–17-year-olds with standard deviations of the errors of estimate of 2.1 kg of fat in females and 3.3 in males. For individuals, estimates may be expected to have errors of ± 5–6 kg (i.e., 2 SD), illustrating the difficulty of applying equations to individuals.

The value of the body mass index (BMI) as an estimate of body fat content or fatness in childhood is not established. Certainly, the rationale is not the same as for adults. In prepubescent children BMI is not independent of height. The obese are frequently taller than the nonobese, and after puberty, the correlation of fatness and BMI may be negative. There are good reference data for stature, weight, arm circumferences, and triceps and subscapular skinfolds for children, and these are likely to remain the common measures of nutritional status.

The elderly. With aging, the density of bone decreases as does the proportion of body potassium and muscle mass with the result that FFM is of lower density. Skinfolds are more compressible so that estimates of body fat are apt to be low. All the evidence is that estimates of criterion variables and of body fat and fatness are less reliable in the elderly. Womersley and Durnin (1977) found skinfolds to be no better than W/S^n in women over 30 years and to have higher SEE in women 40–68 years. Similarly, Jackson et al. (1980) found SEE to rise in women over 40 years. Lohman (1981) reports a pooled SEE of density from skinfolds in three studies of middle-aged women to be 10.8 $kg{\cdot}m^{-3}$. These are not elderly subjects, but the trend is illustrated.

The obese. The estimation procedures described cannot be expected to estimate body composition well at the extremes of the population. Even though efforts were made by the investigators to get wide ranges, the numbers of obese subjects are small. Further errors arise because skinfolds may be difficult to measure in the obese, and weight gain changes the composition of the FFM and the relationship between the criterion variable and fatness. The accentuated limitations of skinfold measurements in the obese have been listed by Kuczmarski et al. (1987) and Bray and Gray (1988).

Quetlet's index, W/S^2, kg m^{-2}, has been a key index in the assessment of obesity in population groups. The ranges of W/S^2 associated with minimum, increased, and markedly increased mortality and morbidity have been identified and used in the management and treatment of obesity (Garrow, 1981).

Bray and Gray (1988) recommend circumferences rather than skinfolds as intra- and interobserver variability are less, and circumferences can be measured in all subjects but skinfolds cannot. Weltman et al. (1987) have produced validated equations from mean abdominal circumference in obese men. SEE were 2.9%Fat and 2.9 kg FM. The correlations were low, reflecting the curtailed ranges of specific groups.

Changing nutritional status. In clinical settings and exercise programmes, it may be more important to assess accurately the change in body fat or composition than the absolute levels. Many of the changes are small compared with the error of the method and may be preceded by changes in clinical signs. Cohn et al. (1981) found estimates of fat from skinfolds to be much lower than those from body potassium, body water, body density, or body nitrogen and to be poorly correlated with fat from the other methods in cancer patients. Burkinshaw (1982) reports that the precision of the measurement of skinfold thicknesses and the accuracy of estimation of body composition using standard estimation procedures were as good in surgical patients as in healthy controls; this may not hold for wasted or edematous patients. With only short-term changes in fat content, estimates from skinfold thickness have a precision of 0.8 kg FM and have been shown to out-perform more sophisticated isotopic methods (Almond et al., 1984).

Other ethnic groups. The density of FFM is greater in blacks than in whites due in part to the denser, heavier skeletal mass. Hugg et al. (1982) however found reasonable concordance between observed and predicted densities from equations developed on white subjects in nonathletic, college-aged black men. This is unexpected in the light of fat-patterning differences between ethnic groups. Jones et al. (1976) found differences in the relationships between skinfolds and density for Europeans and Indians. Durnin and Womersley's equations have been applied with some success to Papua New Guineans (Norgan, 1982). Given that many of these subjects are at the end of the range for fatness, it is to be expected that estimation will be less accurate. This will apply to other lean groups such as athletes.

Athletes. Physical performance is closely related to body composition in many sports, and there have been many studies of athletes. Most of the conclusions are not directly relevant to the assessment of nutritional status, although athletes are not without their nutritional problems. However, athletes have been the subjects in some of the larger and better cross-validation surveys (Thorland et al., 1984; Sinning and Wilson, 1984; Sinning et al., 1985). These results suggest that in athletes and possibly other lean subjects, the quadratic equations are more generalised than the log or linear equations. Given the limited age and density range in the studies, the advantage may be greater than it appears. In the meantime, the fact that some linear equations performed well, e.g., Sloan's equation in men, and some quadratic equations did less well, e.g., that used by Jackson et al. with three skinfolds in women, suggests that further cross-validation studies along the lines of these exemplary studies, including other groups in the population, are required.

Conclusions and Recommendations

Why do we want to estimate body fat and fatness? Is the information more useful than simple measures of adiposity? Garrow (1981) suggests that a convenient, valid method for measuring fatness would not immediately replace the body mass index in the field of obesity, as the hazards of obesity are linked to weight-for-height data but not yet to fatness. Also, some of the differences in errors of the different methods may be only 1%–2%Fat, and there is no evidence relating such small differences to morbidity and mortality. However, fatness data are being included in prospective mortality studies and are proving to be a better risk factor than relative weight. Roche et al. (1981) suggest that both fatness and fat content be graded as there may be separate associations between each and disease, social effects, and performance.

Many of the methods described give estimates that are accurate for the population but not for the individual. This is unfortunate as in the assessment of nutritional status the focus is usually on the individual. In young adults, middle-aged men, and possibly women and youths too, density, %Fat and FM can be estimated with an acceptable error of estimate from quadratic or logarithmic equations using the sum of three or more skinfolds. Alternatively, because density is estimated more accurately than %Fat and FM and sources of reference data of unselected populations have been identified (Roche, 1984), density itself may be utilised as a measure of fatness. In infants, young children, and the elderly, it is inadvisable to estimate %Fat and FM from skinfolds or W/S^2. Instead, the simple indices can be used directly. Roche et al. (1981) suggest that triceps skinfold be used to grade %Fat from limited data except for men where W/S^2 performs better. To grade FM, W/S^2 can be used except in boys, where subscapular skinfold is better. Individual data can be compared with reference data from national surveys and a percentile rank used to grade fatness.

Advances in research design and statistical analysis have allowed progress in developing general equations for estimating body density. The improvement has not been in the accuracy of estimating %Fat but in widening the applicability of the general equations. It is becoming clearer which equations best estimate fatness. In the future, fewer equations will be used, but these will be better equations. Even so, some populations, e.g., athletes and patients, may require individual equations, but these too must be cross-validated. A significant increase in the validity of estimates of fatness will come when anthropometric variables are related to %Fat and FM derived from multicomponent models of body composition incorporating estimates of body density, total body water, and mineral.

New anthropometric techniques, in the classical sense of the term anthropometry, may not be forthcoming in the field of body composition. However, other techniques with related characteristics of simplicity, cheapness, acceptability, etc. have been developed, e.g., bioelectrical impedance analysis (Lukaski, 1987b). The application of validation principles established over the years for anthropometry will benefit the newer methodology.

ANTHROPOMETRIC ASSESSMENT OF FAT DISTRIBUTION AND FAT PATTERNING

The terms *distribution* and *patterning* are used synonymously, but there is much to be said for adopting the convention that fat distribution is used for binary or trinary comparisons of anatomically distinct regions and fat patterning is reserved for recognisable configurations of a large array of standardised fat thicknesses.

Fat distribution and patterning can be described in two ways: There is subcutaneous fat patterning, the distribution of fat on the surface and the internal: external distribution. In addition, fat patterning may be absolute, what is seen and measured, or relative, a current pattern that appears after differences due to the amount of fat at each site have been removed mathematically. The absolute fat pattern varies with the amount of subcutaneous fat and is, in this respect, obviously linked to nutritional status. The relative fat pattern is regarded as independent of level of fatness, perhaps more determined by genetic factors and less affected by environmental factors. As the separate risks to health of the two types are only beginning to be described, the assessment of both types is described and to be recommended.

Subcutaneous Fat Distribution and Patterning

Absolute fat distribution and patterning. This is commonly described by a ratio of two skinfolds to compare the fat distribution of two areas, e.g., subscapular:triceps, trunk:limb distribution. This method is popular because of its simplicity, but it is important to include a lower leg site (Kaplowitz et al., 1987). Single sites may not, however, adequately characterise a limb or segment, and the use of ratios is confusing. Taking several skinfolds in each region overcomes this problem, but the expression of the data is complex and usually takes the form of graphical profiles, which are difficult to compare, or a ratio of sum of trunk skinfolds to limb skinfolds, which results in a loss of information.

Relative fat distribution and patterning. Standardisation of skinfolds, giving each an equal weighting independently of size, i.e., fatness, can be achieved by Z-scoring (Norgan and Ferro-Luzzi, 1986). With several skinfolds, multivariate analysis such as principal component analysis (Mueller and Reid, 1979) has consistently enabled centripetal fat patterning to be described (Baumgartner et al., 1986). This method also identifies a universal component of fatness and allows calculation of individual component scores from which age and sex differences in fat patterning have been described (Norgan, 1987a).

The pioneering work of Vague (1956) provides an ancestry to the study of fat distribution and patterning and disease. His indices of masculine differentation and brachio:femoral adipo:muscular ratio have not proved popular. Several of the skinfold sites are difficult to measure and have poor repeatability. Much of his work was on the obese and diabetic, and its relevance to populations as opposed to patients is not known.

Although there is much evidence linking subcutaneous fat distribution and patterning to disease or risk of disease, most interest in this area is in the internal:external fat distribution.

Internal:External Fat Distribution

The recent evidence that waist:hip circumference ratio (WHC ratio) is a strong predictor of subsequent mortality in men and women and the observation of metabolic differences in adipocytes from different regions have led to increased interest in the internal:external fat distribution, and the intra-abdominal fat. The rationale of the WHC ratio as a measure of internal:external fat distribution is that the waist circumference is correlated with abdominal fatness and metabolic complications. The waist circumference is size dependent so the ratio of waist:hip is used to correct for body size. Reference data on WHC ratio of men are available (Jones et al., 1986b). Waist:thigh ratio is an alternative index, but the measurement of thigh circumference may be less acceptable to women. However, the precision can be expected to be higher, and waist:thigh circumference ratio is a better estimator of abdominal fatness in women than WHC ratio (Seidell et al., 1987).

How well does the WHC ratio assess intra-abdominal fat? Ashwell et al. (1985) found a significant correlation between the ratio and the proportion of intra-abdominal fat in computed tomography scans at the level of the umbilicus (L4) in women. However, this explained only 37% of the variance. Seidell et al. (1987) have developed multiple regression equations which allow the estimation of intra-abdominal and subcutaneous abdominal adipose tissue areas from circumferences, skinfolds, body mass index (W/S^2) and age. R^2 ranged from 0.79 to 0.84. The criterion method was computed tomography. Sjöström et al. (1985) have put forward equations for calculating visceral adipose tissue volumes from transverse and sagittal diameters of the body at the lumbar 4–5 level in women and from diameters plus skinfolds in men.

The anthropometric estimation of intra-abdominal adipose tissue contains all the drawbacks and sources of error found in the assessment of body fatness. There will be no simple procedure of general validity for estimating fat distribution and patterning. The experiences gained in the body composition field provide lessons for those working on fat patterning and distribution (Norgan, 1987b).

REFERENCES

Almond DJ, King RFGJ, Burkinshaw L, Oxby CB, McMahon MJ (1984): Measurement of short-term changes in the fat content of the body: A comparison of three methods in patients receiving intravenous nutrition. Br J Nutr 52:215–225.

Ashwell M, Cole TJ, Dixon AK (1985): Obesity: New insight into the anthropometric classification of fat distribution shown by computed tomography. Br Med J 290:1692–1694.

Baumgartner RN, Roche AF, Guo S, Lohman TG, Boileau RA, Slaughter MH (1986): Adipose tissue distribution: The stability of principal components by sex, ethnicity and maturation stage. Hum Biol 58:719–735.

Boileau RA, Lohman TG, Slaughter MH (1985): Exercise and body composition of children and growth. Scand J Sports Sci 7:17–27.

Bray GA, Gray DJ (1988): Anthropometric measurements in the obese. In Lohman et al. (eds): "Anthropometric Standardization Reference Manual." Champaign, Ill: Human Kinetics, pp 131–136.

Brown WJ, Jones PRM (1977): The distribution of body fat in relation to habitual activity. Ann Hum Biol 4:537–550.

Brozek J, Keys A (1951): The evaluation of leanness–fatness in Man: Norms and interrelationships. Br J Nutr 5:194–206.

Burkinshaw L (1982): Measurement of human body composition in vivo. In Orton CG (ed): "Progress in Medical Physics, Vol 2." New York: Plenum Press, pp 113–137.

Chien S, Peng MT, Chen KP, Huang TF, Chang C, Fang HS (1975): Longitudinal studies on adipose tissue and its distribution in human subjects. J Appl Physiol 39:825–830.

Cohn SH, Ellis KJ, Vartsky D, Sawitsky A, Gartenhaus W, Yasumura S, Vaswani AN (1981): Comparison of methods of estimating body fat in normal subjects and cancer patients. Am J Clin Nutr 34:2839–2847.

Davies PSW, Jones PRM, Norgan NG (1986): The distribution of subcutaneous and internal fat in man. Ann Hum Biol 13:189–192.

Drinkwater DT, Martin AD, Ross WD, Clarys JP (1986): Validation by cadaver dissection of Matiegka's equations for the anthropometric estimations of anatomical body composition in adult humans. In Day JA (ed): "Perspectives in Kinanthropometry." Champaign, Ill: Human Kinetics, pp 221–227.

Durnin JVGA, Womersley J (1974): Body fat assessed from total body density and its estimation from skinfold thickness: Measurements on 481 men and women aged from 16 to 72 years. Br J Nutr 32:77–97.

Garrow JS (1981): "Treating Obesity Seriously: A Clinical Manual." Edinburgh: Churchill Livingstone.

Garrow JS (1983): Indices of adiposity. Nutr Abstr Rev 53:697–708.

Himes JH (1980): Subcutaneous fat thickness as an indicator of nutritional status. In Greene LS, Johnston FE (eds): "Social and Biological Predictors of Nutritional Status, Physical Growth and Neurological Development." New York: Academic Press, pp 9–32.

Himes JH, Roche AF, Webb P (1980): Fat areas as estimates of total body fat. Am J Clin Nutr 33:2093–2100.

Hugg JE, Schutte EJ, Townsend EJ, Blomquist CG, Malina RM (1982): Prediction of body density from skinfold data on young Black males. Am J Phys Anthropol 52:197–198.

Jackson AS (1984): Research design and analysis of data procedures for predicting body density. Med Sci Sports Exerc 16:616–620.

Jackson AS, Pollock ML (1976): Factor analysis and multivariate scaling of anthropometric variables for the assessment of body composition. Med Sci Sports 8:196–203.

Jackson AS, Pollock ML (1978): Generalised equations for predicting body density in men. Br J Nutr 40:497–504.

Jackson AS, Pollock ML, Ward A (1980): Generalised equations for predicting body density of women. Med Sci Sports Exerc 12:175–182.

Johnston FE (1982): Relationships between body composition and anthropometry. Hum Biol 54:221–245.

Johnston FE, Paolone AN, Taylor HL, Schell LM (1982): The relationship of body fat weight, determined densitometrically, to relative weight and triceps skinfold in American youths, 12–17 years of age. Am J Phys Anthropol 57:1–6.

Jones PRM, Bharadwaj H, Bhatia MR, Malhotra MS (1976): Differences between ethnic groups in the relationship of skinfold thicknesses to body density. In Bhatia B, Chhina GS, Singh B (eds): New Delhi: Inter Print, pp 373–376.

Jones PRM, Davies PSW, Norgan NG (1986a): Ultrasonic measurements of subcutaneous adipose tissue thickness in Man. Am J Phys Anthropol 71:359–362.

Jones PRM, Hunt MJ, Norgan NG, Brown TP (1986b): Waist–hip circumference ratio and its relation to age and overweight in British men. Hum Nutr: Clin Nutr 40C:239–247.

Kaplowitz HJ, Mueller WH, Selwyn BJ, Malina RM, Bailey DA, Mirwald RL (1987): Sensitivities, specifities, and positive predictive values of simple indices of body fat distribution. Hum Biol 59:809–825.

Katch FI, Behnke AR, Katch VL (1979): Estimation of body fat from skinfolds and surface area. Hum Biol 51:411–424.
Katch FI, Katch VL (1980): Measurement and prediction errors in body composition assessment and the search for the perfect prediction equation. Res Q Exerc Sports 51:249–260.
Katch FI, McArdle WD (1973): Prediction of body density from simple anthropometric measurements in college-age men and women. Hum Biol 45:445–454.
Kuczmarski RJ, Fanelli MT, Koch GG (1987): Ultrasonic assessment of body composition in obese adults: Overcoming the limitations of the skinfold caliper. Am J Clin Nutr 45:417–724.
Lohman TG (1981): Skinfolds and body density and their relation to body fatness: A review. Hum Biol 53:181–225.
Lohman TG (1984): Research progress in validation of laboratory methods of assessing body composition. Med Sci Sports Exerc 16:596–603.
Lohman TG (1986): Applicability of body composition techniques and constants for children and youths. Exerc Sports Sci Rev 14:325–357.
Lohman TG (1988): Anthropometry and body composition. In Lohman et al. (eds): "Anthropometric Standardization Reference Manual." Champaign, Ill: Human Kinetics, pp 125–129.
Lohman TG, Roche AF, Martorell M (1988): "Anthropometric Standardization Reference Manual." Champaign, Ill: Human Kinetics.
Lukaski HC (1987a): Methods for the assessment of human body composition: Traditional and new. Am J Clin Nutr 46:537–556.
Lukaski HC (1987b): Use of the tetrapolar bio-electrical impedance method to assess human body composition. In Norgan NG (ed): "Human Body Composition and Fat Distribution." Wageningen, Holland: Euro-Nut, pp 143–155.
Martin AD, Ross WD, Drinkwater DT, Clarys JP (1985): Prediction of body fat by skinfold caliper: Assumptions and cadaver evidence. Int J Obes 9(suppl 1):31–39.
Matiegka J (1921): The testing of physical efficiency. Am J Phys Anthropol 4:223–230.
Mueller WH, Malina RM (1987): Relative reliability of circumferences and skinfolds as measures of body fat distribution. Am J Phys Anthropol 72:437.
Mueller WH, Reid RM (1979): A multivariate analysis of fatness and relative fat patterning. Am J Phys Anthropol 50:199–208.
Mukherjee D, Roche AF (1984): The estimation of percent body fat, body density and total body fat by maximum R^2 regression equations. Hum Biol 56:79–109.
Norgan NG (1982): Human energy stores. In Harrison GA (ed): "Energy and Effort." London: Taylor and Francis, pp 139–158.
Norgan NG (1987a): Fat patterning in Papua New Guineans: Effects of age, sex and acculturation. Am J Phys Anthropol 74:385–392.
Norgan NG (ed) (1987b): "Human Body Composition and Fat Patterning. Euro-Nut Report No. 8." Wageningen, Holland: Euro-Nut.
Norgan NG, Ferro-Luzzi A (1982): Weight–height indices as estimators of fatness in men. Hum Nutr:Clin Nutr 36C:363–372.
Norgan NG, Ferro-Luzzi A (1985): The estimation of body density in men: Are general equations general? Ann Hum Biol 12:1–15.
Norgan NG, Ferro-Luzzi A (1986): Simple indices of subcutaneous fat patterning. Ecol Food Nutr 18:117–123.
Pollock ML, Jackson AS (1984): Research progress in validation of clinical methods of assessing body composition. Med Sci Sports Exerc 16:606–613.

Roche AF (1984): Anthropometric methods: New and old, what they tell us. Int J Obes 8:509–523.
Roche AF, Siervogel RM, Chumlea WC, Webb P (1981): Grading body fatness from limited anthropometric data. Am J Clin Nutr 34:2831–2838.
Ross WD, Eiben OG, Ward R, Martin AD, Drinkwater DT, Clarys JP (1986): Alternatives for the conventional methods of human body composition and physique assessment. In Day JA (ed): "Perspectives in Kinanthropometry." Champaign, Ill: Human Kinetics, pp 203–220.
Ross WD, Ward R (1984): "The O-Scale System." Vancouver, B.C.: Rosscraft.
Seidell JC, Oosterlee A, Thijssen MAO, Burema J, Deurenberg P, Hautvast JGAJ, Ruijs JHJ (1987): Assessment of intra-abdominal and subcutaneous abdominal fat: Relation between anthropometry and computed tomography. Am J Clin Nutr 45:7–13.
Sinning WE, Dolny DG, Little KD, Cunningham LN, Racaniello A, Siconolfi SF, Sholes JL (1985): Validity of 'generalised' equations for body composition analysis in male athletes. Med Sci Sports Exerc 17:124–130.
Sinning WE, Hackney AC (1985): Body composition estimated by girths and skeletal dimensions in male and female athletes. In Day JA (ed): "Perspectives in Kinanthropometry." Champaign, Ill: Human Kinetics, pp 239–244.
Sinning WE, Wilson JR (1984): Validity of 'generalised' equations for body composition analysis in women athletes. Res Q Exerc Sports 55:153–160.
Siri WF (1961): Body composition from fluid spaces and density: Analysis of methods. In Brozek J, Henschel A (eds): "Techniques for Measuring Body Composition." Washington, DC: National Academy of Sciences, pp 223–243.
Sjöström L, Kvist H, Tylen K (1985): Methodological aspects of measurements of adipose tissue distribution. In Vague J, Bjorntorp P, Guy-Grand B, Rebuffe-Scrive M, Vague P (eds): "Metabolic Complications of Human Obesities." Amsterdam: Excerpta Medica, pp 13–19.
Sloan AW (1967): Estimation of body fat in young men. J Appl Physiol 23:311–315.
Thorland WG, Johnson GO, Tharp JD, Fagot TG, Hammer RW (1984): Validity of anthropometric equations for the estimation of body density in adolescent athletes. Med Sci Sports Exerc 16:77–81.
Vague J (1956): The degree of masculine differentiation of obesities: A factor determining predisposition to diabetes, atherosclerosis, gout, and uric acid calculous disease. Am J Clin Nutr 4:20–34.
Weltman A, Seip RL, Tran ZV (1987): Practical assessment of body composition in adult obese males. Hum Biol 59:523–535.
Wilmore JH (1983): Body composition in sport and exercise: Directions for future research. Med Sci Sports Exerc 15:21–31.
Wilmore JH, Behnke AR (1974): "Evaluation and Regulation of Body Build and Composition." Englewood Cliffs, NJ: Prentice-Hall, pp 53–81.
Womersley J, Durnin JVGA (1977): A comparison of the skinfold method with extent of 'overweight' and various weight–height relationships in the assessment of obesity. Br J Nutr 38:271–284.

Anthropometric Assessment
of Nutritional Status, pages 213–231

13
Genetic Aspects of Anthropometric Dimensions Relevant to Assessment of Nutritional Status

CLAUDE BOUCHARD
Physical Activity Sciences Laboratory, Laval University, Ste-Foy, Québec G1K 7P4, Canada

INTRODUCTION

This chapter deals with the role of genotype in the variation observed in anthropometric dimensions that are thought to be useful in the assessment of nutritional status. We know that bone, skeletal muscle, and adipose tissue, among other tissues, can be greatly affected by long-term exposure to nutritional stresses such as undernutrition or excess energy intake. Some characteristics of these tissues can be directly measured by the appropriate anthropometric measurements. Others can only be indirectly assessed through anthropometric techniques, but it may be sufficient to allow for rapid diagnosis and for prescription of a treatment, particularly under field conditions.

In addition to the proper equipment, the use of a good measurement methodology, and the availability of relevant reference values, the use of anthropometric dimensions in the assessment of nutritional status requires an understanding of the potential sources of variation. One has to be aware, of course, of the sources of error variance pertaining to these measurements. But, perhaps more important, the user should be familiar with the variety of factors that may contribute to intraindividual and interindividual differences over time in anthropometric phenotypes. These factors include age, gender, maturity status during the growing years, energy intake, nutrient intake and absorption, habitual energy expenditure, level of physical activity, climate, various diseases, and others. In addition, one must recognize that anthropometric phenotypes are also influenced by the genotype of the individual, perhaps in many ways.

The fact that anthropometric phenotypes can be influenced by a variety of factors plus their quantitative nature imposes some special constraints on the study of their genetically determined variation. By definition, an anthropometric phenotype is measured on a continuous metric scale, and its variation, in any given individual, is the result of a complex network of interactions, some dependent, others independent of the genotype. Such phenotypes are usually referred to as *multifactorial traits*, and their genetic analysis requires some special study designs and analytical strategies. They will be briefly described in the next section. This chapter will focus on the genetics of height, weight, body mass index (BMI), bone length, bone breadth, skinfold thicknesses, fat mass, fat-free mass, estimated muscle size in limbs, and physique.

VARIOUS GENETIC EFFECTS FOR A MULTIFACTORIAL PHENOTYPE

The multifactorial anthropometric phenotype can in theory be affected by an array of genetic and nongenetic sources of variation. Some of these sources are listed in Table 1. In this chapter, our interest lies primarily in the additive genetic effect, i.e., the heritability, of the anthropometric phenotype. However, it is also quite informative to have data on other kinds of genetic effects: maternal or paternal effect, X-linked or Y-linked effect, sex-limited effect, major gene effect or genetic pleiotropism within a given tissue (e.g., bones). Unfortunately, these other genetic effects have not been studied systematically for the anthropometric phenotypes. Often these other genetic effects may turn out to be components of the additive genetic effect per se.

Variation in a given anthropometric phenotype *(P)* can be described in terms of the major components of the following equation (Bouchard, 1986, 1987, 1988):

$$P = G + E + G \times E + e$$

in which G represents the additive genetic effect, E the environmental and lifestyle influences, $G \times E$ the genotype–environment or lifestyle interaction

TABLE 1. Potential Sources of Variation for an Anthropometric Phenotype Measured at a Given Age

Category	Source of variation
Genetic	Additive genetic effect
	Nonadditive genetic effect
	Paternal or maternal genetic effect
	X-linked or Y-linked effect
	Sex-limited effect
	Major gene effect
	Genetic pleiotropism
Nongenetic	Measurement error
	Nutritional status
	Physical activity level
	Disease state (or past diseases)
	Age or maturity status
	Gender
Interaction between the genotype and the nongenetic conditions.	

effect, and e the sources of error. The G effect is generally obtained from one of three types of study design: a familial, a twin or an adoption study design. As a rule, these studies assume that $e = G \times E = 0$. In other words, the situation illustrated in Figure 1 is assumed to prevail, and variations in P are ascribed to linear and additive effects of G and E.

Under these circumstances, the G effect is thought to represent the extent of the additive genetic effect in the total P variance. The G effect is therefore a population parameter expressing the relative contribution of genetic variation to the interindividual differences seen for P under the average environment (nongenetic) conditions. The knowledge of G for a given anthropometric P has no predictive value as to the genetic characteristics of a given individual.

An acceptable estimate of the G effect for a given anthropometric phenotype requires a complex data base and is not a simple task. Ideally, one would like to have data on all types of two- and three-generation relatives including adoption data, twins reared together and apart, and families of identical twins. Large sample sizes would be desirable in order to obtain reliable estimates of G and other parameters. Needless to say, data currently available seldom meet these stringent requirements and, thus, any estimates of heritability for anthropometric phenotypes must be viewed with caution. In practice, we find in the literature mainly correlation data among relatives from one of the study de-

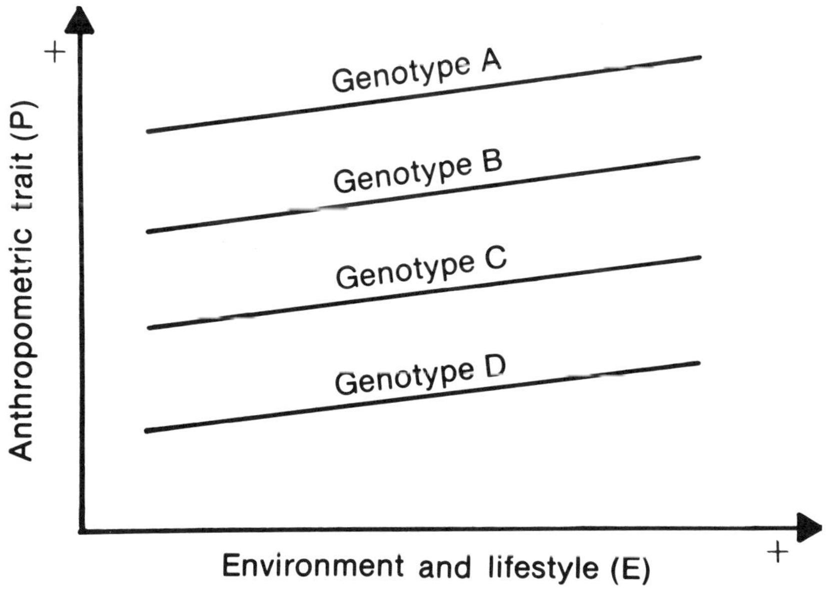

Fig. 1. Variation in a given anthropometric measurement (P) when $G \times E = e = 0$. In the present case, $P = G + E$. (Reproduced from Bouchard, 1988, with permission of the publisher.)

signs identified above, with little based on more recent methods from the field of genetic epidemiology (Bouchard and Pérusse, 1988).

We have, however, shown that the assumption that $G \times E = 0$ was seldom met for a series of phenotypes presenting a relationship with nutritional status (Bouchard, 1987; Bouchard and Tremblay, 1985; Poehlman et al., 1986). Figure 2 describes a situation that is probably closer to reality (Bouchard, 1988). In this case, changes in P associated with variation in E are not identical for all genotypes. In other words, the response of the anthropometric phenotype to alterations in nutritional status are not always predictable and are determined, to a certain extent, by the genetic characteristics of the individual.

The remaining sections of the chapter will summarize some of the published and unpublished data concerning, first, the heritability of anthropometric phenotypes and, second, the presence or absence of a $G \times E$ effect for the same traits.

HERITABILITY OF ANTHROPOMETRIC DIMENSIONS

Height, Weight, and BMI

Studies have consistently demonstrated that, although human stature is mainly determined by genotype, it remains susceptible to environmental influences, especially malnutrition. Reviewing the early twin studies of Dahlberg

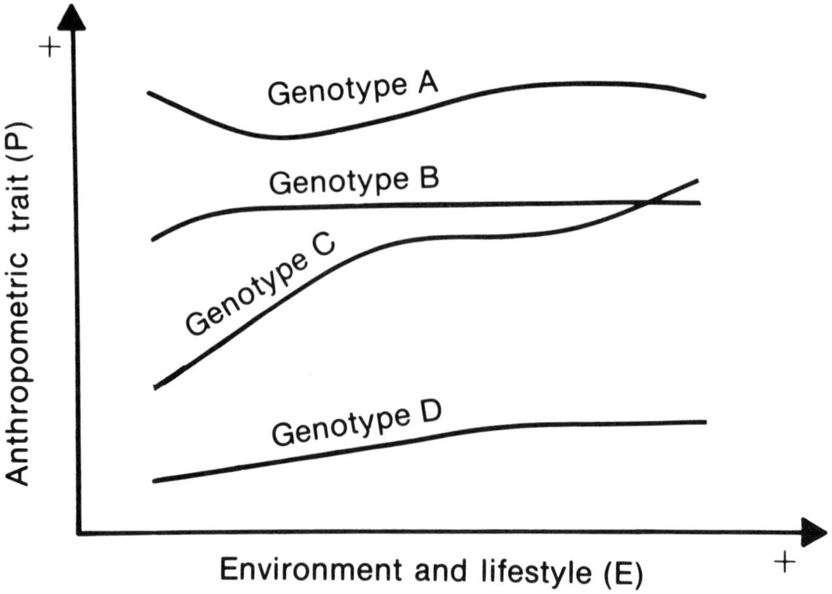

Fig. 2. Variation in a given anthropometric measurement *(P)* when $e = 0$. In this case, $P = G + E + G \times E$. (Reproduced from Bouchard, 1988, with permission of the publisher.)

(1926) and Holzinger (1929), Tanner (1953) concluded that about 90% of the variability in height was genetically determined. Vandenberg (1962) compared the results from six different twin studies. Because several twin studies have considered stature, and data are reported in different ways by the investigators, the reported variances, correlations, and F-ratios from 19 samples of twins have all been translated into heritability estimates (Bouchard and Lortie, 1984). Reanalysis of these data indicated that the heritability of body height ranged from 0.69 to 0.96, with a mean coefficient of 0.85 and a standard deviation of 0.07.

The parent–child correlation remains rather stable throughout childhood (Garn, 1966; Tanner and Israelsohn, 1963; Tanner et al., 1970). It declines slightly circumpubertally (Furusho, 1968; Welon and Bielicki, 1971) and then increases during the latter phase of growth (Furusho, 1968; Garn, 1966). Parent–child correlations must be interpreted in the light of the fact that the correlation lessens as the difference in age between parent and child increases (Furusho, 1974).

On the other hand, when the height of parents and children is correlated at the same chronological age, the variation in the coefficient with time is not apparent (Furusho, 1974). Although full-sibling correlations for stature with both sibs at the same chronological age are more easily obtained than parent–offspring data, the pattern of age-associated variation is not clearly established. Thus, some studies have reported significant changes from birth to maturity (Garn and Rohmann, 1966), while others have observed only a very slight and almost linear increase with age (Furusho, 1972, 1974). A survey of data available on sibs and offspring over 15 years of age gives a mean weighted parent–child correlation of 0.49 for 6,344 pairs and a correlation of 0.53 for 3,412 pairs of full siblings (Bouchard and Lortie, 1984).

Several authors have looked at the contribution of sex-linked genes to the covariation between biological relatives. The most important conclusion is that the major fraction of variance in stature is determined by autosomal genes (Garn, 1966), and that the contribution, if any, of sex-linked genes is small. For a while, consideration was given to the idea that genes on the Y chromosome were responsible for the sexual dimorphism in size (Garn, 1966). This hypothesis, however, was based on individuals with abnormal chromosome complement and was apparently never substantiated in quantitative studies of normal persons. X-associated effects on stature have been discussed more frequently. Some X-linked influences have been concluded from the results of several studies (Garn and Rohmann, 1966; Garn et al., 1969; Livson et al., 1962; Tanner and Israelsohn, 1963; Welon and Bielicki, 1971), while other studies have shown no X-linked variance (Bouchard and Lortie, 1984; Furusho, 1974; Gerylovova and Bouchalova, 1974; Hewitt, 1957b; Suzanne, 1975; Tanner et al., 1970) or no predominant effect of one parent on the variation in stature within families (Eveleth and Tanner, 1976).

The presence of a dominance effect in genetic variance has been of concern to several investigators. The most detailed study of this problem has been reported by Furusho (1974). Using several sets of familial correlations for stature, ranging from parent–child to twin pairs, he partitioned the total phenotypic variance in stature by a least squares method. The dominance effect accounted for only 11% of the phenotypic variance, while the additive genetic effect reached 65%. In other words, 85% of the genetic variance was additive, while only 15% could be imputed to a dominance deviation (Furusho, 1974). However, this effect can as well be interpreted as a common environment effect, which is not the same in all kinds of relatives.

Mueller (1985) has summarized the results of four longitudinal studies that have reported parent–child correlations for body weight. The pattern of these correlations with age is far less consistent than that observed for height. In general, the data suggest a lower heritability value for body weight than for stature. This conclusion is also supported by the data on midparent–natural child and foster midparent–adopted child pairs presented in Table 2. Stature and sitting height and more highly correlated among biological parents and their natural children than among foster parents and their adopted children. The difference is much less evident for body weight. These data clearly suggest a higher genetic effect in stature than in body weight.

The body mass index is a commonly used indicator of obesity when no direct assessment of body fat is available. It must be kept in mind, however, that the BMI is more strictly a measure of "heaviness" relative to height and that it is influenced by body build and fat-free mass as well as fat mass (Bouchard, 1987). The literature dealing with heredity and the BMI has been reviewed elsewhere (Bouchard and Pérusse, 1988). Most of the data suggest that shared lifestyle and environmental conditions are important in determining the familial resemblance observed in BMI. The correlations reported in Table 2 are consistent with this conclusion as we have not found any difference in the resemblance between foster parents–adopted child and biological parents–natural child, composed of individuals living together (Bouchard, 1985; Bouchard and Tremblay, 1985).

TABLE 2. Midparent–Child Interclass Correlations for Selected Anthropometric Phenotypes[a]

Variable	Foster midparent–adopted child (N = 154 sets)	Midparent–natural child (N = 622 sets)
Stature	0.18*	0.51**
Sitting height	0.07	0.47**
Body weight	0.24*	0.34**
BMI	0.29**	0.30**

[a]Scores were adjusted for age and gender effects by generation and normalized.

From Bouchard et al., unpublished data.

*$P < 0.05$.

**$P < 0.01$.

The technique of path analysis has been used in some studies to determine the contribution of genetic factors on stature and BMI (Annest et al., 1983; Bouchard et al., 1988a; Longini et al., 1984; Pérusse et al., 1988). In one of these studies, we used the BETA model (Cloninger et al., 1979) of path analysis, which allows the separation of biological and cultural components of inheritance (Bouchard et al., 1988a; and unpublished data). The results of these analyses are summarized in Figure 3. We found a transmissible variance of about 60% for stature and 35% for BMI, but the genetic component within this transmissible variance was only 40% for height and 5% for BMI. Clearly, there are nongenetic factors operating on these two important anthropometric phenotypes.

Bone Lengths

Segmental and body lengths, typically taken as indicators of long bone lengths, are apparently under a significant degree of genotypic control, probably more so than any other morphological measurement (Howells, 1953; Schreider, 1969; Tanner, 1953). In an early review of twin studies, Vandenberg (1962) reported significant *F*-ratios (variance of DZ, dizygotic, over variance of MZ, monozygotic) for suprasternal height, sitting height, leg length, total arm length, forearm length, foot length, and hand length measurements; only one out of 24 reported *F*-ratios was not statistically significant.

To obtain comparable estimates of the genetic contribution to these traits, heritability coefficients from 12 twin samples were computed from the published variances, correlations, or *F*-ratios. A total of 33 broad heritability coefficients could thus be obtained. The arithmetic mean is 0.80 with a standard deviation of 0.10. As in the case of stature, the heritability values for composite indicators of length from twin data are generally high. Suprasternal height has a mean coefficient of 0.84 (± 0.10). Sitting height has a mean coefficient of

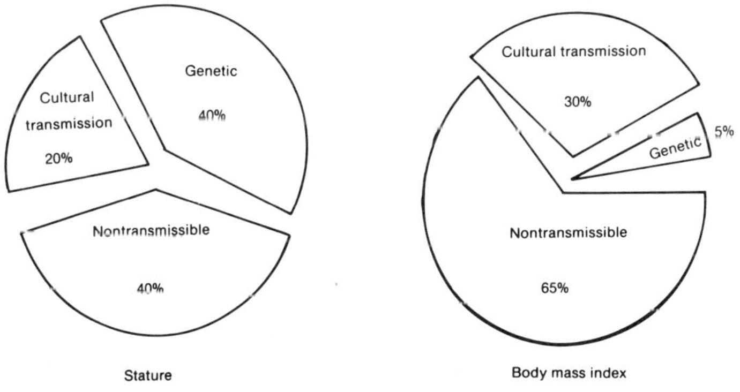

Fig. 3. Total transmissible variance and its genetic component for stature and BMI. (Adapted from Bouchard et al., 1988a, for BMI, and unpublished data for stature.)

0.71 (± 0.29). Total arm length has a coefficient of 0.84 (± 0.04), while foot length reaches a mean value of 0.82 (± 0.02). The most significant results from this survey are probably those concerning the two direct measurements of single long bones, i.e., upper arm length and forearm length. The two mean values are in reasonable agreement with each other and have rather a narrow range (0.62 ± 0.01 to 0.71 ± 0.09) of heritability estimates (Bouchard and Lortie, 1984).

Although less frequent than twin studies, parent–child and full-sib data have also been reported and have been summarized (Bouchard and Lortie, 1984). Considering first the composite criteria of body length and segmental length, mean weighted parent–child correlations ranged from 0.30 for total leg length (n = 784 pairs) to 0.53 for suprasternal height (n = 564 pairs). Mean full-sib weighted correlations tended to be slightly higher, reaching 0.42 for sitting height (n = 1,507 pairs); 0.56 for suprasternal height (n = 300 pairs) and total leg length (n = 355 pairs); and 0.47 for total arm length (n = 332 pairs).

Using the length of the tibia as the dependent variable, Ikoma and Murotani (1976) submitted familial data to quantitative genetic analysis in order to estimate additive and dominance components. They concluded that the dominance effect was very small (0.01) for tibial length, in contrast to the additive genetic effect (0.80).

Table 3 summarizes some of our unpublished data for upper arm length (essentially length of the humerus bone) and tibial height. The midparent–child coefficients are about twice as high for the individuals sharing genes by descent and the home environment than for those sharing only the home environment. These data strongly support the hypothesis of a significant genetic effect determining the length of individual long bones.

TABLE 3. Midparent–Child Interclass Correlations for Selected Bone Dimensions[a]

Variable	Foster midparent–adopted child (N = 154 sets)	Midparent–natural child (N = 622 sets)
Upper arm length	0.20**	0.39**
Tibial height	0.29**	0.54**
Femur breadth	0.15*	0.53**
Ankle breadth	0.08	0.49**
Humerus breadth	0.25**	0.62**
Wrist breadth	−0.03	0.44**
Biacromial breadth	0.01	0.43**
Biiliac breadth	0.13	0.42**

[a]Scores were adjusted for age and gender by generation and normalized. From Bouchard et al., unpublished data.

*$P < 0.05$.

**$P < 0.01$.

There is also some statistical support in favor of a genetic pleiotropic effect in bone length. Using eight indicators of bone length measured in 208 pairs of 10-year-old sibs, we were able to demonstrate that one factor accounted for 92% of the variation in skeletal length measurements after adjustment for environment and familial indices (Bouchard et al., 1980a). This study suggested that skeletal lengths of the body were highly influenced by a single genetic system.

Bone Breadths

Although it is commonly thought that there is more stringent genetic regulation of linear skeletal dimensions (Osborne and DeGeorge, 1959; Schreider, 1969) than of breadth and mass of the skeleton, the latter are not without a substantial genetic variance. Garn (1962), for example, suggested that the bone-related mineral mass of the human body could be under significant genetic control, as illustrated by the higher mineralization in both sexes of black races. Another line of evidence submitted by Garn (1962) was that 12-year-old male monozygotic (MZ) twins are more alike than male dizygotic (DZ) twins in both the midshaft cortical and medullary thicknesses of the tibia. Hewitt (1957a) has shown that breadth of bone obtained from an x-ray film of the calf in sib pairs, 6 months–5 years of age, tended to exhibit a higher genetic determination than other tissues. Smith et al. (1973) have reported on the mass and width of the radius obtained through a photon absorption method in 71 young and 70 adult twin pairs. In both the growing children and the adult twin pairs, the intrapair variance of MZ twins was significantly lower than the DZ variance for both bone mass and radius width. Thus, the intrapair variance for the 23 juvenile DZ pairs reached 0.0052 g/cm^2 for bone mass and 0.0011 cm for the bone width, while the variance in 48 MZ pairs attained only 0.0013 g/cm^2 ($P < 0.001$) and 0.0006 cm ($P < 0.05$) for bone mass and width, respectively.

The genetic determination of skeletal breadth has been studied primarily through anthropometric techniques. Vandenberg (1962) has summarized data from six twin studies and, in general,the F-ratios of DZ variance to MZ variance are significant, suggesting the presence of substantial genetic variance. From data reported in nine twin samples (Clark, 1956; Dahlberg, 1926; Osborne and DeGeorge, 1959; Vandenberg and Strandskov, 1964; Venerando and Milani-Comparetti, 1973; Vogel and Wendt, 1956; Von Verschuer, 1954), the mean heritability coefficients for biacromial and biiliac diameters are 0.64 ($\pm$ 0.22) and 0.60 ($\pm$ 0.13), respectively, while chest breadths have moderately low values (0.34 and 0.52). Few studies have reported on wrist breadth, ankle breadth, and bicondylar diameters of the humerus and femur, and the available data tend to indicate a fairly high degree of heritability. A total of 31 coefficients yielded a mean heritability of 0.60 ($\pm$ 0.18).

Parent–child and full-sib correlations have also been published for some breadth measurements. On the basis of approximately 1,000 parent–child pairs, mean weighted correlations of 0.34 and 0.41 have been computed for biacromial and biiliac diameters respectively. For the same 2 variables, the average sib–sib correlations were 0.44 and 0.46. Average parent–child correlations reached 0.32 for the bicondylar diameter of the humerus and 0.34 for bicondylar diameter of the femur. Full-sib coefficients for these two bone breadths were 0.35 and 0.52, respectively. In general, the full-sib correlations tended to be higher than the parent–child values. Furthermore, the data reviewed do not provide any evidence in support of a clear sex-linked genetic effect (Bouchard and Lortie, 1984).

Recent data from our laboratory are summarized in Table 3. Six indicators of skeletal breadths were obtained in 154 sets of foster midparent–adopted child and 622 sets of midparent–natural child individuals. The correlations are essentially zero for four of the six measurements in the foster midparent–adopted child sets but consistently above 0.4 in the biological midparent–natural child. These results suggest the presence of a rather strong genetic effect in bony breadths, an effect that seems to be even stronger than what was observed for bone lengths in the same subjects (Table 3).

An earlier study has suggested that the pleiotropic effect of a single genetic system was evident across a series of skeletal breadth measurements (Bouchard et al., 1980a). A more recent report based on photon absorptiometry in DZ and MZ twins also finds evidence for genetic determinants of bone mass and also concludes that a single gene or set of genes determines bone mass at all sites assessed in the study, namely, one forearm site, one lumbar spine site, and three femoral sites (Pocock et al., 1987). Moreover, it has been suggested at least in one study that the same genes were contributing to some extent to both bony lengths and breadths as revealed by a bivariate path analysis of twin data for stature and biiliac breadth (Kramer et al., 1986).

Subcutaneous Fat

Skinfold measurements at various sites of the body can be used to estimate the amount of subcutaneous fat. From recent reviews (Mueller, 1983; Bouchard and Pérusse, 1988), it seems that parent–child correlations ranging from 0.15 to 0.25 and sibling correlations ranging from 0.20 to 0.40 are typical for individual skinfolds. Typically, correlations are higher for DZ twins (0.4–0.5) and highest for MZ twins (0.8–0.9).

A more reliable estimator of the amount of subcutaneous fat can be obtained from the sum of several skinfolds, particularly if they are distributed over the trunk and the upper and lower extremities. Such data were available for our 154 sets of foster midparent–adopted child and 622 sets of biological midparent–natural child individuals and are presented in Table 4. Correlations are similar in both sets for all thicknesses, suggesting that sharing genes had little to do with the absolute amount of subcutaneous fat. However, one finds that the regional distribution of subcutaneous fat is probably influenced by the genotype as revealed by the coefficients of 0.26 and 0.42 for the sets of adopted and biological relatives, respectively (trunk to extremity skinfold ratio).

These observations were borne out by the BETA path analysis data that we

TABLE 4. Midparent–Child Interclass Correlations for Skinfold Measurements[a]

Variable	Foster midparent–adopted child (N = 154 sets)	Midparent–natural child (N = 622 sets)
Triceps	0.32**	0.29**
Biceps	0.31**	0.30**
Medial calf	0.24*	0.31**
Subscapular	0.38**	0.35**
Suprailiac	0.36**	0.47**
Abdominal	0.33**	0.25**
Extremity skinfolds	0.31**	0.31**
Trunk skinfolds	0.38**	0.34**
Sum six skinfolds	0.36**	0.31**
Trunk/extremity ratio	0.26**	0.42**

[a]Scores were adjusted for age and gender by generation and normalized. Adapted from Bouchard, 1985, 1987.
*$P < 0.05$.
**$P < 0.01$.

recently reported (Bouchard et al., 1988a). A total transmission effect across generations of about 40% was found with this technique, a transmission effect comparable to what has been reported by other investigators who obtained total transmissibility ranging from about 0.4 to 0.55 (Byard et al., 1984; Devor et al., 1986; Pérusse et al., 1988). However, the additive genetic component in our study reached only about 5% in our study, demonstrating that most of the transmission effect had little to do with the genotype (Bouchard et al., 1988a). In other words, most of the individual differences in skinfold thicknesses are independent of the genotype and are associated with the determinants of energy balance, i.e., habitual energy intake and total habitual energy expenditures.

Fat Mass

To the best of our knowledge, only one study has been reported on the genetic effect in fat mass and percent body fat measured with one of the accepted direct methods (Bouchard et al., 1988a). In this research, we had underwater weighing measurements of body density in a relatively large number of individuals belonging to nine different kinds of relatives by descent or by adoption. Using the BETA analytical procedure, we were able to conclude that about half of the variance, after adjustment for age and gender, in fat mass or percent body fat was associated with a transmissible effect, but that only 25% of the variance was an additive genetic effect (Fig. 4). Given our observations on the low heritability of subcutaneous fat, it is not unreasonable to suggest that the genetic effect seen in fat mass is caused by the deep fat or visceral fat component of fat mass.

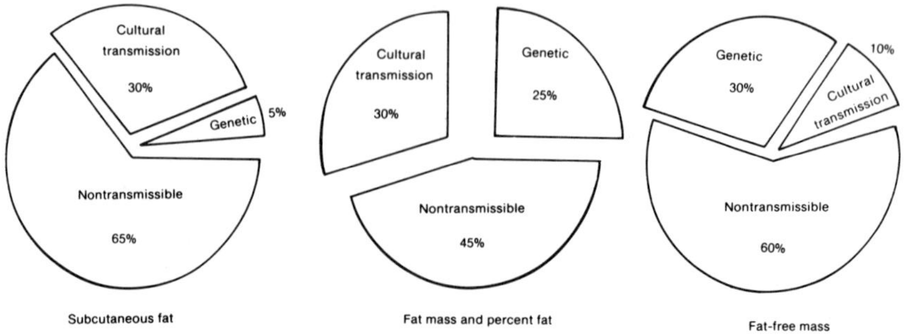

Fig. 4. Total transmissible variance and its genetic component for subcutaneous fat, total body fat and fat-free mass. (Adapted from Bouchard et al., 1988a.)

Muscle Mass

As for fat mass, little has been reported for muscle mass or fat-free mass. Figure 4 also summarizes our findings about the heritability of fat-free mass derived from underwater weighing measurements (Bouchard et al., 1988a). We found that the genetic effect for fat-free mass reached about 30% of the age- and gender-adjusted variation in the phenotype.

Quite often nutritional assessment of muscle mass is attempted from anthropometric indicators such as limb circumferences corrected for skinfold thicknesses. Such data were available in the sets of midparent–natural child and foster midparent–adopted child described above. We have used the upper arm circumference corrected for the triceps skinfold and the calf circumference corrected for the contribution of the medial calf skinfold as described earlier by Brozek (1961). These correlations for both estimated muscle diameters are presented in Table 5. The correlations are not significantly different from zero for both variables in the relatives by adoption, but they reached .30 in the biological relatives. These results are quite compatible with our observations on the heritability of fat-free mass, which clearly indicate that the genotype contributes significantly to variations in lean tissues and most likely muscle size or mass.

Physique

One approach to the study of the genetics of anthropometric indicators relevant to the assessment of nutritional status is to consider overall assessment of physique such as in somatotyping. Parnell (1958) has presented data of significance for the discussion of heredity of body type in children. Parnell's own system of somatotyping distinguishes anthropometrically the components of fatness, muscularity, and linearity. From the comparison of anthropometric somatotypes in children and their parents, he found about 75% concordance between the physique ratings. The index of stature/weight$^{1/3}$ (ponderal index) supposedly reflects a continuum of linearity in physique, and is used

TABLE 5. Midparent–Child Interclass Correlations for Estimated Muscle Size[a]

Variable[b]	Foster midparent–adopted child (N = 154 sets)	Midparent–natural child (N = 622 sets)
Upper arm muscle diameter	.09	.30*
Calf muscle diameter	.10	.29*

[a]Scores were adjusted for age and gender by generation and normalized.
[b]Estimated muscle diameter = circumference (cm) ÷ π minus skinfold (mm) × 10.
From Bouchard et al., unpublished data.
*$P < 0.001$.

in somatotype systems to estimate the ectomorphic component of physique. The mean value for the heritability coefficients of the ponderal index from three twin series was computed and reached 0.53 (± 0.19) (Bouchard and Lortie, 1984). In an early study, we obtained data in parent–child and biological sibs for ectomorphy and suggested that heritability of this physique component ranged from about 0.35 to 0.50 (Bouchard et al., 1980b). Mesomorphy and endomorphy were assessed in the Heath and Carter system for 208 pairs of 10-year-old biological siblings. Heritability reached 0.50 for endomorphy and 0.42 for mesomorphy (Bouchard et al., 1980b).

More recently, we were able to obtain the anthropometric somatotype components of the Heath and Carter system in foster parents and their adopted child(ren) as well as in biological parents and their natural child(ren). Some of these data are summarized in Table 6. No difference was observed between the two sets for endomorphy, while only a slight advantage (0.33 versus 0.26) was seen in favor of the biological relatives for ectomorphy. In contrast, the

TABLE 6. Midparent–Child Interclass Correlations for Somatotype Components[a]

Variable	Foster midparent–adopted child (N = 154 sets)	Midparent–natural child (N = 622 sets)
Endomorphy	0.37**	0.35**
Mesomorphy	0.19*	0.41**
Ectomorphy	0.26**	0.33**

[a]Scores adjusted for age and sex effects by generation and normalized.
From Bouchard et al., unpublished data.
*$P < 0.05$.
**$P < 0.01$.

midparent–natural child correlation was strikingly higher than the foster midparent–adopted child coefficient for the mesomorphy component. These results suggest that the degree of mesomorphy may turn out to be inherited to a larger extent than the other somatotype components. The lack of a significant genetic effect for endomorphy is consistent with our finding of a genetic transmission of only about 5% for the amount of subcutaneous fat and BMI (see above).

HEREDITY AND ADAPTATION TO CHANGES IN NUTRITIONAL STATUS

Let us now turn our attention to a special genetic effect, one that is often known as the genotype *(G)* and environment *(E)* interaction effect or $G \times E$. The $G \times E$ effect results from the fact that all individuals (or genotypes) do not respond similarly to changes in E (see Fig. 2 above). First, one may ask whether there are differences in the response of anthropometric indicators to a standardized nutritional stress. We have documented this issue in a series of experiments using either chronic exposure to a positive energy balance or chronic exposure to a negative energy balance. One of these studies involved five young males who were exposed to an energy deficit of 1,000 kcal (4.2 MJ) per day, 6 days a week, for a period of 100 days. The energy deficit was caused by exercise twice a day, 55 minutes per session, on the cycle ergometer at 58% (mean value) of $\dot{V}O_2$ max, and the total deficit was 84,000 kcal for each subject over the duration of the experiment. Figure 5 shows the individual weight loss

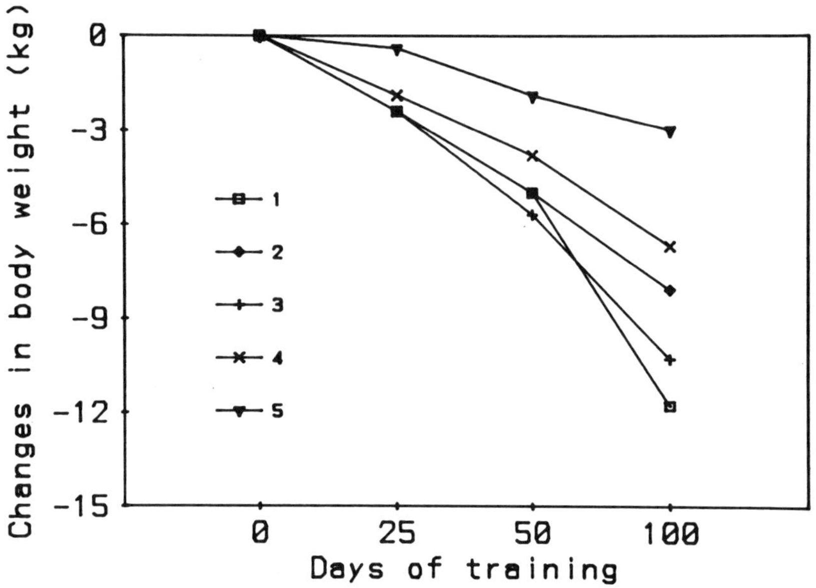

Fig. 5. Weight loss in five subjects submitted to a total energy deficit of 84,000 kcal through regular exercise over a period of 100 days. (Modified from Bouchard et al., 1990.)

over time in these subjects. One can clearly see that even though they all lost body weight, there were large differences in the response to the nutritional stress.

One way to assess the role of genotype in the adaptation to a chronic nutritional stress is to apply exactly the same treatment to the two members of each pair of several sets of identical twins. The comparison of the variation within and between pairs, and thus the genotypes, allows testing of the hypothesis of a $G \times E$ effect in response to the treatment. We have applied this design in many studies and have shown quite conclusively that a substantial portion of the individual differences in the response to a nutritional stress was genetically determined (Bouchard, 1987; Bouchard et al., 1988b).

For instance, six pairs of male MZ twins were subjected to a 1,000 kcal/d caloric surplus during 22 consecutive days (Poehlman et al., 1986). There were considerable interindividual differences in the response of anthropometric indicators to the overfeeding treatment, but these variations were not randomly distributed. For instance, an intraclass correlation of 0.88 was found for the changes in fat mass, indicating a high intrapair resemblance in the response to the treatment (Fig. 6). These data indicate that some individuals are more

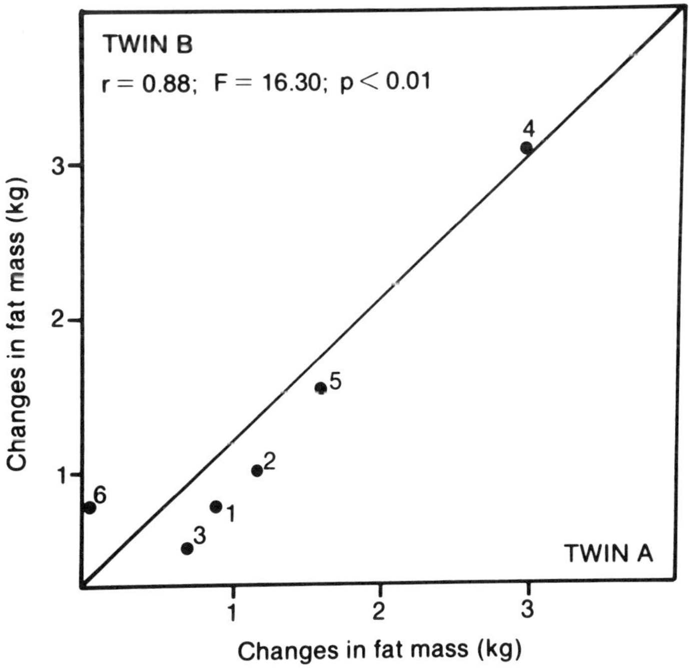

Fig. 6. Intrapair resemblance in fat mass increase caused by a 1,000 kcal per day overfeeding treatment for 22 consecutive days in six pairs of male identical twins. (Adapted from Bouchard and Pérusse, 1988; Bouchard et al., 1988b.)

at risk than others to gain fat when exposed to caloric affluence, and that this risk is largely genotype dependent.

IMPLICATIONS OF THESE DATA

The data reviewed or presented here indicate that there are some anthropometric dimensions with very low or no heritability. BMI, endomorphy, and skinfold thickness or amount of subcutaneous fat fall into that category. On the other hand, a significant genetic effect has been observed or inferred for regional fat distribution, total fat mass, fat-free mass, estimated muscle size, mesomorphy, and bone lengths and breadths. A significant genetic effect implies only that variations in the anthropometric phenotype are determined, in the population under study, by genetic factors to the extent of the size of the heritable component. It is therefore a population parameter which is not very helpful in interpreting the observations made on a given individual. It is, however, as useful as other population parameters, in the sense that it informs about the forces operating in the phenotype variance.

More informative is the $G \times E$ component. Unfortunately, there is a paucity of data concerning this effect in humans submitted to a variety of nutritional stresses. The experiments needed to quantify and understand the impact of the genotype in the adaptation to a given stress are always very difficult to execute and at times impossible to undertake for obvious ethical reasons. The data that we have been able to generate indicate clearly, however, that the $G \times E$ effect is ubiquitous, particularly in the response to nutritional stresses. There are high-responders and low-responders, or high-gainers and low-gainers, depending on the treatment, and the responder or gainer status is determined by the genotype to a large extent. From preliminary data that we have been able to gather, it seems as if the responder status (e.g., for adipose tissue) was not a good predictor of the sensitivity to treatment in other tissues (e.g., for lean tissues). This may of course increase the complexity of the research into the genetic elements associated with variation in adaptive capacity to nutritional stresses.

REFERENCES

Annest JL, Sing CF, Biron P, Mongeau JG (1983): Familial aggregation of blood pressure and weight in adoptive families, III: Analysis of the role of shared genes and shared household environment in explaining family resemblance for height, weight and selected weight/height indices. Am J Epidemiol 117:492–506.

Bouchard C (1985): Inheritance of fat distribution and adipose tissue metabolism. In Vague J, Björntorp P, Guy-Grand B, Rebuffé-Scrive M, Vague P (eds): "Metabolic Complications of Human Obesities." Amsterdam: Elsevier, pp 87–96.

Bouchard C (1986): Genetics of aerobic power and capacity. In Malina RM, Bouchard C (eds): "Sport and Human Genetics." Champaign, Ill: Human Kinetics, pp 59–88.

Bouchard C (1987): Genetics of body fat, energy expenditure and adipose tissue metabolism. In Berry EM, Blondheim SH, Eliahou HE, Shafrir E (eds): "Recent Advances in Obesity Research: V." London: John Libbey, pp 16–25.

Bouchard C (1988): Human variation in anthropometric dimensions. In Lohman TG, Roche AF, Martorell R (eds): "Anthropometric Standardization Reference Manual." Champaign, Ill: Human Kinetics, pp 103–105.

Bouchard C, Demirjian A, Malina RM (1980a): Genetic pleiotropism in skeletal lengths and breadths. In Ostyn M, Beunen G, Simons J (eds): "Kinanthropometry II. Vol 9, International Series On Sport Sciences." Baltimore: University Park Press, pp 78–87.

Bouchard C, Demirjian A, Malina RM (1980b): Heritability estimates of somatotype components based upon familial data. Hum Heredity 30:112–118.

Bouchard C, Lortie G (1984): Heredity and endurance performance. Sports Med 1:38–64.

Bouchard C, Pérusse L (1988): Heredity and body fat. Annu Rev Nutr 8:259–277.

Bouchard C, Pérusse L, Leblanc C, Tremblay A, Thériault G (1988a): Heredity, human body fat and fat distribution. Int J Obesity 12:205–215.

Bouchard C, Tremblay A (1985): Genetics of body composition and fat distribution. In Norgan NG (ed): "Human Body Composition and Fat Distribution." London: Euro-Nut, pp 175–188.

Bouchard C, Tremblay A, Després JP, Poehlman ET, Thériault G, Nadeau A, Lupien P, Moorjani S, Dussault J (1988b): Sensitivity to overfeeding: the Québec experiment with identical twins. Prog Food Nutr Sci 12:45–72.

Bouchard C, Tremblay A, Nadeau A, Dussault J, Deprés JP, Thériault G, Lupien PJ, Serresse O, Boulay MR, Fournier G (1990): Long-term exercise training with constant energy intake. 1: Effect on body composition and selected metabolic variables. Int J Obesity 14:57–73.

Brozek J (1961): Body measurements including skinfold thickness, as indicators of body composition. In Brozek J, Henschel A (eds). "Techniques for Measuring Body Composition." Washington, DC: National Research Council.

Byard PJ, Sharma K, Russell JM, Rao DC (1984): A family study of anthropometric traits in a Punjabi community, II: An investigation of familial transmission. Am J Phys Anthropol 64:97–104.

Clark PJ (1956): The heritability of certain anthropometric characters as ascertained from measurements of twins. Am J Hum Genet 8:49–54.

Cloninger CR, Rice J, Reich T (1979): Multifactorial inheritance with cultural transmission and assortative mating, II: A general model of combined polygenic and cultural inheritance. Am J Hum Genet 31:176–198.

Dahlberg G (1926): "Twin Births and Twins from a Hereditary Point of View." Stockholm: Tidems Tsyckeri.

Devor EJ, McGue M, Crawford MH, Lin PM (1986): Transmissible and nontransmissible components of anthropometric variation in the Alexanderwohl Mennonites, II: Resolution by path analysis. Am J Phys Anthropol 69:83–92.

Eveleth PB, Tanner JM (1976): "Worldwide Variation in Human Growth." Cambridge: Cambridge University Press.

Furusho T (1968): On the manifestation of genotype responsible for stature. Hum Biol 40:437–455.

Furusho T (1972): Genetic study on growth of stature. Jpn J Hum Genet 17:249–272.

Furusho T (1974): Genetic study on stature. Jpn J Hum Genet 19:1–25.

Garn SM (1962): The genetics of normal human growth. In Gedda (ed): "De Genetica Medica." Rome: Mendel Institute, Vol 2, pp 415–434.

Garn SM (1966): Body size and its implication. In Hoffman LW, Hoffman ML (eds): "Review of Child Development Research 2." New York: Sage Foundation, pp 529–561.

Garn SM, Hertzog KP, Rohmann CG (1969): Evidence for X-linkage of tibial length and body length. Am J Phys Anthropol 31:187–190.
Garn SM, Rohmann CG (1966): Interaction of nutrition and genetics in the timing of growth and development. Pediatr Clin North Am 13:353–359.
Gerylovova A, Bouchalova M (1974): The relationship between children's and parent's heights in the age range 0–6 years. Ann Hum Biol 1:229–232.
Hewitt D (1957a): Sib resemblance in bone, muscle and fat measurements of the human calf. Ann Hum Genet 22:213–221.
Hewitt D (1957b): Some familial correlations in height, weight and skeletal maturity. Ann Hum Genet 22:26–35.
Holzinger K (1929): The relative effect of nature and nurture influences on twin differences. J Educ Psychol 20:241–248.
Howells WW (1953): Correlations of brothers in factor scores. Am J Phys Anthropol 11:121–140.
Ikoma E, Murotani N (1976): A genetic study on the length of tibia. Ann Hum Genet 39:475–483.
Kramer AA, Green LJ, Croghan IT, Buck GM, Ferer R (1986): Bivariate path analysis of twin children for stature and biiliac diameter: Estimation of genetic variation and co-variation. Hum Biol 58: 517–525.
Longini IM, Higgins MW, Hinton PC, Moll PP, Keller JB (1984): Genetic and environmental sources of familial aggregation of body mass in Tecumseh, Michigan. Hum Biol 56: 733–757.
Livson N, McNeill D, Thomas K (1962): Pooled estimates of parent–child correlations in stature from birth to maturity. Science 138: 818–820.
Mueller WH (1983): The genetics of human fatness. Yearbook Phys Anthropol 26: 215–230.
Mueller WH (1985): The genetics of size and shape in children and adults. In Falkner F, Tanner JM (eds): "Human Growth. A Comprehensive Treatise. Vol 3., Methodology. Ecological, Genetic, and Nutritional Effects on Growth." New York: Plenum Press, pp 145–168.
Osborne RH, DeGeorge FV (1959): "Genetic Basis of Morphological Variation." Harvard: Harvard University Press.
Parnell RW (1958): "Behaviour and Physique." London: Arnold.
Pérusse L, Leblanc C, Bouchard C (1988): Inter-generation transmission of physical fitness in the Canadian population. Can J Sports Sci 13:8–14.
Pocock NA, Eisman JA, Hopper JL, Yeates MG, Sambrook PN, Eberl S (1987): Genetic determinants of bone mass in adults. A twin study. J Clin Invest 80: 706–710.
Poehlman ET, Tremblay A, Després JP, Fontaine E, Pérusse L, Thériault G, Bouchard C (1986): Genotype-controlled changes in body composition and fat morphology following overfeeding in twins. Am J Clin Nutr 43: 723–731.
Schreider E (1969): Biométrie et génétique. Biométrie Hum 4:65–85.
Smith, DM, Nance WE, Kang KW, Christian JC, Johnston CC (1973): Genetic factors in determining bone mass. J Clin Invest 52: 2800–2808.
Suzanne C (1975): Genetic and environmental influences on morphological characteristics. Ann Hum Biol 2: 279–287.
Tanner JM (1953): Inheritance of morphological and physiological traits. In Sorsby A (ed): "Clinical Genetics." St Louis: CV Mosby, pp 155–174.
Tanner JM, Goldstein H, Whitehouse RH (1970): Standards for children's height at ages 2–9 years allowing for height of the parents. Arch Dis Child 45: 755–762.
Tanner JM, Israelsohn WJ (1963): Parent–child correlations for body measurements of

children between the ages of one month and seven years. Ann Hum Genet 26: 245–259.

Vandenberg SG (1962): How stable are heritability estimates? A comparison of heritability estimates from six anthropometric studies. Am J Phys Anthropol 20:331–338.

Vandenberg SG, Strandskov HH (1964): A comparison of identical and fraternal twins on some anthropometric measures. Hum Biol 36:45–52.

Venerando A, Milani-Comparetti M (1973): Heredity versus environment in biomechanics. In Cerquiglini S, Venerando A, Wartenweiler J (eds): "Biomechanics III." Basel: Karger, pp 151–155.

Vogel F, Wendt GG (1956): Zwillingsuntursuchung uber die erblichkeit einiger anthropologischer masse und konstitutionsindices. Z Menschliche Vererbung Konstitutionslehre 33:425–446.

Von Verschuer O (1954): "Wirksame Faktoren im Leben des Menschen." Wiesbaden: F Steiner.

Welon Z, Bielicki T (1971): Further investigations of parent–child similarity in stature as assessed from longitudinal data. Hum Biol 43:517–525.

Anthropometric Assessment
of Nutritional Status, pages 233–257

14
Maternal Anthropometry During Pregnancy, Pregnancy Weight Gain, and Pregnancy Outcome

LINDA S. ADAIR AND EILENE Z. BISGROVE
Carolina Population Center, University of North Carolina, Chapel Hill, North Carolina 27514

INTRODUCTION

Maternal nutritional status during pregnancy is one of the most important determinants of fetal growth. Through its effects on birth weight, nutritional status of the mother also influences perinatal mortality, neonatal morbidity, and postnatal growth. In addition, the health and future reproductive success of the mother may be strongly influenced by nutritional factors in a current pregnancy. One important component of maternal nutritional status that bears significantly on pregnancy outcome is energy balance, which is reflected in the size of body fat stores. Anthropometric assessment of nutritional status is valuable because it provides information about fat stores as well as other aspects of maternal body size and composition that affect pregnancy outcomes.

Anthropometric assessment of nutritional status during pregnancy relies on measures of stature, prepregnancy weight (PPW), weight gain during pregnancy (PWG), skinfold thicknesses, and limb circumferences. Some measures reflect a woman's nutritional status or energy stores as she enters pregnancy (height, PPW), while others reflect changes in her nutritional status over the course of pregnancy (skinfolds, circumferences, PWG). The latter are attributable to changes in maternal energy stores, development of maternal reproductive tissue, increased blood volume and extracellular fluid, and fetal growth.

COMPONENTS OF WEIGHT GAIN IN NORMAL PREGNANCY

To get a better sense of what kind of information is provided by anthropometric assessment, it is useful to describe the components of weight gain during a normal pregnancy.

Studies of normal pregnancy are complicated by a number of problems. First, the definition of what constitutes a "normal" pregnancy may be unclear, and may change over time. For example, what was considered a normal weight gain in developed countries during the 1950s and 1960s differs from what is considered a normal weight gain in the 1980s. This is due primarily to the earlier feared consequences of excessive weight gains and deliberate recommendations to curtail them. Second, in a number of studies, women's diets have been purposefully manipulated. Third, most data are from retrospective studies or from studies begun after a pregnancy is in progress. This is a particularly noteworthy problem. Data on PPW of the mother are usually based on recall, and are subject to inaccuracies. Use of weight measured after a pregnancy has been identified introduces bias by incorporating maternal body changes that occur in the early weeks of pregnancy.

Despite these shortcomings, the obstetric literature provides a reasonable view of what to expect in normal pregnancy. Based on a compilation of studies in developed countries, Hytten and Chamberlain (1980) estimate that the average healthy primigravida eating to appetite gains about 12.5 kg during pregnancy. But changes range from weight losses to gains of 23 kg or more. Although the incidence of complications rises at the extremes of this range, there is a wide variability in the changes which are compatible with healthy outcomes.

Mean weights of 2,868 British normotensive primigravidae from the 13th week of pregnancy plotted across time demonstrated a gentle sigmoid curve (Thomson and Billewicz, 1957). A compilation of studies showed rate of weight gain accelerating rather sharply from 16 through 32 weeks and then gradually slowing until term (see Fig. 1). Average weight gains by quarters of

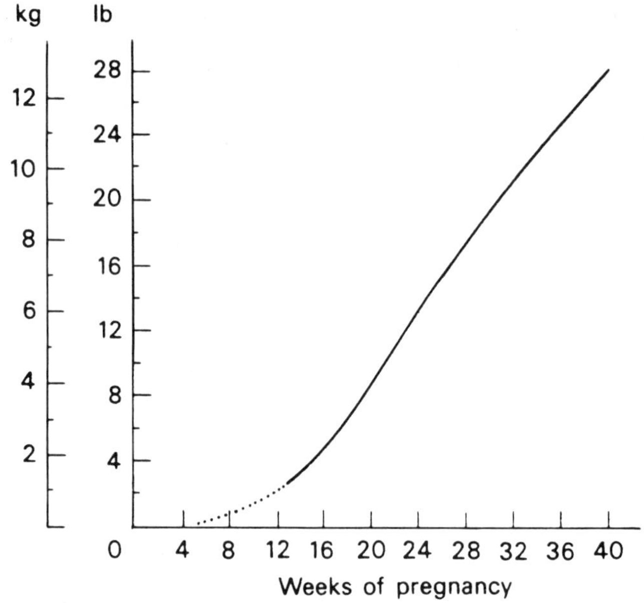

Fig. 1. Mean weight gain in pregnancy of 2,868 normotensive primigravidae. (Reproduced from Hytten and Chamberlain, 1980, with permission of the publisher.)

pregnancy are 650 g at 10 weeks, 4 kg at 20 weeks, 8.5 kg at 30 weeks, and 12.5 kg at term (Hytten and Chamberlain, 1980).

It is important to note that total PWG is affected by the length of gestation and, therefore, studies which relate PWG to outcomes should account for gestational age. Alternatively, PWG can be expressed as a rate of gain between specified time points during pregnancy.

PWG can be compartmentalized into products of conception and maternal tissues changes. Products of conception include the fetus, placenta, and amniotic fluid, whereas the maternal component includes uterus, breasts, blood volume, total body water, and fat stores. Direct measurement of these separate components during pregnancy is not possible. Most information on components of PWG is based on either cross-sectional data from autopsies, miscarriages, and hysterectomies or indirect estimates such as tracer dilution for total body water or skinfold measures of maternal body fat. Factorial approaches often leave some component unmeasured. For example, postpartum weighing of the fetus and placenta allows calculation of "net PWG" as the sum of total PWG minus the sum of products of conception but does not account for amniotic fluid.

Products of Conception

Changes in weight of the products of conception are summarized in Table 1. Products of conception represent about 8%–9% of total PWG at 10 weeks, 20% at 20 weeks, 30% at 30 weeks, and nearly 40% at term (Hytten and Chamberlain, 1980).

Most fetal growth curves are derived from cross-sectional data and show that weight follows a sigmoid curve with maximum rate of increase during the third quarter and deceleration near term (Fig. 1). The contribution of the fetus to total PWG in the first half of pregnancy is small. At term, however, the fetus represents a larger contribution to PWG than any other single component. Average weight of full-term infants of well-nourished mothers is 3,400 g, or about 27% of total PWG.

Placental weight increases in a more gradual sigmoid fashion than fetal weight (see Fig. 2). Placental weight increases from about 20 g at 10 weeks to about 650 g (5% of total PWG) at 40 weeks (see Table 1; Hytten and Leitch, 1971; McKeown and Record, 1953; Hosemann, 1949). Differences in estimates of placental weight reflect the method of delivery, the time at which the umbilical cord is tied, and whether membranes are trimmed off and blood clots systematically removed (Hytten and Chamberlain, 1980). Amniotic fluid is difficult to measure. Most estimates are based on volumes measured during hysterectomy early in pregnancy or on cesarean deliveries later in pregnancy. Lind and Hytten (1972) found that amniotic fluid volume increases during the first half of pregnancy in direct relation to fetal weight. During the second half of pregnancy, increases are independent of fetal weight and highly variable. Maximum fluid volume of about 900 mL is attained by 36 weeks, followed by a fairly rapid decrease to 800 mL at term and 500 mL by 42 weeks.

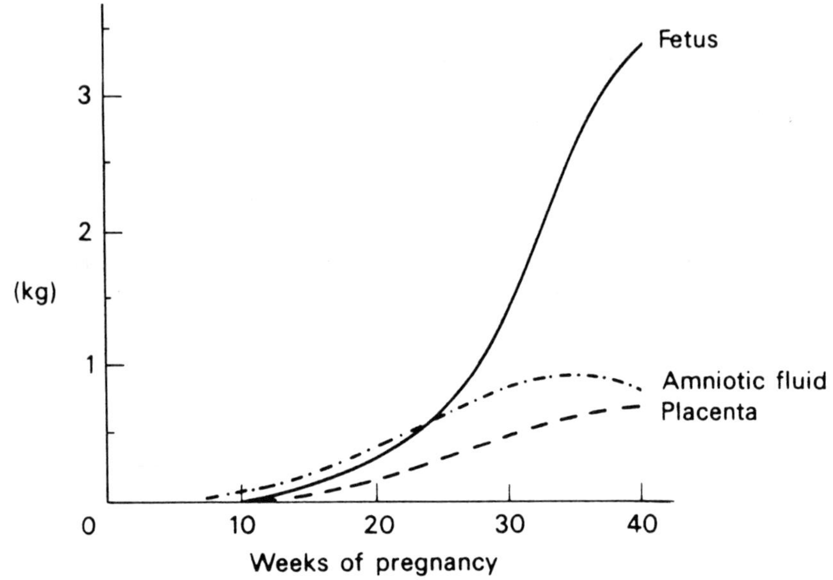

Fig. 2. The pattern of weight increase in amniotic fluid, placenta, and fetus. (Reproduced from Hytten and Chamberlain, 1980, with permission of the publisher.)

Maternal Components of Weight Gain

Maternal components of weight gain are summarized in Table 1. In well-nourished women, more than 60% of PWG is maternal rather than fetal, and is due to growth of the uterus and breasts, increased maternal fat stores, and expansion of blood volume and fluid. Some of these components can be isolated, and estimates of changes during pregnancy can be made. For others, such as total body water and total body fat, increases in the mother cannot be separated from increases in the fetus.

Growth of the uterus is difficult to quantify, and most data come from surgically removed tissue or autopsies. Overall, uterine weight increases in normal pregnancy amount to about 1 kg. Changes in breast tissue are also difficult to quantify. Estimates are based on mastectomy or on water displacement and are subject to considerable error. Also, the nonpregnant breast is so variable that estimation of increases due to pregnancy is difficult. Average increases in breast weight amount to about 400 g. Fat content of breast is thought to be about 3% of the glandular tissue increase, or about 12 g.

Changes in maternal body composition reflect fluid and solid constituents. Blood volume changes as a result of increases in both plasma and red cells. Changes are highly variable, but are positively correlated with birth weight. Blood volume is also related to parity and season (Retief and Brink, 1967;

TABLE 1. Components of Pregnancy Weight Gain: Increases by Quarter of Pregnancy and as a Percentage of Total Pregnancy Weight Gain

	Length of pregnancy (weeks)							
	10		20		30		40	
	g	%	g	%	g	%	g	%
Products of conception								
Fetus	5	0.8	300	7.5	1,500	17.6	3,400	27.2
Placenta	20	3.1	170	4.3	430	5.1	650	5.2
Amniotic fluid	30	4.6	350	8.8	750	8.8	800	6.4
Total	55	8.5	820	20.6	2,680	31.5	4,850	38.8
Maternal components								
Uterus[a]	140	21.5	320	8.0	600	7.1	970	7.8
Breasts	45	6.9	180	4.5	360	4.2	405	3.2
Blood	100	15.4	600	15.0	1,300	15.3	1,250	10.0
Extracellular fluid[b]	0	0	30	0.7	80	0.9	1,680	13.4
Fat stores[c]	310	47.7	2,050	51.3	3,480	40.9	3,345	26.8
Total	595	91.5	3,180	79.5	5,820	68.4	7,650	61.2
Total pregnancy weight gain	650		4,000		8,500		12,500	

Data from Hytten and Leitch (1971).
[a]Blood free increase above nonpregnant weight.
[b]With no edema or leg edema only.
[c]Weight increase not accounted for, assumed to be depot fat.

Dieckmann and Wegner, 1934). Estimated increases by quarter of pregnancy are presented in Table 1.

Total body water, representing intracellular plus extracellular fluid increases steadily throughout pregnancy.[1] Due to large interindividual differences and lack of serial data, estimates of mean changes in normal pregnancy have not been definitive.

A major concern in measuring body composition is the effect of edema, or the accumulation of excess interstitial fluid. Edema alters the percentage of water in nonadipose tissue and subsequently affects estimates of both total body water and fat. Edema also affects direct measures of extracellular water and alters skin compressibility, thereby affecting indirect measures of body composition such as skinfolds and limb circumferences.

Edema during pregnancy is not only common but, at lower degrees, may have a more physiological than pathological significance. From a retrospective

[1]Total body water estimates use a variety of tracers, the most reliable of which is deuterium oxide. Methods which use antipyrine appear to grossly overestimate total body water during pregnancy, particularly if edema is present.

study of 24,079 single pregnancies without hypertensive complications, Thomson et al. (1967) found some evidence of edema in nearly 40% of the women. In 20% of the edematous women, the edema was localized in the legs and ankles only, while the remaining 80% had more generalized edema. Edema of the lower extremities only was found to be associated with a total water increase of 2.5–3 L, while generalized edema was associated with increased body water of about 5 L at term (Hytten et al., 1966).

The solid body constituents of primary concern during pregnancy are fat and protein. It is generally agreed that protein storage does not occur apart from that which is represented in maternal reproductive tissue and the products of conception. Fat storage does occur to a considerable degree during pregnancy, and is a critical indicator of maternal energy balance.

Once all other components of PWG have been accounted for, the remaining portion of PWG is assumed to represent maternal fat stores. Estimates of fat accumulation during pregnancy based on underwater weighing or deuterium oxide fit well with the theoretical picture of fat accumulation provided by Hytten and Leitch (1971). They describe a net fat gain in well-nourished women of about 3.5 kg by 30 weeks of pregnancy (see Table 1). More than half of the total increase is accomplished by the midpoint of pregnancy. As the fetus makes its final growth spurt in the last 10 weeks, maternal storage of fat slows down. In undernourished women, fat may be mobilized to meet increased energy demands for fetal growth and maternal maintenance in the last trimester of pregnancy. For women with generalized edema, fat gain at term is considerably lower than in nonedematous women. Edematous women appear to gain more water at the expense of fat, particularly in the final few weeks of pregnancy (Hytten and Leitch, 1971).

It should be noted that some of the indirect and often circuitous methods traditionally used to estimate maternal body fat may be inappropriate during pregnancy if they are based on assumptions about the water content of tissue. More direct techniques, such as the use of selectively absorbed tracers, may be inappropriate depending on whether the tracers are able to cross the placenta.

Estimates of maternal subcutaneous fat can be made by measuring skinfold thicknesses at selected body sites. However, skinfold thicknesses during pregnancy may not as accurately reflect total body fat as they do for nonpregnant individuals. While subcutaneous fat thicknesses are highly correlated with body density and total body water in nonpregnant subjects (Himes et al., 1980), these relationships have not been explored in pregnant women.

Skinfold measurements have the advantage of considering only maternal tissue, and can be taken in the field without complicated equipment. A number of studies have examined changes in skinfold thicknesses during pregnancy. Figure 3 shows results from a study of 84 healthy women measured at seven sites (triceps, biceps, scapula, costal, suprailiac, midthigh, and kneecap). The overall pattern is of increasing skinfold thickness over the abdomen, back, and thighs up to about 30 weeks accompanied by no increase or even slight decreases at peripheral sites (Taggart et al., 1967). It is important to note that

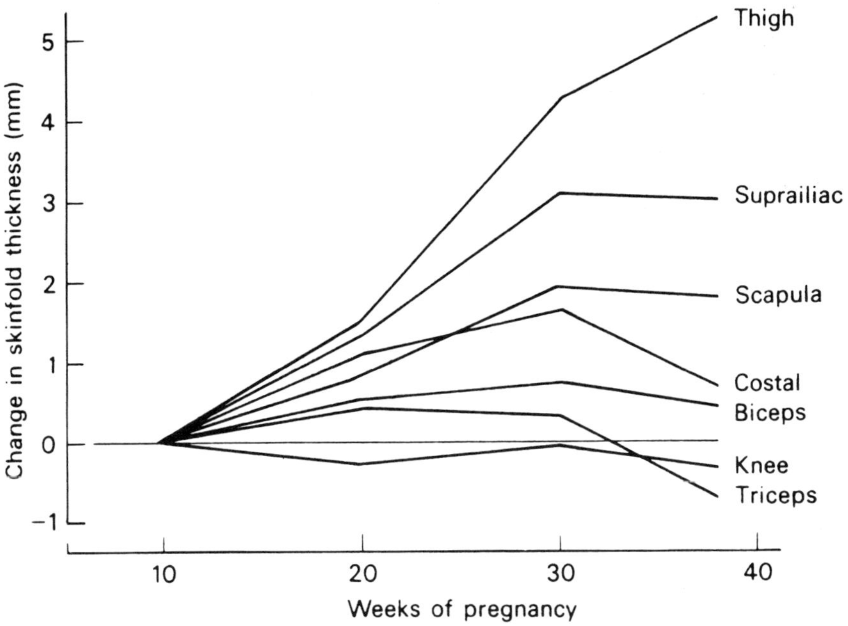

Fig. 3. Increase in skinfold thicknesses at seven sites during pregnancy. (From the data of Taggart et al., 1967; reproduced from Hytten and Chamberlain, 1980, with permission of the publisher.)

during pregnancy skin compressibility may be altered by edema or hormone-based changes in connective tissues and these changes may affect skinfold measures. This problem has not been addressed in the literature.

Studies in low-income populations where women's nutritional status before and during pregnancy varies more widely have yielded conflicting pictures of how skinfolds change. Arroyo et al. (1978) measured 57 Mexican women divided into low and high weight-for-height groups using the seven sites listed above. The most pronounced changes (both increases and decreases) occurred at central sites between weeks 24 and 30 of pregnancy. Both weight groups contained a number of cases in which there were no changes or even reductions in total skinfold thicknesses; however, the proportion of reductions was significantly larger for the low-weight group (32%) than for the high-weight group (19%). The picture was further clouded by the fact that high-weight women who showed the greatest decrease in total skinfolds had the highest mean weight for height, while the low-weight women who lost subcutaneous fat had the lowest weight for height. The authors conclude that women's nutritional status at the beginning of pregnancy and energy balance during pregnancy interact to determine accumulation of subcutaneous fat. Adair et al. (1983), in their study of rural Taiwanese women, found highly variable patterns of change in triceps and subscapular skinfold thicknesses. Overall, increases at both sites were observed during the first two trimesters of pregnancy, followed by declines in the third trimester. Fat was accumulated at the subscapular site earlier in pregnancy, and less fat was lost later at this site. In contrast, mean triceps skinfold thickness measured just before birth was less than the mean prepregnancy value. From a sample of 813 rural African women with energy intakes averaging 1,500 to 1,600 calories, Jansen et al. (1984) found low second trimester weight gains (2.2 kg) to be associated with significant decreases in arm circumference and triceps and biceps skinfolds between the second and third trimesters.

Patterns of fat deposition and mobilization during pregnancy reflect maternal energy balance. Differences in those patterns may represent alternative adaptive strategies contingent on the availability of dietary energy and whether nutritional stress is chronic or acute.

Clearly, major changes in the maternal body and the products of conception occur during pregnancy. A critical question is, what do anthropometric assessments tell us about these physiological changes? How well do they reflect nutritional status during pregnancy?

MATERNAL ANTHROPOMETRY AND PREGNANCY OUTCOME

The importance of anthropometric indicators of nutritional status during pregnancy can best be assessed by looking at how they affect selected pregnancy outcomes. What follows is a discussion of the relationship of PWG and maternal anthropometric variables to infant birth weight, gestational age, and perinatal mortality.[2]

Maternal Stature

Stature reflects maternal genetic factors, skeletal maturity (in the case of adolescent pregnancy), and nutritional history. Maternal genetic effects on fetal growth may be direct (for example, the fetus inherits genes for tall stature) or indirect (the fetal environment may differ in tall versus short mothers). Indirect genetic effects and poor nutritional history resulting in short maternal

[2]A particularly valuable source of information on the determinants of intrauterine growth and gestational duration is a monograph by Kramer (1988). This is a review of literature published from 1970 to 1984, and includes (along with a wide variety of other topics) assessments of the effects of maternal stature, PPW and PWG. All references were evaluated and rated on appropriate methods, including general aspects of research design and adequate controls for confounding variables. Wherever possible, summary calculations of the effects of particular variables on pregnancy outcome were made from studies which satisfactorily met the preestablished methodological standards (e.g., kg of PWG/g birth weight). References to these secondary analyses are included where appropriate.

stature may limit fetal growth by imposing physical restrictions on growth of the maternal reproductive organs and the fetus.

Numerous studies have documented an association between maternal height and pregnancy outcomes. However, since height is strongly correlated with weight, it is important to determine whether the effect of maternal height is direct or mediated through weight. For example, Thomson's (1959) frequently cited work shows a decline in the incidence of prematurity with increasing maternal stature in a large sample of Aberdeen, United Kingdom, women, but does not account for the potential confounding effects of PPW or PWG. No significant independent effect of maternal height on gestational age or prematurity has been shown in studies that do control for weight.

There is, however an independent effect of maternal height on birth weight. In the majority of studies which adequately control for confounding variables (namely, gestational age of the infant, maternal PPW, PWG, and smoking during pregnancy), the effect is positive (Niswander and Jackson, 1974; Lazar et al., 1975; Miller and Merritt, 1979; Winikoff and Debrovner, 1981; Bhargava et al., 1983; Luke et al., 1981; Bhatia and Tyagi, 1984). The effect of height tends to be relatively small after accounting for PWG and PPW, particularly in developed countries (cf. Weis and Jackson, 1969; Rush et al., 1972). Kramer (1988) determined an average effect of 7.8 g of birth weight/cm maternal height. Several studies from developing countries show effects of greater magnitude. Among Indian women who delivered in a university hospital, Bhatia and Tyagi (1984) reported a 10.7 g/cm effect of maternal height on birth weight. After controlling for maternal arm fat and muscle area at 30 weeks of pregnancy, Adair and Popkin (1988) found a significant positive effect of maternal height on birth weight and length in a community-based study of nearly 2,000 Filipino mothers and infants. Similarly, an independent contribution of maternal height to birth weight was found in the Guatemalan study of Habicht et al. (1973). In contrast, no effect of maternal stature on birth weight was found in an urban Peruvian sample of nearly 5,000 women studied by Frisancho et al. (1977). Short and tall mothers with comparable subcutaneous fat and upper arm muscle area just prior to delivery gave birth to infants of similar size. The authors concluded that variations in stature alone have minimal effects on prenatal growth

Short maternal stature represents a risk factor for low birth weight (LBW) and intrauterine growth retardation (IUGR) as well as obstetrical complications that increase perinatal mortality (Thomson, 1959; Camilleri, 1981; Kappel et al., 1987). In a detailed study of determinants of pregnancy outcome risk groups based on birth weight and body proportions, Adair and Popkin (1988) have shown short maternal stature to be a significant determinant of proportionate growth retardation in Filipino infants. Miller and Merritt (1979) also reported a significant effect of maternal stature on infant crown–heel length and head circumference. Theirs is a five-year study based on births in a large U.S. university hospital.

Differences in the reported effects of maternal stature on pregnancy outcome may be attributed to several factors. First, studies vary with respect to the confounding variables included in multivariate analyses. Second, the populations under study may differ with respect to how well maternal stature represents genetic versus environmental factors. The direct and weight-mediated effects of stature on birth weight may differ according to why a women is short. In poorly nourished populations, short maternal stature is likely to be the result of a poor nutritional history, and not a good reflection of the mother's (and thus her infant's) genotype.

Maternal Weight Before or During Pregnancy

PPW of the mother, expressed relative to height, is assumed to reflect maternal nutritional stores available to meet the increased needs of pregnancy. The woman with low PPW, and thus low energy stores, must be able to meet her own needs as well as fetal needs for growth and development solely by increased dietary intake. When this is not accomplished, adverse effects on pregnancy can be expected. A number of strategies have been used to define weight for height as an indirect measure of body fat stores. These include indices such as the Quetelet (wt/ht^2) or ponderal (wt/ht^3) index, and weight expressed as a percentage of ideal weight for a given height defined in a reference standard. If such expressions accurately reflect energy stores, and energy stores are the component of maternal body composition that affects pregnancy outcomes, one would expect them to be more strongly related to pregnancy outcome than in PPW alone. But the value of expressing PPW relative to height has been questioned by Garn and Pesick (1982). Using data on 44,725 pregnancies from the U.S. Perinatal Collaborative Study, they found that indices of relative weight were no more effective than PPW alone in predicting infant birth weight. In fact, based on a comparison of product-moment correlations and analyses of birth weight by decile of weight or each index, birth weight and birth weight variability were better related to PPW than to any index of weight relative to height. Other studies have not included such comparisons and generally control for maternal height when addressing the relationship of PPW to pregnancy outcomes. Regardless of how it is defined, low PPW is strongly related to a number of pregnancy outcomes, including gestational age, birth weight, and perinatal mortality.

Several U.S. studies have shown an elevated risk of preterm delivery among women with low PPW for height (Meyer et al., 1976; Kaminski et al., 1973; Edwards et al., 1979). A clearer association is found between PPW and birth weight. Women with low PPW tend to have lighter babies (Peckham and Christianson, 1971; Simpson et al., 1975; Eastman and Jackson, 1968; Niswander et al., 1969; Ounsted and Scott, 1981). Kramer (1988) has estimated an average PPW effect on birth weight of 9.5 g/kg maternal PPW. Miller and Merritt (1979) also found a significant effect of PPW on head circumference in full-term infants: The incidence of low occipital-frontal circumferences was significantly elevated in infants born to mothers with low PPW for height. Increased perinatal mortality is also related to low maternal PPW expressed as an index of ponderosity (Naeye 1983; based on Perinatal Collaborative Study data).

PPW interacts significantly with PWG so that its independent effects are difficult to determine. This issue will be discussed in greater detail in the section on PWG.

Pregnancy Weight Gain

PWG consists of four major components: maternal reproductive tissue; increased maternal blood volume and extracellular fluid; the fetus, placenta, and amniotic fluid; and maternal fat stores. Fat stores are the component of primary concern as a maternal nutritional determinant of infant outcomes. Except in cases where marked edema develops, differences in the amount of maternal fat deposited account for much of the variability in PWG between individuals. The size of other components of PWG (e.g., blood volume, the fetus and placenta) is more biologically constrained.

PWG is the most frequently measured indicator of maternal nutritional status during pregnancy. It reflects generalized changes in many body dimensions as evidenced by its high correlations with maternal skinfolds and body diameters and circumferences (e.g., upper arm, calf, and chest) (Lechtig et al., 1978).

The relationship of PWG to birth weight has been recognized for a long time and provides the rationale for numerous dietary recommendations designed to regulate weight gain. The purposeful restriction of dietary intake to limit the size of the fetus and ensure an easier delivery is a practice found in many parts of the world. In traditional societies, such restrictions may take the form of culturally regulated food taboos during pregnancy. In the United States, restricting weight gain during pregnancy was an accepted obstetric practice up to the early 1970s (Gormican et al., 1980). Restrictions were based on several mistaken assumptions: One was that limited weight gain reduces the incidence of preeclampsia, a second is that the fetus is the "perfect parasite," able to meet its needs irrespective of maternal nutritional status. Niswander and Jackson (1974) have even suggested that the higher incidence of LBW and perinatal mortality in the United States compared with several northern European countries can be partly attributed to lower PWG in American women. In developed countries, most LBW is accounted for by prematurity rather than IUGR. Low PWG is associated with both LBW and IUGR. For example, Miller and Merritt (1979), in their study of women delivering in a large university hospital in Kansas, showed that compared with those with adequate or high PWG, women with low PWG (< 7 kg) were much more likely to have preterm or IUGR infants. In developing countries, low PWG associated with maternal undernutrition during pregnancy is recognized as a major determinant of LBW and IUGR.

In virtually every published study on PWG and birth weight, a strong positive relationship between these two variables has been found. Studies differ markedly with respect to sample size, study design, and how well they control for other factors known to influence birth weight. Even when the most important factors are controlled (e.g., gestational age, maternal height, smoking, and PPW), PWG remains a highly significant determinant of birth weight. In fact it is usually the single most important factor after gestational age. Several studies have quantified the average contribution of PWG to birth weight. For the average woman with adequate prenatal nutrition, the PWG effect on birth weight is 20.3 g/kg (Kramer, 1988; based on Niswander and Jackson; 1974, and Rush et al., 1972).

Several U.S. studies done in the 1960s (Eastman and Jackson, 1968; Niswander et al., 1969) suggested a direct effect of PWG on birth weight. This brought into focus the potential detrimental effects of restricting weight gain. New recommendations were established for "optimal" weight gains during pregnancy based on gains observed to be compatible with the best fetal outcomes, namely birth weights of 3,000–4,500 g, or the lowest perinatal mortality rates (Niswander and Gordon, 1972; Hytten and Leitch, 1971). For example, the National Academy of Sciences recommended an average gain of 24 pounds. Beginning in the 1970s, however, some investigators began to question whether recommendations for weight gain ought to be contingent on maternal energy reserves present at the beginning of pregnancy. In other words, they questioned whether similar weight gains had the same effects on pregnancy outcomes in women who were underweight versus overweight at the beginning of pregnancy.

A large number of U.S. studies have addressed this issue. Most are based on retrospective data gathered from hospital and clinic records. Mothers are classified as underweight, normal, overweight, or obese based on a comparison of height and PPW to a reference standard. The Metropolitan Life Standard is frequently used despite its shortcomings. First, the standard is based only on insured persons, and second, it requires that frame size be determined. The latter is a difficulty for prospective studies, and is usually not possible at all for retrospective studies, most of which simply use average frame size for all subjects.

A consistent finding is that the effect of PWG on pregnancy outcome depends on PPW for height. Miller and Merritt (1979) found a fourfold increase in prematurity and a threefold increase in IUGR among women with both low PPW and low PWG compared to women with average or above average PPW for height. Brown et al. (1981) reported that underweight women with the same PWGs as normal weight women had lighter babies. Similarly, Abrams and Laros (1986) found that a 1 kg maternal weight gain had different effects on birth weight depending on the woman's PPW-for-height status: Each 1 kg of PWG contributed an average of 25.9 g to birth weight among underweight women, but only 17.8 g to birth weight for overweight women. Among obese women, the relationship between PWG and infant birth weight was not statistically significant.

Luke and Petrie (1980) and Luke et al. (1981) also explored relationships of PPW, PWG, and birth weight. Their subjects were black women referred for nutrition counselling through the outpatient clinic of the Columbia Presbyterian Hospital in New York. To avoid the problems associated with inaccurate recall of PPW or use of weight at the first prenatal visit, mean weekly weight gains were calculated from the first visit to the final recorded predelivery weight.[3] Women were classified into rate of gain categories (low $<$ 230 g/wk, medium 230–454 g/wk, high $>$ 455 g/wk). To ascertain PPW and establish weight-for-height groups, the authors still used recalled PPW. Within each PWG group, increased newborn length and weight were associated with higher PPW. Within each PPW-for-height group (based on Metropolitan Life Standards), the incidence of small for gestational age (or IUGR) infants decreased markedly with increasing rates of PWG.

Winikoff and Debrovner (1981) found differences by weight-for-height group in the maternal anthropometric variable that best explains birth weight. Among low weight-for-height women, PWG best explains birth weight, but among intermediate weight-for-height women, PPW best explains birth weight. The authors suggested that the relative effects of genetic and environmental factors on birth weight differ depending on the body type of the mother.

Recently, Hediger et al. (1988) explored the relationship of birth weight to early (before 24 weeks) versus late (24 weeks to term) PWG in a large sample of low-income adolescents in the United States. This type of investigation is important because it differentiates weight gain which is primarily attributable to accumulation of maternal tissue (early PWG) from gains attributable to growth of the fetus (which predominates in the last trimester of pregnancy). They found that inadequate early PWG represents a risk for lower birth weights even when late gains were adequate. This finding has particular importance for supplementation programs which have focused on providing additional food late in pregnancy when fetal demands are high.

The relationship of PPW, PWG, and perinatal mortality was explored by Naeye (1979) in data from the Collaborative Perinatal Project of the National Institute of Neurological and Communicative Disorders and Stroke. He found that optimal weight gains, i.e., those gains associated with the lowest perinatal mortality rates, differed among women who were overweight at the start of pregnancy (optimal gain = 7.3 kg), underweight (optimal gain = 13.6 kg), or normal weight (optimal gain = 9.1 kg). For all three groups, perinatal mortality rates increased when PWG exceeded or fell short of these optimums. With excessive weight gains ($>$14.5 kg), an increased incidence of perinatal mortal-

[3]Note that this method also introduces a bias. Rates of weight gain vary over the course of pregnancy. Maximum rates are achieved between 17 and 24 weeks (Hytten and Chamberlain, 1980). Thus, average gains over the observed period may differ according to when a woman was first measured.

ity was observed independent of complications such as hypertension or gestational diabetes that often accompany excessive gains or maternal obesity. Based on data from the 1980 U.S. National Natality and Fetal Mortality Survey, Taffel (1986) explored the relationship of PWG to fetal deaths. Women with low PWG (< 9.5 kg) were 1.5 times more likely to have pregnancies that terminated in a fetal death compared to women with higher PWG (after controlling for mother's age, prenatal care, gestational age, parity, and smoking). Furthermore, the risks of smoking for fetal death declined as PWG increased. On the other end of the weight gain spectrum, Taffel also noted a small rise in fetal deaths associated with excessive (>16.3 kg) weight gains.

Maternal Postpartum Weight

Ideally, the correlation of PWG with birth weight should only consider the maternal components of weight gain. In practice, this is difficult, since the components cannot be measured directly. Several investigators have tried to deal with this problem by considering maternal postpartum weight. Immediate postpartum weight continues to reflect some PWG components other than increased fat stores, but is still a good reflection of the mother's net energy stores at the end of pregnancy. Luke and Petrie (1980) found increased birth weight to be associated with heavier maternal postpartum weight in underweight and normal weight women (classifications based on a comparison of postpartum weight to the Metropolitan Life Standards). In overweight women, a negative association of postpartum weight with birth weight was found. Several studies in India also show positive relationships of maternal postpartum weight and infant birth weight (Bhargava et al., 1983; Bhatia and Tyagi, 1984).

Measures of Fatness and Muscularity

Upper arm circumference (UAC) and skinfold thicknesses are well recognized as important indicators of nutritional status. Estimates of arm muscle and fat area can be derived when UAC and triceps skinfold thickness are known.

A number of studies have described changes in maternal skinfolds over the course of pregnancy (see earlier section on skinfolds), but relatively few have looked at the relationship of skinfolds or fat areas to pregnancy outcomes. This is surprising in light of the fact that such measurements provide more direct information about maternal energy reserves than does PPW or PWG, both of which summarize maternal and nonmaternal components. It is generally assumed that adequate maternal energy stores contribute significantly to good pregnancy outcomes. Thus, a positive relationship between skinfold thicknesses or fat area and outcomes such as birth weight is anticipated. Results from studies in several different populations are consistent with this expectation. For example, Butte et al. (1981) found birth weight of Navajo infants to be significantly related to maternal upper arm and calf circumferences and triceps and subscapular skinfold thicknesses during pregnancy. Bissenden et al. (1981) studied a small group of Asian women in Birmingham. They found that reduced increments in triceps and biceps skinfolds during the second and third trimesters of pregnancy represented a risk factor for small for gestational age infants. Similarly, Viegas et al. (1987), studying a slightly larger sample of Asian women (n = 81) in Birmingham, found that changes in triceps skinfolds during the second trimester of pregnancy were highly effective predictors of poor fetal growth. The second trimester of pregnancy is ordinarily the time when most maternal fat deposition takes place. Viegas et al. suggest that second trimester changes in triceps skinfolds reflect maternal energy balance at a time in pregnancy that is particularly important for fetal growth.

The relationship of maternal energy stores to birth weight has been questioned by Briend (1985) based on a study of over 2,400 deliveries in a poor African periurban community. A stepwise multiple regression revealed that when maternal weight was controlled, triceps skinfold thickness was negatively correlated with birth weight. Briend concluded that birth weight is regulated by some unknown factor related to lean body mass rather than to energy reserves. This is consistent with findings reported by Frisancho et al. (1977), who looked at the relationship of maternal anthropometric variables and pregnancy outcomes in a sample of nearly 5,000 mothers and infants from Lima, Peru. Mothers were divided into fat and lean categories based on their triceps skinfold thicknesses and into groups representing high and low muscularity based on upper arm muscle area just prior to delivery. Fat mothers had significantly fatter, but not longer or heavier, newborns. In other words, greater maternal fat reserves were not reflected in fetal linear growth or increased birth weight. However, mothers with high muscle area had heavier and longer infants than mothers with low muscle area. Muscle area was interpreted by the authors as a measure of protein reserves. The authors concluded that increased maternal protein reserves rather than energy reserves enhance fetal linear growth and birth weight.

In their study of rural Guatemalan women, Lechtig et al. (1978) found no correlation of birth weight with maternal skinfold thicknesses at the end of pregnancy or with monthly changes in skinfolds during pregnancy. In a multivariate analysis, once maternal weight at the end of pregnancy was accounted for, no association of birth weight and any other maternal anthropometric variable was found. However, maternal height and head and arm circumference together were as good as weight at the end of pregnancy in predicting birth weight.

The independent contributions to pregnancy outcomes of different maternal anthropometric variables are difficult to ascertain because of the high correlation between these variables. Table 2 presents data from a large sample of Filipino women measured during pregnancy. Pearson correlation coefficients of several maternal anthropometric variables show their strong interrelations. The variables are not only highly correlated, but share joint determinants as well. In this same population, Adair and Popkin (1988) found low maternal fat reserves (measured by arm fat area at 30 weeks of pregnancy) to be a significant determinant of proportionate growth retardation. Also, there

TABLE 2. Maternal Anthropometric Variables at 30 Weeks of Pregnancy: Pearson Correlations in a Sample of 3,326 Filipino Women

	Height	Weight	Triceps	UAC	Fat area	Muscle	BMI
Height	1.00	0.52	0.21	0.15	0.17	0.18	0.03
Weight		1.00	0.64	0.79	0.72	0.65	0.87
Triceps skinfold			1.00	0.75	0.98	0.32	0.66
Upper arm circumference				1.00	0.86	0.86	0.81
Arm fat area					1.00	0.49	0.73
Arm muscle area						1.00	0.66
Body mass index							1.00

was a significant positive effect of arm fat area weight and length of the infant at birth. This latter effect was found using a multiple regression model, with birth weight and length as independent variables, and (among others) maternal height, arm fat and muscle area, caloric intake, parity, smoking, and gestational age as independent variables. However, when the mother's weight was included in the model along with height, the effect of maternal fat area on birth weight was negative, a result consistent with that reported by Briend (1985). But, when more sophisticated analytic techniques were used to control for joint determination (endogeneity) of the key variables, the negative effect of arm fat area on birth weight disappeared. This result strongly points out the need for more sophisticated methods to sort out the independent contribution to birth weight of maternal energy reserves, muscularity, and stature. Most research to date has not adequately addressed this issue.

Fundal Height

Fundal height, the distance from the upper border of the pubic symphysis to the top of the uterus, is a useful indicator of fetal growth and can be used as a screening tool for IUGR. Fundal height is thus not a true indicator of maternal nutritional status, but it is a valuable anthropometric tool for predicting poor outcomes. At 12 weeks, the fundus normally lies just above the symphysis, at 16 weeks it is halfway between the symphysis and the umbilicus, at 20 weeks it is at the umbilicus, and at 36 weeks it reaches to just below the ensiform cartilage. From 20 to 30 weeks, fundal height in cm is roughly equivalent to gestational age. Fundal height is routinely measured in most obstetric practices and clinics in the United States and is gaining increasing use as a screening tool in developing countries (Huffman et al., 1985). Belizan et al. (1978) established fundal height standards on a sample of Argentine women delivering normal infants of known gestational age. Of 44 low-weight neonates (weighing less than the 10th percentile established for the hospital), 38 had mothers in whom at least one fundal height measurement during pregnancy fell below the established fundal height 10th percentile. Of 95 neonates with adequate birth weight, 85 had mothers with fundal height above the 10th percentile. Thus, fundal height has a sensitivity of 86% and a specificity of 90% for predicting IUGR. A similar study was conducted in Oxford using a local standard based on women delivering full-term infants with birth weight between the 5th and 90th percentiles of weight for gestational age (Quaranta et al., 1981). Based on two consecutive or three isolated measures indicating fundal height below the 10th percentile, sensitivity for predicting IUGR was found to be 70% for weeks 32–40, and specificity ranged from 75% to 95%.

Special Conditions

Two maternal conditions are worthy of special note, particularly for developed countries. These are maternal obesity and pregnancy in adolescence.

Obesity. Maternal obesity represents a significant obstetric risk factor. It is often associated with a cluster of conditions which pose health threats to both mothers and infants. These include low PWG (less than 5.4 kg), hypertension, preeclampsia, gestational diabetes, multiple gestation, infant macrosomia (birth weight over 4,500 g), and elevated maternal mortality (Maeder et al., 1975; Gross et al., 1980; Kleigman and Gross, 1985; Johnson et al., 1987). The prevalence of pregnancy complications and poor infant outcomes among obese mothers is difficult to compare across studies for several reasons. First, there is no consistency in the definition of obesity. In some cases, the definition is based on an absolute weight (e.g., 90 kg), while in others it is based on weight expressed as a percentage of ideal weight for height in comparison with a reference standard. Different cutoff points may be established. For example, one study may consider as obese women who weigh more than 120% of ideal weight for height, while another study establishes the cutoff at 135%. Second, some studies fail to separate the independent effects of obesity on infant outcomes from effects that are due to the most common maternal complications of obesity, namely hypertension and gestational diabetes.

Overweight and obese women tend to gain less weight during pregnancy and are at increased risk of very low PWG (Taffel, 1986; Harrison et al., 1980). Kleigman and Gross (1985) estimated that 10%–40% of obese women in the United States (defined as PPW in excess of 90 kg) lose weight or gain less than 5.4 kg during pregnancy. The strong relationship between PWG and birth weight found in normal and underweight women tends to break down among heavy women. For example, several studies have reported no significant relationship of PWG to birth weight among overweight or obese women (Luke et al., 1981; Abrams and Laros, 1986). In one case, a negative relationship was found between mean birth weight and postpartum weight in overweight women (Luke et al., 1981). Each 10% increase in postpartum weight among these women (whose weights were 160% or more above ideal based on Metropolitan Life Standards) was associated with a 29.8 g decrease in mean birth weight. A stronger relationship between PPW and birth weight exists in obese women. Despite lower PWG, they are much less likely than normal or underweight women to give birth to IUGR infants, and in general tend to have babies who are heavier at birth. Garbaciak et al. (1985) examined the effects of obesity on pregnancy outcome by a retrospective analysis of 9,667 University of Illinois Hospital records. Compared with normal weight women, obese women (PPW greater than 120% of ideal weight for height based on the Metropolitan Life Tables) with no other antenatal complications required cesarean deliveries more often and gave birth to infants with significantly higher mean birth weight. But there were no effects on perinatal mortality attributable to maternal weight alone.

The independent effect of obesity on infant outcomes is small. Consequences for the mother may be more severe. Pregnancy may cause the expression of or exacerbate maternal health problems associated with obesity, most notably diabetes and hypertension. These conditions in turn adversely affect infant outcomes.

Adolescence. Adolescents represent an age group at high risk of poor pregnancy outcomes, particularly LBW (National Research Council, 1977; Institute of Medicine, 1985). Because they have yet to complete their own growth and development, the relationship of anthropometric indicators of nutritional status during pregnancy to birth outcomes may differ between adolescents and adults. This issue was addressed by Frisancho et al. (1983) in a sample of 12–25-year-olds giving birth at the Maternity Hospital of Lima, Peru. Young mothers (less than 17 years old) with the same weights, muscularity, and fatness had smaller babies than their older counterparts. A similar effect was found for PWG. The same PWG resulted in smaller infants born to mothers less than 17 versus over 17, when other factors (such as PPW and height) were controlled. Gynecologic age was not controlled in these analyses. Similar results were obtained in the U.S. Perinatal Collaborative Study (Naeye, 1981). Mothers aged 10–16 had smaller infants than older mothers with the same PWG and PPW. This suggests that the same level of nutritional status produces different outcomes in adolescents versus adult women. Additional research which addresses the role played by differences in maturity of the adolescent is needed. Nonetheless, special care needs to be taken to ensure adequate PWG in the adolescent.

SUMMARY

Anthropometric assessment of nutritional status during pregnancy focuses on maternal energy reserves reflected by PPW, weight gain, and skinfold thicknesses during pregnancy and by postpartum weight. PPW or PPW for height indicates the state of those reserves as a woman enters pregnancy. The low energy stores of underweight women place them at increased risk of delivering low-weight infants. Weight gain during pregnancy encompasses changes in maternal energy stores along with the products of conception, maternal reproductive organs, and blood. PWG is positively associated with birth weight except among obese women. PWG should be judged relative to maternal nutritional status at the beginning of pregnancy; underweight women need to gain more during pregnancy to match the outcomes of women who began pregnancy with adequate energy stores. Skinfold measurements and postpartum weight are useful indicators of energy stored during pregnancy because, unlike PWG, they reflect maternal changes rather than a composite of maternal and fetal changes. Most studies show a clear positive relationship of some measure of energy stores and good postnatal outcomes except among obese women.

DISCUSSION

A number of important, but as yet unanswered, theoretical issues are raised by the studies presented above. A key question concerns the importance of maternal energy stores. This is the aspect of maternal nutritional status best addressed by anthropometric assessments during pregnancy. Are good pregnancy outcomes possible in the absence of significant maternal energy stores? Is there a direct relationship between birth weight and maternal PPW or PWG? It has generally been assumed that PPW and PWG reflect the state of maternal energy balance, and that high values of these variables indicate the presence of adequate energy stores. Furthermore, it has been assumed that maternal energy stores are in fact the aspect of maternal nutritional status during pregnancy that have the greatest bearing on pregnancy outcomes. Both of these assumptions may be questioned. First, more research is needed to quantify the relationship of fat accumulation during pregnancy to total PWG. The often cited estimates of fat accumulation during pregnancy (Hytten and Leitch, 1971) are based on the ideal pregnancy. We need to know more about changes in maternal energy reserves and their relationship to PWG across a wide range of PWG. This would require methods which adequately isolate changes in the maternal body from changes in the products of conception. Second, the precise role played by maternal energy reserves (to the extent that they have been adequately quantified) relative to other aspects of maternal body composition is not entirely understood. Some controversy remains in the literature about the relationship of energy reserves to pregnancy outcome. This controversy may stem, in part, from the difficulties of isolating the independent effects of different aspects of maternal body composition.

For purposes of argument, let us accept that PPW and PWG represent adequate proxies for energy reserves. Clearly, there is a strong positive relationship between PPW, PWG (and thus presumably energy stores), and birth weight. But this relationship may not be simple or direct. The effects of these variables on pregnancy outcomes, particularly birth weight, may depend upon the relative energy demands of the mother versus the fetus. Luke et al. (1981) offer a theoretical explanatory framework. Energy demands on the mother during pregnancy include the costs of maintaining her own metabolism, meeting fetal needs for growth and maintenance, and a component which Luke et al. describe as a correction for metabolic defects. The latter includes the effects of low maternal energy stores at the beginning of pregnancy. Energy is supplied by dietary intake, and when needed, by reserves reflected by maternal PPW. PPW categories (underweight, normal, and overweight) represent depleted, adequate, or excessive reserves, respectively. In the underweight woman with low PWG, the only source of energy available is that which is supplied exogenously. Fetal growth under these circumstances is likely to be impaired, particularly when food availability is limited or energy demands of physical activity are high. The importance of energy stores early in pregnancy is highlighted by the work of Hediger et al. (1988), which shows that inadequate early PWG has a negative effect on birth weight even when later PWG is adequate. Similarly, Papoz et al. (1981) found that fetal growth is more dependent on available stores early in pregnancy than on subsequent energy intakes. Low total PWG represents both failure of the mother to augment her energy reserves in the form of body fat and small fetal size. In women with adequate PPW or fat stores, energy demands during pregnancy can be met by calling upon energy stores. Favorable pregnancy outcomes can be expected, even if energy stored during pregnancy is minimal. In the case of overweight women, stores are sufficient to support good pregnancy outcomes even with pregnancy weight losses or very low gains.

This framework applies to adolescent pregnancy as well. In the very young mother, additional energy is needed to support growth and development of the mother as well as the fetus. Thus additional weight must be gained in the adolescent compared with the older mother in order to achieve the same effect on birth weight.

What are the practical implications? For the obstetrician, recommendations on optimal weight gains during pregnancy should take energy stores of the mother prior to pregnancy into consideration. This approach is represented in a paper by Rosso (1985) in which a chart to monitor PWG is based on adequacy of maternal PPW for height (see Fig. 4).

A target of 120% of standard weight for height is established for the end of pregnancy. To maximize fetal growth, Rosso suggests that the average woman needs to increase her weight by 20%. The underweight woman needs to gain relatively more during pregnancy to reach the target, while the overweight woman needs to gain relatively less (a minimum gain of 7 kg is recommended for the woman who begins pregnancy with a PPW greater than 120% of standard). The usefulness of the chart was evaluated among low-income women of New York and women from Santiago, Chile. When the target weight was attained, mean birth weights were higher than when the target was not attained.

For the health professional interested in screening for maternal risk factors associated with poor pregnancy outcomes, several anthropometric indicators may be useful. For risk assessment during pregnancy, one would ideally like to know PPW, how much weight has been gained since the beginning of pregnancy, and how much energy has been stored. In the absence of reliable information on PPW (a situation common in field studies in developing countries), information about rates of weight gain or changes in skinfold thicknesses would be valuable. However, these assessments require several visits. It may be desirable to assess risk based on information that can be collected at a single visit. To this end, Gueri et al. (1982) have developed a reference table

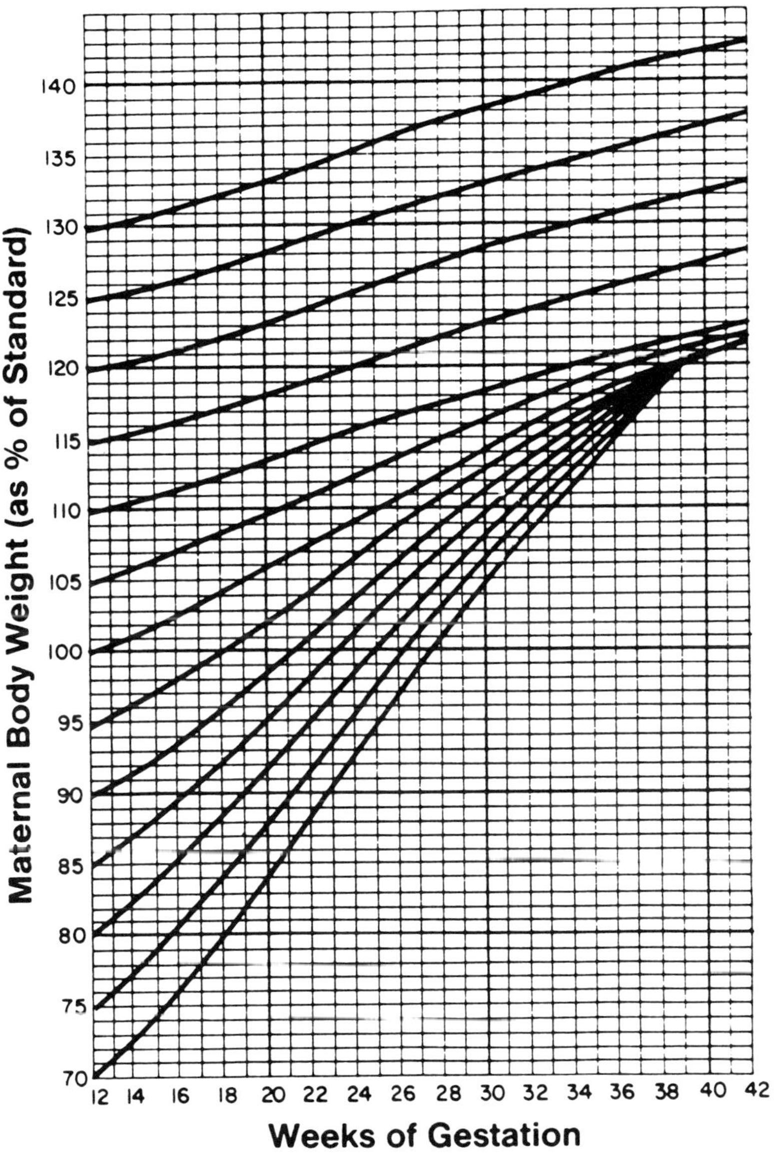

Fig. 4. Chart to monitor weight gain during pregnancy taking into consideration pre-pregnancy weight and height. (Reproduced from Rosso, 1985, with permission of the publisher.)

of weight for height by week of pregnancy that does not require information about PPW. They tested this reference table in Dominica, and found it to be a useful tool for the prediction of a woman's chances of delivering a LBW infant.

Overall, most research suggests that failure to augment maternal energy stores during pregnancy increases chances of poor pregnancy outcomes. Thus, maternal anthropometric assessments which accurately reflect low energy reserves either at the beginning or during the course of pregnancy are valuable tools for identifying those women at increased risk of poor outcomes. For prematurity and increased perinatal mortality, these include low PPW and PWG. For low birth weight, however, low PPW, low PWG, and low increments in skinfold thicknesses during the second and third trimesters of pregnancy represent important risk factors.

The effects of maternal nutritional status during pregnancy on infant outcomes is a subject that has been extensively researched. Many important questions in this area have been answered. However, several additional topics are relatively unexplored. For example, more information is needed on the effects of nutritional status during pregnancy on the mother. Significant issues include long-term effects on maternal health and reproductive success. Failure to store energy in a current pregnancy may affect the success of lactation, and contribute to the maternal depletion syndrome which is associated with repeated or closely spaced pregnancies in undernourished women. In developed countries, excessive weight gain during pregnancy represents a different set of risks, including those associated with obesity. Thus, the anthropometric assessment of nutritional status during pregnancy is important not only for assessing risk of poor health outcomes in the infant, but also for learning more about long-term maternal health.

REFERENCES

Abrams BF, Laros RK (1986): Prepregnancy weight, weight gain and birth weight. Am J Obstet Gynecol 154:503–509.

Adair LS, Popkin B (1988): Birth weight, maturity and proportionality in Filipino infants. Hum Biol 60(2):319–339.

Adair LS, Pollitt E, Mueller WH (1983): Maternal anthropometric changes during pregnancy and lactation in a rural Taiwanese population. Hum Biol 55(4):771–787.

Arroyo P, Garcia D, Lirena C, Quiroz SE (1978): Subcutaneous fat accumulation during pregnancy in a malnourished population. Br J Nutr 40:485–489.

Belizan JM, Villar J, Nardin JC, Malamud J, DeVicuna L (1978): Diagnosis of intrauterine growth retardation by a simple clinical method: Measurement of uterine height. Am J Obstet Gynecol 131:643–666.

Bhargava V, Chatterjee M, Prakash A, Bharia B, Mishra A (1983): Fetal growth variations, I: Influence of maternal size and nutrition on identification of fetal growth retardation. Indian Pediatr 20:549–559.

Bhatia BD, Tyagi NK (1984): Maternal determinants of birth weight: A multivariate analysis. Indian Pediatr 21:365–371.

Bissenden JG, Scott PH, King J, Hallum J, Mansfield HN, Wharton BA (1981): Anthropo-

metric and biochemical changes during pregnancy in Asian and European mothers having light for gestational age babies. Br J Obstet Gynecol 88:999–1008.
Briend A (1985): Do maternal energy reserves limit fetal growth? Lancet 1:38–40.
Brown JE, Berdan KW, Splett P, Robinson M, Harris LJ (1981): Influence of pregnancy weight gain on the size of infants born to underweight women. Obstet Gynecol 57:13–17.
Butte NF, Calloway DH, Van Duzen JL (1981): Nutritional assessment of pregnant and lactating Navajo women. Am J Clin Nutr 34:2216–2228.
Camilleri AP (1981): The obstetric significance of short stature. Eur J Obstet Gynecol Reprod Biol 12:347–356.
Dieckmann WJ, Wegner CR (1934): The blood in normal pregnancy. Arch Int Med 53:71–86.
Eastman NJ, Jackson E (1968): Weight relationships in pregnancy. Obstet Gynecol Survey 21:1003–1025.
Edwards LF, Alton IR, Barrada MI, Hakanson EY (1979): Pregnancy in the underweight woman. Am J Obstet Gynecol 135:297–302.
Frisancho AR, Klayman JE, Matos J (1977): Influence of maternal nutritional status on prenatal growth in a Peruvian urban population. Am J Phys Anthropol 46:265–274.
Frisancho AR, Matos J, Flegel P (1983): Maternal nutritional status and adolescent pregnancy outcome. Am J Clin Nutr 38:739–746.
Garbaciak JA, Richter M, Miller S, Barton JJ (1985): Maternal weight and pregnancy complications. Am J Obstet Gynecol 152:238–245.
Garn SM, Pesick SD (1982): Relationship between various maternal body mass measures and size of the newborn. Am J Clin Nutr 36:664–668.
Gormican A, Valentine J, Satter E (1980): Relationships of maternal weight gain, prepregnancy weight and infant birth weight. J Am Diet Assoc 77:662–667.
Gross T, Sokol RJ, King KC (1980): Obesity in pregnancy: Risks and outcome. Obstet Gynecol 56:446–450.
Gueri M, Jutsum P, Sorhaindo B (1982): Anthropometric assessment of nutritional status in pregnant women: A reference table of weight-for-height by week of pregnancy. Am J Clin Nutr 35:609–611.
Habicht JP, Yarbrough C, Lechtig A, Klein RE (1973): Relationships of birth weight, maternal nutrition and infant mortality. Nutr Rep Int 7:533–546.
Harrison GG, Udall JN, Morrow G (1980): Maternal obesity, weight gain in pregnancy and infant birth weight. Am J Obstet Gynecol 136:411–412.
Hediger ML, Scholl TD, Salmon R (1988): Patterns of early weight gain in pregnant teenagers and fetal outcome. Am J Phys Anthropol 75:222. Abstract.
Himes JH, Roche AF, Webb P (1980): Fat areas as estimates of total body fat. Am J Clin Nutr 33:2093–2100.
Hoseman H (1949): Schwangershaftsdauer und Gewicht der Placenta. Arch Gynakologe 173:453.
Huffman SL, Krasovec K (1985): Maternal nutritional risk assessment. Paper presented at the XIII International Congress of Nutrition, Brighton, U.K.
Hytten FE, Chamberlain G (1980): "Clinical Physiology in Obstetrics." Oxford: Blackwell Scientific.
Hytten FE, Leitch I (1971): "The Physiology of Human Pregnancy." 2nd ed. Oxford: Blackwell Scientific.
Hytten FE, Thomson AM, Taggart N (1966): Total body water in normal pregnancy. J Obstet Gynecol Br Comm 73:553.

Institute of Medicine (1985): "Preventing Low Birthweight." Washington, DC: National Academy Press.
Jansen AAJ, Kusin JA, Thiuri B, Lakhani SA, Mannetje W (1984): Machakos project studies No. XXIV: Anthropometric changes during pregnancy in rural African women. Trop Geogr Med 36:91–97.
Johnson SR, Kolberg BH, Varner MW, Rausback LD (1987): Maternal obesity and pregnancy. Surg Gynecol Obstet 164:431–437.
Kaminski M, Goujard J, Rumeau-Rouquette C (1973): Prediction of low birth weight and prematurity by a multiple regression analysis with maternal characteristics known since the beginning of pregnancy. Int J Epidemiol 2:195–204.
Kappel B, Ericksen G, Hansen KB, Hvidman L, Krag-Olsen B, Nielsen J, Videbech P, Wohlert M (1987): Short stature in Scandanavian women. An obstetrical risk factor. Acta Obstet Gynecol Scand 66:153–158.
Kleigman RM, Gross T (1985): Perinatal problems of the obese mother and her infant. Obstet Gynecol 66:299–306.
Kramer MS (1988): "Determinants of Intrauterine Growth and Gestational Duration: A methodological Assessment and Synthesis." Geneva: WHO. Organization.
Lazar P, Dreyfus J, Papiernik-Berkhauer E (1975): Individual correction of birth weight for parental stature with special reference to small-for-date and large-for-date infants. J Perinat Med 3:242–247.
Lechtig A, Martorell R, Delgado H, Yarbrough C, Klein RE (1978): Food supplementation during pregnancy, maternal anthropometry and birth weight and infant birth weight in a Guatemalan Rural Population. Trop Pediatr Environ Child Health 24:217–222.
Lind T, Hytten FE (1972): Fetal control of the fetal fluids. In Holdari AA, Mariona FG (eds): "The Physiological Biochemistry of the Fetus." Springfield, Ill: CC Thomas.
Luke B, Dickenson C, Petrie RH (1981): Intrauterine growth: Correlations of maternal nutritional status and role of gestational weight gain. Eur J Obstet Gynecol Reprod Biol 12:113–121.
Luke B, Petrie RH (1980): Intrauterine growth: Correlation of infant birth weight and maternal post partum weight. Am J Clin Nutr 33:2311–2317.
McKeown T, Record RG (1953): The influence of placental size on foetal growth according to sex and order of birth. Endocrinology 10:73.
Maeder EC, Barno A, Mecklenburg (1975): Obesity: A maternal high-risk factor. Obstet Gynecol 45:669–671.
Meyer MB, Jones BS, Tonascia JA (1976): Perinatal events associated with maternal smoking during pregnancy. Am J Epidemiol 103:464–476.
Miller HC, Merritt TA (1979): "Fetal Growth in Humans." Chicago: Year Book.
Naeye RL (1979): Weight gain and the outcome of pregnancy. Am J Obstet Gynecol 135:3–9.
Naeye RL (1981): Teenaged and pre-teenaged pregnancies: Consequences of the maternal-fetal competition for nutrients. Pediatrics 67:146–150.
Naeye RL (1983): Effects of maternal nutrition on fetal and neonatal survival. Birth 10:109–113.
National Research Council (1977): Relation of nutrition to pregnancy in adolescence. Clin Obstet Gynecol 14:367–392.
Niswander K, Jackson EC (1974): Physical characteristics of the gravida and their association with birth weight and perinatal death. Am J Obstet Gynecol 119:306–313.
Niswander KR, Gordon M (1972): "The Women and Their Pregnancies." Philadelphia: WB Saunders.

Niswander KR, Singer J, Westphal M, Weiss W (1969): Weight gain during pregnancy and pre-pregnancy weight. Obstet Gynecol 33:482–491.

Ounsted M, Scott A (1981): Association between maternal weight, height, weight-for-height, weight gain and birth weight. In Dobbing J (ed): "Maternal Nutrition in Pregnancy: Eating for Two?" London: Academic Press.

Papoz L, Echwege E, Pequignot G, Barrat J (1981): Dietary behavior during pregnancy: The St. Antoine Maternity Hospital study in Paris. In Dobbing J (ed): "Maternal Nutrition in Pregnancy. Eating for Two?" London: Academic Press.

Peckham CH, Christianson RE (1971): The relationship between pre-pregnancy weight and certain obstetric factors. Am J Obstet Gynecol 111:1–7.

Quaranta P, Currell R, Redman CWG, Robinson JS (1981): Prediction of small-for-dates infant by measurement of symphysial-fundal-height. Br J Obstet Gynecol 88:115–119.

Retief FP, Brink AJ (1967): A study of pregnancy anaemia: Blood volume changes correlated with other parameters of hemopoietic efficiency." J Obstet Gynecol Br Commonwealth 74:683–693.

Rosso P (1985): A new chart to monitor weight gain during pregnancy. Am J Clin Nutr 41:644–652.

Rush D, Davis H, Susser M (1972): Antecedents of low birth weight in Harlem, New York City. Int J Epidemiol 1:375–387.

Simpson JW, Lawless RW, Mitchell AC (1975): Responsibility of the obstetrician to the fetus, II: Influence of prepregnancy weight and pregnancy weight gain on birth weight. Obstet Gynecol 45:481–487.

Taffel SM (1986): Association between maternal weight gain and outcome of pregnancy. J Nurse-Midwifery 31:78–86.

Taggart NR, Holliday RM, Billewicz WZ, Hytten FE, Thomson AM (1967): Changes in skinfolds during pregnancy. Br J Nutr 21:439–451.

Thomson AM (1959): Maternal stature and reproductive efficiency. Eugeni Review 51:157–162.

Thomson AM, Billewicz WZ (1957): Clinical significance of weight trends during pregnancy. Br Med J 1:243–247.

Thomson AM, Hytten FE, Billewicz WZ (1967): The epidemiology of oedema during pregnancy. J Obstet Gynecol Br Commonwealth 74:1–10.

Viegas OAC, Cole TJ, Wharton BA (1987): Impaired fat deposition in pregnancy: An indicator for nutritional intervention. Am J Clin Nutr 45:23–28.

Weis W, Jackson EC (1969): Maternal factors affecting birth weight. In "Perinatal Factors Affecting Birth Weight." Washington, DC: PAHO Publ. No. 185.

Winikoff B, Debrovner CH (1981): Anthropometric determinants of birth weight. Obstet Gynecol 58:678–684.

Anthropometric Assessment
of Nutritional Status, pages 259–271

15
Birth Weight as an Indicator of Fetal Nutritional Status

LAURA E. CAULFIELD
Division of Human Development and Nutrition, School of Public Health, University of Minnesota, Minneapolis, Minnesota 55455

INTRODUCTION

Weight at birth is probably the most routinely collected anthropometric measurement. Birth weight data are used by clinicians, researchers, and public health planners for a variety of purposes including establishing newborn energy requirements, screening for high-risk newborns, assessing and monitoring the health and nutritional status of newborn populations, and evaluating the effectiveness of maternal and child health services. Although widely used, few consider the methodological issues related to the use of birth weight data. The purpose of this chapter is to identify theoretical and practical concerns related to the use of birth weight data in assessing fetal nutritional status and to discuss the relevance of these concerns in light of the intended use of the birth weight indicator.

BIRTH WEIGHT AS AN INDICATOR

The weight of the infant at birth is not itself an outcome of interest; however, the weight of an infant at birth is important because it summarizes the processes of fetal growth and development and predicts short- and long-term postnatal health outcomes. Thus, birth weight is both a reflective indicator of fetal nutritional status and a prospective indicator of postnatal health and survival.

The difference between an indicator and an outcome of interest is that the indicator is influenced by factors unrelated to the outcome. For example, although height is a measure of nutritional status in young children, variation in height is also influenced by nonnutritional factors ranging from genetics to the time of day the measurement is taken. Habicht et al. (1979) suggest that these factors can be grouped according to the manner in which they affect the indicator; factors may impair the 1) precision, 2) dependability, or 3) accuracy of the indicator. By understanding how these factors influence the precision, dependability, and accuracy of an indicator, decisions can be made regarding its usefulness for different applications.

Issues involving the role of birth weight as a health indicator of the newborn have been described elsewhere (WHO, 1981; Rasmussen et al., 1985). Therefore, the objective of this chapter is to identify influences on the precision, dependability, and accuracy of birth weight and to discuss how they affect the usefulness of birth weight as an indicator of fetal nutritional status.

Precision

Precision is the degree to which one can determine the correct value of the indicator. Thus, it depends on the characteristics of the measurement process itself. Important concerns in measuring birth weight are the quality of the scales and of the training of the observers. Sources of imprecision include intraobserver and interobserver errors, rounding errors, and digit preference (David, 1980). A potentially common source of error is the failure to subtract the weight of any cloth in which the baby may be wrapped.

Few data exist regarding the precision of birth weight measurements per se. Measurement of body weight in general is considered to be precise (Habicht et al., 1979; Himes, 1989). Habicht et al. (1979) estimate measurement variability (i.e., imprecision) for body weight measured under research conditions to be 20 grams, and to be less than 1% of the total variability of body weight in a population of chronically malnourished children. Even though such measurement variability would constitute a greater percentage of the total variability of birth weight, birth weight data measured under such conditions would be considered quite precise. Birth weight data used for research and programming purposes, however, are usually abstracted from hospital records and birth certificates. To my knowledge, no published estimates of imprecision of birth weight data as routinely measured in hospitals (and recorded on birth certificates) are available. Thus, it is not possible to make a statement regarding the precision of the birth weight indicator as it is most commonly used.

Dependability

An indicator is considered to be dependable if variation in the indicator can be attributed to variation in the underlying outcome of interest—in our case, the nutriture of the fetus. Thus, the dependability of birth weight as an indicator of fetal nutritional status will be compromised to the extent that nonnutritional factors influence variation in birth weight. Five types of nonnutritional influences acting on birth weight are discussed below. They are 1) length of gestation; 2) genetics of fetal growth; 3) circumstances of labor and delivery; 4) maternal parity; 5) timing of the weighing.

Length of gestation. A baby's birth weight is his or her weight at the moment of passing from the intrauterine to the extrauterine environment. In the human, this change occurs across a range of chronological ages (time since conception). The size (weight) of a baby at birth, then, depends on the time spent in utero as well as the rates of growth achieved in utero. Because of this, observed changes in the birth weight distribution of a population may be due to changes in the gestational age distribution of the population and not necessarily to changes in fetal nutritional status per se.

The determinants of length of gestation are not well defined, although environmental and genetic factors affecting the mother and the fetus are clearly involved. To the extent that these factors determine length of gestation without affecting the rate of fetal growth, they too represent a source of undependability of the birth weight indicator.

The fetal growth process itself, however, may influence length of gestation (Wilcox, 1981). If, for example, faster growing fetuses deliver earlier than their slower growing counterparts, then the influence of fetal growth rates in determining length of gestation could explain the flattening and trailing off of the fetal growth curve around 40 weeks of gestation (Usher and McLean, 1974; Wilcox, 1981). If true, gestational age should not be conceptualized as a source of undependability but rather as a mediating variable in the relationship between fetal growth and birth weight.

Errors in the estimation of length of gestation may also affect the dependability of the birth weight indicator. Length of gestation is most commonly measured using the date of the mother's last menstrual period (LMP). There are many sources of error in the estimation of gestation length using such data. It is estimated that even when LMP dates are known with some accuracy, there is an error of ± one week in estimating the gestational age of the fetus (Finnstrom, 1972). Research in this area has been reviewed recently (see Jones et al., 1986).

Genetics of fetal growth. Clearly, size at birth is determined to some degree by maternal and fetal genetics. Breeding experiments and familial aggregation studies have been conducted to estimate the heritability of birth weight, i.e., the percent of the variance in birth weight attributable to maternal and fetal genotypes. Research on the heritability of birth weight has been recently reviewed (Yates, 1988).

It is generally concluded that fetal genotype is relatively unimportant in determining birth weight, accounting for only 8%–18% of the variation in birth weight (Penrose, 1961, Polani, 1974; Yates, 1988). Maternal genotype is thought to contribute approximately 20% of the variation in birth weight with the remaining 62%–72% of the variance due to environmental factors (Polani, 1974; Yates, 1988).

One aspect of the fetal genotype contributing to variation in birth weight is gender. Generally, males weigh 50–150 grams more than females at birth with the magnitude of the between-sex differences in birth weight increasing with increasing length of gestation (Thomson et al., 1968; Hoffman et al., 1974; Bjerkedal et al., 1973; Milner and Richards, 1974). Gender is estimated to account for approximately 2% of the total variation in birth weight (Polani, 1974).

Maternal and fetal genetics may affect size at birth by influencing either fetal growth or the length of gestation. Current thinking (discussed in Gluckman, 1986) suggests that fetal genotype is relatively unimportant in the biological regulation of fetal growth. It is likely that length of gestation is under greater genetic control than rate of fetal growth, but the degree to which fetal and maternal genetics determine length of gestation is not known. Regardless of this, fetal and maternal genetics represent a small source of undependability of the birth weight indicator.

Circumstances of labor and delivery. There are several circumstances of labor and delivery that may affect the dependability of the birth weight indicator. The timing of the clamping of the cord and whether or not the fetus expels meconium during labor and delivery will affect birth weight. The mode of delivery may also be important. Cassady (1971) found that infants delivered by cesarean section had 20% higher total body water than infants delivered vaginally, presumably because infants born vaginally lose body water during labor and delivery. Cheek et al. (1982), however, found no differences in cell hydration between vaginally and cesarean-delivered infants. The relative importance of these sources of undependability is not known, but is presumed to be small.

Obstetric practices such as induction may also affect the dependability of the birth weight indicator. This has been described by Carr-Hill and Pritchard (1985:pp 8–26). Infants delivered following induction are younger and lighter than infants delivered following spontaneous onset of labor. Thus, the proportion of induced births in a population will affect the distribution of birth weights regardless of the state of fetal nutritional status of the population. Further, specific sections of the birth weight distribution may be affected because the decision to induce is not random, but is related to either the growth of the fetus or the duration of gestation.

Maternal parity. First-born infants tend to be lighter than second- and later-born infants, with demonstrated differences in mean birth weight between first- and later-born infants of as much as 200 grams at certain gestational ages (Carr-Hill and Pritchard, 1985:pp 8–26). Because of this, birth weight standards have been developed based on maternal parity (Thomson et al., 1968; Bjerkedal, 1973).

The mechanism by which maternal parity influences birth weight, however, is not understood. Specifically, it is not clear whether the diminished size of first-born infants represents normal or abnormal fetal growth. To the extent that the former is true, the influence of parity on birth weight represents a source of undependability of birth weight as an indicator of fetal nutritional status.

Timing of the weighing. In many field situations, it is difficult to weigh the infant at birth, and the weight of the infant during the first 24–48 hours is often taken as his or her birth weight. All infants, however, lose weight after birth. They lose approximately 2.5%–3.8% of their birth weight during the first 24 hours and approximately 5.0%–6.3% of their birth weight by the end of the first 48 hours (Naish and Edwards, 1952; Furuhjelm, 1954; MacLaurin, 1966;

Cheek et al., 1984). The percentage of weight lost by an infant is influenced by neonatal morbidity and neonatal care procedures (Fleischman, 1982).

The composition of this weight loss is open to debate. Early studies suggested that postnatal weight loss is due to dehydration (MacLaurin 1966; Cassady and Milstead, 1971), but more recent work suggests that such weight loss is due to catabolism (Cheek et al., 1982; van de Wagen et al., 1985). Postnatal weight loss most likely reflects a combination of water and tissue loss. Clearly, the pattern and composition of postnatal weight loss have strong implications for the accuracy of research investigating the nutritional status of the newborn. For the purpose of assessing fetal nutritional status, however, variation in the timing of the weighing of the infant after birth introduces a source of undependability of birth weight regardless of the composition of the weight loss.

Two conclusions can be drawn from this discussion. First, it is clear that many nonnutritional influences are acting on birth weight and potentially rendering it undependable as an indicator of fetal nutritional status. Second, the effect of these influences on the dependability of birth weight depends on its intended use. The dependability of the birth weight indicator relative to its intended uses will be discussed later.

Accuracy

Accuracy is the degree to which changes in the underlying outcome of interest are reflected in changes in the indicator; that is, the degree to which changes in fetal nutritional status are reflected in changes in birth weight. To evaluate the accuracy of birth weight as an indicator, we need to examine the relationship between birth weight and body composition in the newborn.

Birth weight and body composition. It is difficult to measure the body composition of the newborn. Thus, researchers have depended on chemical analyses of small samples of fetuses of varying gestational ages. Because such samples are small and quite selective, it may be erroneous to draw firm conclusions about the body composition of the fetus; however, the results do provide general information.

The body composition of the fetus changes as the fetus matures. At 26 weeks' gestation, the fetus is 86%–88% water, 9% protein, and 1%–3% fat, while at 40 weeks' gestation, the fetus is 68%–76% water, 11%–13% protein, and 11%–15% fat (Fomon, 1967; Ziegler et al., 1976; Fomon et al., 1982; Widdowson, 1981). The bodies of small-for-date newborns contain less fat (% weight), but approximately the same amount of protein as normally grown newborns (Apte and Iyengar., 1972; Cheek et al., 1984). Correspondingly, the bodies of small-for-date newborns contain more water for their body weight than normally grown newborns.

There are notable gender differences in body composition. For their weight, male newborns have more water and protein than female newborns. This is due to the greater fat content of female newborns; at term, female newborns are approximately 14.9% fat as compared with 13.7% fat for male newborns (Fomon et al., 1982).

Clearly, the fastest changing component of the body during the third trimester is fat. Ziegler et al. (1976) estimate that the percentage of fetal weight gain contributed by fat increases from 5% at 24 weeks of gestation to 29% at 40 weeks of gestation. The type of fat deposited also changes during the third trimester; whereas, the majority of the fat deposited before the third trimester is in the form of structural lipids, the majority of the fat deposited during the third trimester is subcutaneous. Subcutaneous fat constitutes approximately 80% of the total fat found in the full-term infant (Widdowson, 1981). Given that fat is the fastest changing component of body composition during the third trimester, comparing the relationship between variation in body fat and body weight should give us insights into the accuracy of birth weight as an indicator of fetal nutritional status.

Correlations between birth weight and measures of body fat are moderate to high. The correlation between birth weight and percent body fat estimated from carcass analysis is 0.95 (Brans et al., 1974). Estimates of the correlation between skinfold thickness measurements and birth weight vary between 0.39 and 0.87 (Garn, 1958; Farr, 1966; Brans et al., 1974; McGowan et al., 1975) with the magnitude of the correlation dependent on the sample of infants and the skinfold site. Consistently across studies, the relationship between birth weight and skinfold thickness is described as positive and linear (Garn, 1958; Gampel, 1965; Farr, 1966; Brans et al., 1974; Oakley et al., 1977; Peterson et al., 1988).

The correlation between body fat (as measured by skinfold thicknesses) and gestational age seems to be fairly low. Most authors provide estimates ranging between -0.01 and 0.37 (Garn, 1958; Farr, 1966; McGowan et al., 1975); however, Brans et al. (1974) estimate the correlation between gestational age and skinfold thickness to be on the order of 0.80–0.84. It has been suggested that because birth weight and gestational age are moderately correlated, the estimated correlation between body fat and gestational age is artifactual (McGowan et al., 1975). The low correlations between gestational age and skinfolds, however, may be explained partially by the curvilinear nature of the relationship between the two variables (Gampel, 1965).

It appears that birth weight is more important than gestational age in describing variation in body fat. In several studies, for example, no difference was found in the mean skinfold thicknesses of groups of infants with similar mean birth weights but differing mean gestational ages (Brans et al., 1974; Enzi et al., 1981; Peterson et al., 1988). Groups of infants with similar mean gestational ages but differing mean birth weights, however, were found to have different mean skinfold thicknesses, with the greater mean skinfold thickness observed for the heavier group (Enzi et al., 1981). Farr (1966), however, found that mean skinfold thickness did decrease, albeit slightly, with increasing mean gestational age within each of three categories of birth weight. Further, the results of Peterson et al. (1988) suggest that gestational age may influence percent body fat, independent of birth weight.

There is disagreement in the literature concerning the functional form of the relationship between birth weight and percent body fat. The data reported by Enzi et al. (1981) suggest that the relationship between birth weight and percent body fat is sigmoidal, such that changes in birth weight at the tails of the distribution are linearly related to changes in percent body fat, while changes in birth weight in the center portion of the distribution are not related to changes in percent body fat. Similarly, Dauncey et al. (1977) found that the relationship between birth weight and percent body fat was linear among newborns weighing less than 2 kilograms, but found no relationship between birth weight and percent body fat among newborns weighing more than 2 kilograms. These results are in contrast to Brans et al. (1974), who described a linear relationship between percent body fat and birth weight.

The results from the literature suggest that body weight and body fat in the newborn are strongly related. Variation in gestational age is also related to variation in body fat, but to a lesser degree. It appears that the degree to which changes in body fat are reflected in changes in birth weight depends on the level of body fat. Thus, the accuracy of birth weight as an indicator of fetal nutritional status depends on the intended use of the indicator.

USES OF BIRTH WEIGHT DATA

In the previous section, we examined factors affecting the precision, dependability, and accuracy of birth weight as an indicator of fetal nutritional status. It was clear from that discussion that the relative importance of these factors will depend largely on the intended use of the indicator. In the following section, we will examine how problems affecting the precision, dependability, and accuracy of birth weight determine its usefulness as an indicator for three different applications.

Probably the most common use of birth weight data is for the development of standards to describe the variation in birth weight in a population. Typically, these standards describe the distribution of birth weights of a population stratified by week of gestation. Further stratification by gender, maternal parity, and parental height (when applicable) removes additional sources of undependability (Thomson et al., 1968; Bjerkedal et al., 1973; Brenner et al., 1976). Such standards are used, for example, 1) to develop curves depicting fetal growth, 2) to identify infants suffering from intrauterine malnutrition, 3) and to monitor the impact of interventions to improve the nutritional status of newborn populations.

Fetal Growth Curve

The assumption underlying the use of birth weight data for developing fetal growth curves is that cross-sectional distributions of birth weight at various weeks of gestation accurately depict the longitudinal process of intrauterine growth. This assumption should be examined in greater detail.

The appropriateness of using birth weight data to describe intrauterine growth depends on whether the observed distribution of birth weights at a specific week of gestation approximates the true distribution of fetal weights, both observed and unobserved at that week of gestation. The unobserved weights belong to babies waiting to be born. This assumption is questionable because the week of gestation at which the weight is observed (i.e., the baby is born) is not determined randomly. As discussed earlier, the length of gestation is determined by a myriad of factors that are not well understood. To the extent that these determinants are measurable, birth weight standards could be adjusted for selection bias to reasonably depict fetal growth.

The degree to which the observed distributions of birth weight suffer from selection bias is not known precisely; however, evidence of its existence is available from several sources. First, the distributions of birth weights of infants delivered before 34–35 weeks of gestation are generally bimodal, while those characterizing later births are approximately normal (David, 1980). Second, results from both human and animal studies suggest that the distributions of weights of babies delivered spontaneously before term are downwardly biased relative to the true distributions of weights at those gestational ages (Fujikura and Niemann, 1967; Weiner et al., 1985). Thus, it may be concluded that the distributions of birth weight observed at shorter lengths of gestation probably do not accurately describe the magnitude and variation of fetal growth present at that time.

The possibility was discussed earlier that the growth of the fetus itself may influence length of gestation. The implication of this relationship is that each fetus has his or her own growth curve, and thus, observed distributions of birth weight across weeks of gestation cannot accurately represent the process of fetal growth (Carr-Hill and Pritchard, 1985:pp 44–58). Given the implications of this relationship, the extent to which fetal growth rates influence gestation length should be investigated.

Prevalence of Intrauterine Malnutrition

A second use of birth weight standards is for assessing the nutritional status of newborn populations and for identifying those newborns suffering from intrauterine malnutrition. Typically, infants whose weights fall below some predetermined cutoff point for their gestational age are considered to be small for date and suffering from intrauterine growth retardation or malnutrition. Various cutoff points have been used: 25th, 10th, 5th, 3rd percentile of the birth weight distribution, or two standard deviations below the mean of the birth weight distribution.

This indicator of malnutrition, however, is undependable because there is no confirmatory evidence that infants whose weights fall below the cutoff value suffered from malnutrition in utero. Some infants are small because their growth was compromised; however, others are merely genetically small.

Conversely, the growth of some infants weighing more than the cutoff point may have been compromised because of malnutrition. Further, although female infants generally weigh less than male infants at birth, they are not more likely to be growth retarded. The same may hold true for first-born infants. Finally, if the distributions of birth weights among preterm infants are downwardly biased estimates of the true distribution, the extent of malnutrition among preterm infants may be underestimated.

Thus, it is important to investigate the relative validity of the various cutoff points used for identifying malnourished infants. Inasmuch as this involves quantifying the accuracy of the indicator, it would seem likely that quantification of the relationship between birth weight and body fat stratified by week of gestation and gender (and also possibly by maternal parity and parental height) would provide a means for selecting an appropriate cutoff point for identifying intrauterine growth retarded newborns. The selection criteria for identifying the appropriate cutoff point, however, will depend on the intended use of the indicator (Habicht et al., 1982; Brownie et al., 1986). It should be noted that previous research has found the 10th percentile of the birth weight distribution to be an appropriate cutoff point for discriminating differences in early postnatal morbidity and mortality risk among newborns in Argentina and Mexico (Balcázar, 1987; Caulfield, 1989).

Evaluation of Programs

A third use of birth weight standards is to evaluate the impact of interventions aimed at improving fetal nutritional status. Research designs for evaluating such interventions involve the distributions of birth weights between two populations, one receiving the intervention, the other acting as a control, or comparing the distributions of birth weights in the same population before and after the initiation of the intervention.

In determining the impact of an intervention, one must demonstrate that any improvements in the birth weight indicator are due to improvements in fetal nutritional status. Thus, the dependability of birth weight is of prime importance. The nature of the research designs employed in evaluation studies do remove many sources of undependability. Many other sources of undependability, however, must be dealt with during the analytic phase of the project.

An important issue affecting the accuracy of birth weight standards for evaluating changes in fetal nutritional statue must also be discussed. When designing interventions to improve fetal nutritional status, one must also know how much, and what kind of improvement, in fetal nutritional status can be expected in a population. To estimate this, one must know the form of the ideal distribution of birth weights for the population, that is, the distribution of birth weights of normally grown fetuses. Do birth weight standards describe the ideal nutritional status of populations? Clearly the answer is no, because standards as currently developed describe only the present situations of specific populations.

Carr-Hill and Pritchard (1985: pp 8–26) describe how failure to consider the nature of the ideal birth weight distribution can lead to erroneous conclusions regarding changes in the fetal nutritional status of populations. In Aberdeen, the birth weight means between the 32nd and 38th week of gestation have been declining over the past 30 years. Although this shift could be interpreted as a worsening of the fetal nutritional status of the population, it is more likely due to improvements in pregnancy outcomes over the 30-year period. For example, as some causes of preterm delivery (before 37 weeks) are prevented, the distributions of birth weight at each week of gestation for preterm infants will change to increasingly reflect a population of infants whose delivery preterm is nonpreventable. If the weights of these infants are lower than the weights of infants whose delivery preterm was prevented, then improvement in the prevention of preterm delivery is a likely explanation for the type of changes in the birth weight distributions observed for the Aberdeen population. From this discussion, it is clear that changes in the birth weight distributions of populations must be interpreted with respect to the ideal distribution of birth weights.

What does the ideal distribution of birth weights look like? The answer is not known, although specific attributes of the distribution can be described. On a practical level, the importance of this problem may be population dependent. The issue may not be very important for many populations in developing countries, for example, because birth weight standards from industrialized nations may provide acceptable guidelines (given some caveats) for the time being. The issue is crucial, however, for populations where significant improvements in fetal nutritional status have already occurred, and further improvements require heavy investments in health and social services. Our current inability to describe the nature of the distribution of ideal birth weights represents a significant problem for researchers attempting to evaluate the effectiveness of various interventions to improve fetal nutritional status in those populations.

SUMMARY

The purpose of the chapter was to discuss theoretical and methodological issues related to the use of birth weight as an indicator of fetal nutritional status. First, factors affecting the precision, dependability, and accuracy of birth weight as an indicator of fetal nutritional status were discussed. Second, the importance of these and other conceptual issues were discussed relative to three intended uses of the birth weight indicator. Although some issues related to the usefulness of birth weight data may not have been mentioned, it is hoped that the material presented in this chapter provides insights into the complexity of the theoretical and methodological issues involved when using birth weight as an indicator of fetal nutritional status.

ACKNOWLEDGMENTS

Preparation of this chapter was supported in part by Grant HD-24684, National Institutes of Health, Bethesda, Maryland.

REFERENCES

Apte SV, Iyengar L (1972): Composition of the human foetus. Br J Nutr 27:305–312.

Balcázar H (1987): "BirthweightMortality Relationships in an Urban Poor Population of Mexico City: Implications for Screening Infants at Risk." Ithaca, NY: Division of Nutritional Sciences, Cornell University. Ph.D. thesis.

Bjerkedal T, Bakketeig L, Lehmann E (1973): Percentiles of birth weights of single, live births at different gestation periods. Acta Paediatr Scand 62:449–457.

Brans Y, Sumners J, Dweck H, Cassady G (1974): A noninvasive approach to body composition in the neonate: Dynamic skinfold measurements. Pediatr Res 8:215–222.

Brenner W, Edelman DA, Hendricks CH (1976): A standard of fetal growth of the United States of America. Am J Obstet Gynecol 126:555–564.

Brownie C, Habicht J-P, Cogill B (1986): Comparing indicators of health or nutritional status. Am J Epidemiol 124(6):1031–1044.

Carr-Hill R, Pritchard C (1985): "The Development and Exploitation of Empirical Birthweight Standards." New York: Stockton Press, ch 2, pp 8–26; ch 5, 44–58.

Cassady G (1971): Effect of caesarean section on neonatal body water spaces. N Engl J Med 285(16):887–881.

Cassady G, Milstead R (1971): Antipyrine space studies and cell water estimates in infants of low birth weight. Pediatr Res 5:673–682.

Caulfield LE (1989): "An Epidemiological Study of the Determinants and Postnatal Health Consequences of Variation in Ponderal Index Among Intrauterine Growth Retarded Newborns." Ithaca, NY: Division of Nutritional Sciences, Cornell University. Ph.D. thesis.

Cheek D, Wishart J, MacLennan AH, Haslam R (1984): Cell hydration in the normally grown, the premature and the low weight for gestational age infant. Early Hum Dev 10:75–84.

Cheek D, Wishart J, MacLennan AH, Haslam R, Fitzgerald A (1982): Hydration in the first 24 h of postnatal life in normal infants born vaginally or by caesarean section. Early Hum Dev 7:323–330.

Dauncey M, Gancy G, Gairdner D (1977): Assessment of total body fat in infancy from skinfold thickness measurements. Arch Dis Child 52:223–227.

David RJ (1980): The quality and completeness of birthweight and gestational age data in computerized birth files. Am J Public Health 70(9):964–973.

Enzi G, Zanardo V, Caretta F, Inelmen EM, Rubaltelli F (1981): Intrauterine growth and adipose tissue development. Am J Clin Nutr 34:1785–1790.

Farr V (1966): Skinfold thickness as an indication of maturity of the newborn. Arch Dis Child 41:301–308.

Finnstrom O (1972): Studies on maturity in newborn infants. Acta Paediatr Scand 61:33–41.

Fomon SJ (1967): Body composition of the male reference infant during the first year of life. Pediatrics 40(5):863–870.

Fomon SJ, Haschke F, Ziegler EE, Nelson SE (1982): Body composition of reference children from birth to age 10 years. Am J Clin Nutr 35:1169–1175.

Fleischman AR (1982): Special problems of the fetus and neonate. In Finberg L, Kravath RE, Fleischman AR (eds): "Water and Electrolytes in Pediatrics." Philadelphia: W.B. Saunders, pp 220–225.

Fujikura T, Niemann WH (1967): Birth weight, gestational age, and type of delivery in rhesus monkeys. Am J Obstet Gynecol 97:76–80.

Furuhjelm U (1954): Loss of weight in the newborn infant during the first week of life. Etud Neonate 3:93–99.

Gampel B (1965): The relation of skinfold thickness in the neonate to sex, length of gestation, size at birth and maternal skinfold. Hum Biol 37:29–37.

Garn SM (1958): Fat, body size and growth in the newborn. Hum Biol 30:265–281.

Gluckman PD (1986): The regulation of fetal growth. In Buttery PJ, Haynes NB, Lindsay DB (eds): "Control and Manipulation of Animal Growth." London: Butterworths, pp 85–104.

Habicht J-P, Meyers LD, Brownie C (1982): Indicators for identifying and counting the improperly nourished. Am J Clin Nutr 35:1241–1254.

Habicht J-P, Yarbrough C, Martorell R (1979): Anthropometric field methods: Criteria for selection. In Jelliffe DB, Jelliffe EFP (eds): "Human Nutrition: A Comprehensive Treatise." New York: Plenum Press, pp 365–387.

Himes JH (1989): The reliability of anthropometric methods and replicate measurements. Am J Phys Anthropol 79:77–80.

Hoffman H, Stark CR, Lundin FE, Ashbrook JD (1974): Analysis of birth weight and gestational age and fetal viability, U.S. births, 1968. Obstet Gynecol Surv 29(9):651–681.

Jones RM, Peters J, Bagnall KM (1986): Anthropometric measures of fetal growth. In Falkner F, Tanner JM (eds): "Human Growth—A Comprehensive Treatise." New York: Plenum Press, pp 255–274.

MacLaurin J (1986): Changes in body water distribution during the first two weeks of life. Arch Dis Child 41:286–291.

McGowan A, Jordan M, MacGregor J (1975): Skinfold thickness in neonates. Biol Neonate 25:66–84.

Milner RDG, Richards B (1974): An analysis of birth weight by gestational age of infants born in England and Wales, 1967 to 1971. J Obstet Gynaecol Br Cwlth 81:956–967.

Naish FC, Edwards PW (1952): Initial weight-loss: A preliminary enquiry. Arch Dis Child 27:445–448.

Oakley J, Parsons RJ, Whitelaw AGL (1977): Standards for skinfold thickness in British newborn infants. Arch Dis Child 52:287–290.

Penrose LS (1961): Genetics of Growth and Development of the Foetus. In Penrose LS (ed): "Recent Advances in Human Genetics." Boston: Little, Brown and Company, pp 56–75.

Peterson S, Gotfredsen A, Knudsen FU (1988): Lean body mass in small for gestational age and appropriate for gestational age infants. J Pediatr 113:886–889.

Polani PE (1974): Chromosomal and other genetic influences on birth weight variation. In: "Size at Birth." CIBA Foundation Symposium No. 27 (new series). Amsterdam: Elsevier, pp 127–160.

Rasmussen KM, Mock NB, Habicht J-P (1985): "The Biological Meaning of Low Birthweight and the Use of Data on Low Birthweight for Nutritional Surveillance." Cornell Nutritional Surveillance Program, Working Paper Series, No. 43, Ithaca, NY: Cornell University.

Thomson AM, Billewicz WZ, Hytten FE (1968): The assessment of fetal growth. J Obstet Gynaecol Br Cwlth 75:903–916.

Usher RH, McLean F (1974): Normal fetal growth and the significance of fetal growth retardation. In Davis JA, Dobbing J (eds): "Scientific Foundations of Paediatrics." London: Heineman Medical Books, pp 69–79.

van de Wagen A, Okken A, Sweens J, Zijlstra WG (1985): Composition of postnatal wieght loss and subsequent weight gain in small for date newborn infants. Acta Paediatr Scand 74:57–61.

Weiner C, Sabbagha RE, Vaisrum N, Depp R (1985): A hypothetical model suggesting suboptimal intrauterine growth in infants delivered preterm. Obstet Gynecol 65:232–326.

Widdowson EM (1981): Changes in body composition during growth. In Davis JA, Dobbing J (eds): "Scientific Foundations of Paediatrics." London: Heineman Medical Books, pp 330–342.

Wilcox AJ (1981): Birthweight gestation and the fetal growth curve. Am J Obstet Gynecol 131(8):863–867.

World Health Organization (1981): "Uses of Birthweight Data in Public Planning and Practice (MCH/BW/81.1)." Report of a meeting held April 28–May 2, 1980, in Geneva, Switzerland. Cornell Nutritional Surveillance Program Report R9, Ithaca, NY: Cornell University.

Yates J (1988): The genetics of fetal and postnatal growth. In Cockburn F (ed): "Fetal and Neonatal Growth." New York: Wiley, pp 1–10.

Ziegler E, O'Donnell A, Nelson SE, Fomon SJ (1976): Body composition of the reference fetus. Growth 40:329–341.

Anthropometric Assessment
of Nutritional Status, pages 273–286

16
A Fresh Look at Anthropometric Classification Schemes in Protein-Energy Malnutrition

DONALD S. McLAREN
Department of Preventive Ophthalmology, Institute of Ophthalmology, London EC1V 9EJ, United Kingdom

INTRODUCTION

A specialised treatise such as this that deals exhaustively with every aspect of the subject of anthropometric assessment of nutritional status provides an opportunity, perhaps the first, for detailed consideration of the various schemes of classification of protein-energy malnutrition (PEM) employing the techniques of anthropometry that have been put forward over the years.

It should prove both interesting and instructive to trace the developments that have taken place up until the present day. Consideration will be given to the various purposes that have been in the minds of those who have devised the different schemes. Attention will also be paid to the practical limitations that have operated in certain circumstances, necessitating compromise proposals rather than the ideal.

Little more than a decade ago it would almost certainly have been assumed without further thought by editor, author, and reader alike that the term PEM referred exclusively to the major malnutrition problem of childhood in the third world. Today it can be taken for granted that all concerned recognise that PEM is to be found in children and adults alike wherever, and for whatever reason, energy and protein requirements of the body are not being met over a period of time. Consequently there are large numbers of hospitalised medical and surgical patients with PEM (Bistrian et al., 1976; Hill et al., 1977). Their classification, which has until now proved considerably problematic (McLaren, 1988), will be reviewed later.

Some classification schemes of PEM incorporate biochemical and/or immunologic indicators along with anthropometric ones. This will limit their application to those situations where laboratory facilities are available. However, there is this to be said in favor of their inclusion; they introduce another, complementary, form of assessment and in some instances reflect more directly energy-protein status than does anthropometry.

Use and Misuse of Classification Schemes

It is not generally appreciated that classification schemes that are based on isolated, cross-sectional observations (and all currently in use are of this nature) can strictly speaking apply only to population groups and not to individuals. All biological data, including those related to nutritional status such as somatic measurements, have a wide normal range. Classification implies the application, to some extent arbitrary, of cutoff points to create categories in relation to a reference standard which is itself constructed from data pertaining to a large healthy population which exhibits a wide variation of values among individuals.

That this should be necessarily so should be evident when it is remembered that the reference standard is expressed in terms such as centile distribution; as a standard deviation score (*Z*-score); or as a percentage of the reference median (WHO Working Group, 1986). Expression of data from any study population must be in similar terms for comparison.

A simple example may make this important point clear. A healthy male infant aged 6 months weighs 6.2 kg. At this age the 50th centile male value on the NCHS standard is 7.8 kg (the 5th centile is 6.2 kg; the 95th centile is 9.4 kg). Without knowing which centile the infant has previously been following, it is impossible to characterise him at this point: 5th centile implies 100%; 50th centile 79%; and 95th centile only 66% standard weight/age. If the Gómez classification (see below) were to be applied (inappropriately), the case would be labeled as "1st° PEM." If the previous status had been different, it could equally well have been "2nd° PEM" (on the 95th centile) or "normal" (on the 5th centile). The errors that can result in this way may be large; they cannot be ignored.

It is therefore not legitimate to label individual cases in this way on the basis of a single observation, and this applies not just to weight/age but to any similar indicators. If this principle is accepted and followed, then the circumstances in which PEM can be legitimately classified on the basis of cross-sectional data are restricted to population groups. The latest WHO Working Group report (1986) on the subject confirms this by stating "assessment of an individual from a single measurement is inevitably insensitive because of the wide range of intra-individual variation." It probably does not make the point as clearly as needs to be done, and hopefully has been done here, as it is evident that the advice is not being followed, and erroneous classification of individuals is constantly being made.

The WHO report identifies the following uses for classification: 1) overall assessment of a population; 2) identification of target groups or areas for priority action; 3) nutritional surveillance; 4) monitoring of nutritional status; 5) evaluating the impact of programmes; 6) sequential measurements for studying the effects of seasonal changes; and 7) emergency situations (to screen those requiring priority attention). Some of these uses in which individual cases are identified do not qualify strictly speaking for reasons stated above.

THE GÓMEZ CLASSIFICATION

It would appear that Bowditch (1891) almost a century ago was the first to make comparison of the growth of fairly large numbers of children, using for weight and height the method of percentile grades that had been introduced by Galton and which remains current practice.

It was more than 50 years later that the Mexican pediatrician Gómez (1946) constructed weight/age charts with curves on them to represent 1st, 2nd, and 3rd degree PEM. The original paper and several thereafter were in Spanish and attracted little attention, but it was versions of the classification in English a decade or so later (Gómez et al., 1955; Gómez et al., 1956) that have led to this classification being "still the most widely used for nutrition surveys" in the recent words of Frenk (1985), one of its originators.

Table 1 shows the Gómez classification as originally proposed. In the words of Gómez and his colleagues (Gómez et al., 1955), "this classification of malnutrition was adopted by the Hospital Infantil de México in order to simplify the nomenclature of a large group of diverse and confusing ailments, the common basis of which is deficient nutrition." It is not usually realised that the "standard" referred to above is no more than the cross-sectional data on an unspecified number of well-nourished Mexican children hospitalised for conditions other than malnutrition. In this connection also it should be pointed out that the famous Harvard growth standards, which still form the basis of nutritional assessment in many developing countries, were developed from cross-sectional measurements on only about 100 children who were considered to be healthy by a simple physical examination. No attempt was made to exclude those who were overweight. It is only in recent years with the adoption by WHO of the NCHS standard that a firmer foundation is being given to international anthropometry.

Two modifications were made to the Gómez classification. Bengoa (1962) pointed out that abundant edema disguises or may even cancel out any weight deficit, and its mere presence in a malnourished child is accepted as 3rd degree. Jelliffe (1966) proposed shorter percentile intervals in which each phase agrees approximately with one SD.

TABLE 1. Gómez Classification of PEM[a]

Severity	Standard (Harvard) (% Expected weight for age)
Normal	>90
Mild (1st degree)	89–75
Moderate (2nd degree)	74–60
Severe (3rd degree)	<60

[a]In a later modification all cases with nutritional edema, irrespective of weight, were included in 3rd degree.

THE PEM PYRAMID

The next step was the appreciation by McLaren (1966) and Jelliffe (1969) that PEM was not adequately categorised by a three-tier system as in the Gómez classification but that it consisted of forms as well as degrees. This concept is well portrayed in the nutritional pyramid of Jelliffe (1959; see Fig. 1).

Not only are there three degrees of PEM (1st, 2nd, and 3rd degree or mild, moderate, and severe), but the severe degree with clinical manifestations can be divided up into marasmus, marasmic kwashiorkor and kwashiorkor). The three degrees of PEM are characterised by growth failure throughout; biochemical changes emerge in the 2nd degree and worsen in the 3rd degree; clinical signs are confined to the 3rd degree. Evidence for this concept was obtained in studies of severely malnourished children in Jordan (McLaren et al., 1967). A simple scoring system for classifying severe PEM was developed (Table 2) based on a combination of anthropometric, biochemical, and clinical indicators. It has been used quite extensively for the purpose for which it was intended: the classification of hospital cases of PEM.

This system has been criticised for including both edema and serum albumin on the basis that they are closely interrelated. Although the importance of the plasma oncotic pressure exerted by albumin in contributing to the maintenance of intravascular fluid is well known, there is evidence that other factors may be largely responsible for edema in kwashiorkor (Golden, 1982). If this proves to be so, the criticism would lose its validity.

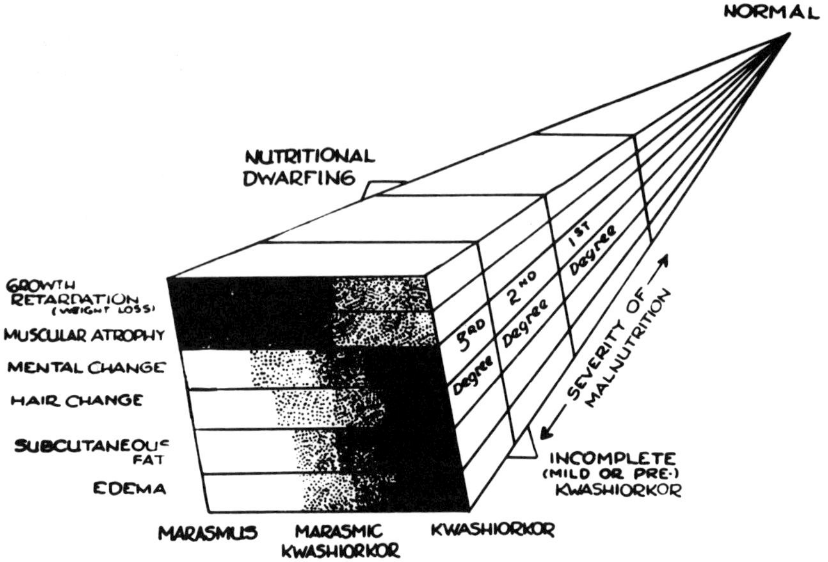

Fig. 1. The nutritional pyramid of protein-energy malnutrition. (Reproduced from Jelliffe, 1959, with permission of the publisher.)

TABLE 2. Scoring System for Severe Forms of PEM[a]

Signs present		Points
Edema		3
Dermatosis		2
Edema plus dermatosis		6
Hair Change		1
Hepatomegaly		1
Serum albumin (or serum total protein) (g/100 mL)		
<1.00	(<3.25)	7
1.00–1.49	(3.25–3.99)	6
1.50–1.99	(4.00–4.74)	5
2.00–2.49	(4.75–5.49)	4
2.50–2.99	(5.50–6.24)	3
3.00–3.49	(6.25–6.99)	2
3.50–3.99	(7.00–7.74)	1
>4.00	(>7.75)	0

From McLaren et al., 1967.
[a]Score = sum of points; 0–3 = marasmus (67.5% or less expected weight by Harvard standard); 4–8 = marasmic kwashiorkor; 9–15 = kwashiorkor.

THE "WELLCOME" CLASSIFICATION

This scheme (FAO/WHO Expert Committee, 1971; see Table 3) was proposed by a group convened by the Wellcome Trust. It is still in use although conceptually it has been superseded. Like the simple scoring system, it is primarily concerned with identifying the different forms of severe PEM and uses only weight/age and the presence or absence of edema for this purpose. For

TABLE 3. "Wellcome" Classification of PEM

	Body weight as % of standard[a]	Edema	Deficit in weight for height[b]
Underweight child	80–60	0	Minimal
Nutritional dwarfing	< 60	0	Minimal
Marasmus	< 60	0	+ +
Kwashiorkor	80–60	+	+ +
Marasmic kwashiorkor	< 60	+	+ +

From FAO/WHO Expert Committee, 1971.
[a]Standard taken as 50th percentile of the Harvard values. See Nelson WE (1964): "Textbook of Pediatrics" 8th edition. Philadelphia: WB Saunders, pp 48–53.
[b]Weight for height $= \frac{\text{Weight of patient}}{\text{Weight of normal subject of same height}} \times 100.$

the first time it attempts to tackle the problem of separating "active" and "inactive" PEM by the use of weight/height, although this is not part of the indicators used.

This classification has several defects (McLaren, 1971). Besides using weight 3 age, with the attendant difficulties to be mentioned below, it confuses classification by degree and type of PEM. For example, the only difference between kwashiorkor and marasmic kwashiorkor in the scheme is the lower weight in marasmic kwashiorkor, thus implying that marasmic kwashiorkor is a more severe and advanced degree of PEM. There is no evidence for this; in Jordanian children there were no differences between the mean weights of children with marasmus, marasmic kwashiorkor, and kwashiorkor (52.5%, 54.7%, and 51.6% of standard; McLaren et al., 1967).

CRITICISMS OF CLASSIFICATIONS USING WEIGHT/AGE

The most serious disadvantage is that they are incapable of distinguishing between "active" and "chronic" PEM. A child that has been malnourished in the past but has made a good recovery will have a weight deficit for its age but may have an appropriate weight for its smaller size. The classifications evolved to address this issue are discussed below.

Age may not be known with any accuracy, especially after the first year of life. It assumes that all children should have the same weight at any given age, irrespective of their "size" as reflected for example by length. Finally, weight is influenced considerably by body composition. The density of adipose tissue is about 0.90, while that of lean body mass approximates to 1.10. Failure to gain or loss of these tissues in different proportions will not be indicated by so crude a measurement as body weight. Furthermore, extracellular water increases, absolutely as well as relatively, during progression towards the kwashiorkor end of the PEM spectrum, and this may obscure some of the weight deficit due to loss of cellular mass. This has been known to have the effect during monitoring of weight gain in a health clinic of lulling the observer into a false sense of security which is only dispelled when a precipitous weight loss occurs as a consequence of an intercurrent infection.

CLASSIFICATION OF PEM BY THE UNSKILLED

A weighing machine requires careful use and proper transport, maintenance, and calibration. Length or height measures are not generally available for field use. Very simple tools, with minimal requirements for their use, can provide valuable information under routine clinic and field conditions, especially in emergency situations.

Probably the first of these was the QUAC stick for height related to arm circumference used in relief operations in Nigeria and Bangladesh (Arnhold, 1969). This and the mid-upper arm circumference alone (Zerfas, 1975) divided children into two broad categories of "normal" and "malnourished." The ratio midarm circumference/head circumference (Kanawati and McLaren, 1970) is independent of age and similar for the sexes between 3 and 48 months, when the incidence of PEM is highest. It correlates very closely with weight/age; Table 4 shows a classification based on these two simple tape measurements that has proved of value in the field.

It is the nature of arbitrary classifications, and that is all that the anthropometric systems for PEM can be, to attract at best an evanescent popularity (Ziman, 1976). A number of systems have sunk virtually without trace, although they may have been put to good use at the time. This may be said for the somatic index (Kanawati et al., 1970), which combined weight, height, midarm circumference, and head circumference measurements and was used, among other things, to separate families in the same environment who had children growing poorly or well.

A goal well worth reaching, but which has never been attained, is to place anthropometry on a percentage scale, as a somatic quotient, comparable to and for comparison with the intelligence quotient (IQ) or developmental quotient (DQ) of the child psychologists (McLaren and Kanawati, 1972). In view of the fact that numerous studies have shown that impairment of intellectual development is the most important long-term consequence of PEM, this concept should receive the serious attention it deserves.

WASTING AND STUNTING

The importance of differentiating between "active" and "chronic" PEM from the points of view of diagnosis (classification), prognosis, and prevention seems to have drawned upon three groups of workers at about the same time (Seoane and Latham, 1971; Waterlow, 1972; McLaren and Read, 1972). Although there were some differences in approach, it was generally agreed that weight/age is the best available indicator of *wasting*, or "active," PEM and height/age of *stunting*, or "chronic" PEM.

The weight/height/age classification of McLaren and Read (1975) lends itself to graphic presentation of both wasting and stunting and can also be used for overweight and obesity (Fig. 2).

The latest review of the subject by a WHO Working Group (1986) recommends the NCHS population as a reference for international use and in the

TABLE 4. Midarm Circumference/ Head Circumference Ratio Classification of Malnutrition in Children 3 Months to 4 Years of Age

Ratio	Classification
>0.310	Nutritionally healthy
0.310–0.280	Mild PEM
0.279–0.250	Moderate PEM
<0.250	Severe PEM

From Kanawati and McLaren, 1970.

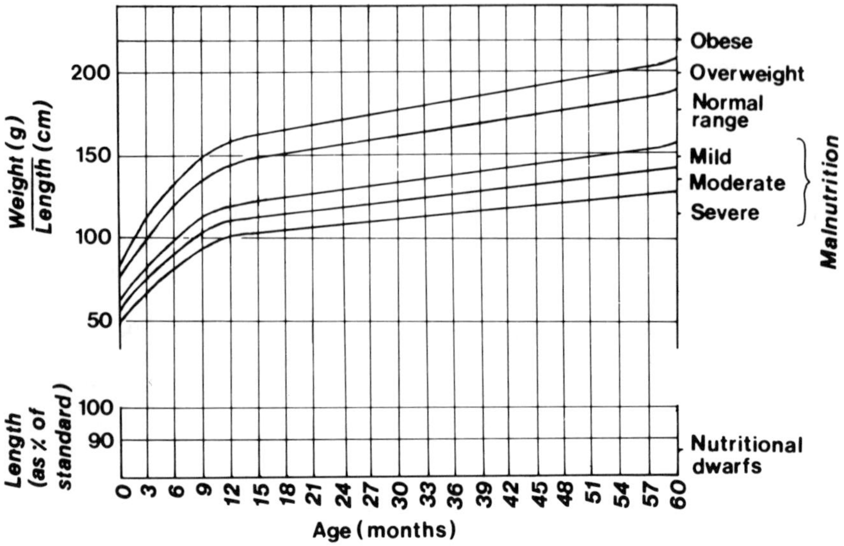

Fig. 2. Chart for assessment of nutritional status and classification of protein-energy malnutrition according to weight/height/age and height/age. (Reproduced from McLaren and Read, 1975, with permission of the publisher.)

analysis of data preference is given to the use of standard deviation (SD) scores and to the presentation of whole distributions.

Table 5 (Keller et al., 1976) shows how a classification such as this can be used to make comparisons between similar groups of children in different countries. Nabarro and McNab (1980) developed a colored wall chart for use

TABLE 5. Two-by-Three Classification[a]

Country	Height for age (%)	Weight for height 80	80–119	120 +
Togo	<90	8.1	14.7	0.0
	90 +	19.9	57.4	0.0
Philippines	<90	3.7	31.7	0.3
	90 +	7.5	56.7	0.4
Yugoslavia	<90	0.0	0.0	0.0
	90 +	1.4	97.3	1.4

From Keller et al., 1976.

[a]% of child populations aged 1–2 years from three countries as stunted, not stunted, wasted, not wasted, and obese.

by "minimally trained health workers to identify children who are so wasted that they require immediate nutritional help."

Cole et al. (1981) later criticised the classifications of Waterlow and McLaren and proposed the use of weight/height^2/age. W/H^2 is, of course, Quetelet's index or body mass index (BMI), the currently most popular index for the classification of obesity in adults. It has also been advocated for this purpose in children (Rolland-Cachera et al., 1982) and has been applied in undernutrition in adults (see below). It has been shown to be the best form of expression of weight/height interrelationships in minimising the influence of height on weight. For this reason it would seem to be preferable to weight/height to classify wasting in children.

SOME OTHER ISSUES

Distance and Velocity Charts

As was pointed out recently (Brook et al., 1986), the keeping of velocity charts of a child's growth is a much better way of detecting growth failure than is the customary recordings made on a distance chart. At present neither type of chart is in general use in the third world. A realistic objective there is the much wider use of distance charts such as the Road to Health Chart. A recent survey in parts of Asia revealed that there are many deficiencies in their day-to-day use (Gopalan, 1987).

Growth at Birth

The WHO Working Group (1986) gave some attention at the end of its report to birth weight. Low birth weight has long been defined, by WHO, as a birth weight less than 2,500 g. However, there are good reasons for suggesting that weight alone, as seen already for older children, is too crude an indicator to reflect accurately growth when body composition, especially adipose tissue mass, can vary so greatly (McLaren 1987a). Maternal undernutrition is a significant cause of intrauterine growth retardation in developing countries (Chiswick, 1985). Other somatic measurements are now beginning to be used to classify newborns according to nutritional status. For example, the mid-arm circumference/head circumference classification has been applied to newborns (Sasanour et al., 1986; Georgieffer et al., 1986).

PEM Classification and Mortality

Of all the possible uses of assessment and classification of PEM, the greatest interest has been shown in the ability of anthropometric indicators to predict a fatal outcome. This is not the place to review the subject in detail, but summarisation of experience in 11 studies (Sommer and Loewenstein, 1975; Shah et al., 1976; Kielmann and McCord, 1978; Chen et al., 1980; Bairagi, 1981; Trowbridge and Sommer, 1981; Kasango Project Team, 1983; Bairagi et al., 1985; Briend et al., 1986, 1987; Smedman et al., 1987) shows that arm circumference alone was the indicator most highly correlated with mortality in more than half the studies in which it was used. Weight/age was a good indicator, better than height/age. Perhaps surprisingly, in none of the studies where it was used did weight/height perform well in this regard.

A useful parallel can be drawn between the arm circumference as a predictor of child mortality and the so-called prognostic nutritional index (PNI) that has been found to correlate closely with the outcome after surgery (Buzby et al., 1988; see below). In both cases the association with the prognosis is close in statistical terms, but it is unlikely that the explanation is provided solely by nutritional status.

PEM IN ADULTS

Weight Loss

In clinical practice the presence, degree, and time scale of any weight loss should be an integral part of routine history taking. Morgan and colleagues (1980) investigated the assessment of weight loss from the use of observed weight, recalled weight, and predicted weight. The classic work of Studley (1936) more than 50 years ago in which he showed for the first time how a simple indicator like weight loss could predict surgical risk has been reviewed recently (Buzby, 1986). The nearest to a classification using weight loss as the basis is the graph showing what are termed severe, significant, and minimal weight loss developed by Blackburn et al. (1977).

Body Mass Index

This index, weight/height^2, is increasingly being used as an indicator of overweight and obesity (Table 6). Its use in anorexia nervosa has been advocated (Llewellyn-Jones and Abraham, 1984). Although it involves very simple measurements and a small calculation, its use can be criticised (Macdonald 1986; Garn et al. 1986; McLaren, 1987b). As was pointed out above for the young child, so even more so for the adult, it is wrong to assume, as is done in the BMI, that everyone of the same sex and height has the same ideal body weight. This ignores the marked differences in body build that exist in health. The BMI is deceptively easy to use in practice, but its use obscures important differences.

TABLE 6. Body Mass Index (BMI) Weight/Height^2 Classification of Obesity

Classification	BMI
Grade III	>40
Grade II	30–40
Grade I	25–29.9
Not obese	<25

Prognostic Nutritional Index

This system (PNI) was developed by Mullen and his group (Buzby et al., 1988) as a linear model predictive of increased morbidity and mortality following surgery. In this model serum albumin in g/dL (A); triceps skinfold thickness mm (TSF); serum transferrin in mg/dL (TFN); and delayed hypersensitivity response (DH) are used in the formula: PNI % = 158 − 16.6(A) − 0.78(TSF) − 0.2(TFN) − (DH) Thus for example, a well-nourished patient with 4.8 g/dL (A); 14mm (TSF); 250 mg/dL (TFN); and 2 (DH) has a PNI of 158.0 − 152.2, or a 5.8% chance of complications. A malnourished patient with all indices abnormal, e.g., 2.8 (A); 9 (TSF); 180 (TFN); and 1 (DH) has a PNI of 158 − 95.3, or a 62.7% chance of complications.

Many factors other than PEM influence serum albumin and transferrin, which are highly correlated (McLaren, 1988), and, as was mentioned earlier when discussing arm circumference and mortality, this is not really a nutritional index. This is not to underestimate its value, but it can lead to misunderstanding and misinterpretation. Very recently (Buzby et al., 1988) a cooperative trial of the effects of TPN in malnourished surgical patients has been initiated. If the PNI is used to monitor the results of this purely nutritional intervention it would be inappropriate. Harvey et al. (1978) introduced a similar index but wisely called it a hospital prognostic index. It is based on a discriminant function composed of serum albumin, delayed hypersensitivity tests, sepsis, and diagnosis.

Adult Marasmus and Hypoalbuminemic Malnutrition

Alone among those who have worked with PEM in hospitalized patients, Blackburn and Bistrian (Bistrian, 1977; Bistrian et al., 1975) have attempted to classify severe adult PEM into different forms. It is generally agreed that the vast majority of cases are marasmic in type, but some in which sepsis and stress play a large part were earlier termed by them as kwashiorkor-like syndrome; but hypoalbuminemic malnutrition is more acceptable, as the patients have only the low serum albumin in common with childhood kwashiorkor. This subject has been reviewed in detail recently (McLaren, 1988).

CONCLUSIONS

For both children and adults with PEM a fully satisfactory classification system has yet to be developed. In the meantime it is important that workers in the field choose their methods with care and use them appropriately. Where circumstances make it possible, the supplementation of anthropometry with biochemical and/or immunologic methods is advisable. There is need for a wider appreciation that body weight is a crude measurement, suitable for use in classification only under the most basic circumstances. Precision in nutritional anthropometric classification awaits replacement of such measurements as birth weight, weight/age, weight/height, and weight/height^2 by indicators that relate to body composition.

REFERENCES

Arnhold R (1969): The QUAC stick: A field measure used by the Quaker Service Team, Nigeria. J Trop Pediatr 15:243–247.

Bairagi R (1981): On validity of some anthropometric indicators as predictors of mortality. Am J Clin Nutr 34:2592–2594.

Bairagi R, Chowdhury MK, Kim YJ, Curlin GT (1985): Alternative anthropometric indicators of mortality. Am J Clin Nutr 42: 296–306.

Bengoa JM (1962): Recent trends in the public health aspects of protein-calorie malnutrition. Geneva: WHO Tech Rep Ser No 245, pp 552–561.

Bistrian BR (1977): Interaction of nutrition and infection in the hospital setting. Am J Clin Nutr 30:1228–1232.

Bistrian BR, Blackburn GL, Scrimshaw NS (1975): Cellular immunity in semi-starved states in hospitalized adults. Am J Clin Nutr 28:1148–1155.

Bistrian BR, Blackburn GL, Vitale J (1976): Prevalence of malnutrition in general medical patients. JAMA 235:1567–1570.

Blackburn GL, Bistrian BR, Maini BS (1977): Nutritional and metabolic assessment of the hospitalized patient. J Parenter Enteral Nutr 1:11–22.

Bowditch HP (1891): The growth of children, studied by Galton's method of percentile grades. Twenty-second Annual Report of the State Board of Health of Massachusetts, Boston.

Briend A, Dykewicz C, Graven K (1986): Usefulness of nutritional indices and classifications in predicting death of malnourished children. Br Med J 293:373–375.

Briend A, Wojtyniak B, Rowland MGM (1987): Arm circumference and other factors in children at high risk of death in rural Bangladesh. Lancet 2:725–728.

Brook CGD, Hindmarsh PC, Healy MJR (1986): A better way to detect growth failure. Br Med J 293:1186.

Buzby GP (1986): Prospective overview to nutrition/metabolism classic. Nutr Int 2:167.

Buzby GP, Mullen JL, Matthews OL (1988): A randomized clinical trial of total parenteral nutrition in malnourished surgical patients: The rationale and impact of previous clinical trials and pilot study on protocol design. Am J Clin Nutr 47:357–365.

Chen LC, Chowdhury AKMA, Huffman SL (1980): Anthropometric assessment of energy protein malnutrition and subsequent risk of mortality among preschool age children. Am J Clin Nutr 33:1836–1845.

Chiswick ML (1985): Intrauterine growth retardation. Br Med J 291:845–848.

Cole JJ, Donnet ML, Stanfield JP (1981): Weight-for-height indices to assess nutritional status—a new index on a slide-rule. Am J Clin Nutr 34:1935–1943.

FAO/WHO Expert Committee (1971): Eighth Report. WHO Tech Rep Ser No 477, Geneva.

Frenk S (1985): Protein-energy malnutrition. In Arneil GC, Metcoff J (eds): "Pediatric Nutrition." London: Butterworths, pp 153–193.

Garn SM, Leonard WR, Hawthorne VM (1986): Three limitations of the body mass index. Am J Clin Nutr 44:996–997.

Georgieff MK, Sasanour SR, Mammel MC, Pereira GR (1986): Mid-arm circumference/head circumference ratios for identification of symptomatic LGA, AGA, and SGA newborn infants. 83:316–321.

Golden MHN (1982): Protein deficiency, energy deficiency, and the oedema of undernutrition. Lancet 1:1261–1265.

Gómez F (1946): Desnutrición. Bol Med Hosp Infant 3:543–551.

Gómez F, Galván RR, Cravioto J, Frenk S (1955): Malnutrition in infancy and childhood, with special reference to kwashiorkor. Adv Pediatr 7:131–169.

Gómez F, Galván RR, Frenk SS (1956): Mortality in second and third degree malnutrition. J Trop Pediatr 2:77–83.

Gopalan C (1987): Nutrition problems and programmes in South East Asia. New Delhi, WHO Regional Office for South East Asia.

Harvey KB, Ruggiero JA, Regan CS (1978): Hospital morbidity-mortality risk factors using nutritional assessment. Clin Res 26: 581A.

Hill GL, Blackett RL, Rickford I (1977): Malnutrition in surgical patients: An unrecognized problem. Lancet 1:689–692.

Jelliffe DB (1959): Protein-calorie malnutrition in tropical pre-school children: A review of recent knowledge. J Pediatr 54:227–256.

Jelliffe DB (1966): "The Assessment of the Nutritional Status of the Community." WHO Monograph Ser. No. 53. Geneva: WHO.

Kanawati AA, Haddad N, McLaren DS (1970): Arm circumference as a public health index of protein-calorie malnutrition of early childhood. J Trop Pediatr 15:233–237.

Kanawati AA, McLaren DS (1970): Assessment of marginal malnutrition. Nature 228:573–575.

Kasango Project Team (1983): Anthropometric measurement of young children's nutritional status as an indicator of subsequent risk of dying. J Trop Pediatr 29:69–75.

Keller W, Donoso G, DeMaeyer EM (1976): Anthropometry in nutritional surveillance: A review based on results of the WHO collaborative study on nutritional anthropometry. Nutr Abstract Rev 46:591–609.

Kielmann AA, McCord C (1978): Weight-for-age as an index of risk of death in children. Lancet 1:1247–1250.

Llewellyn-Jones D, Abraham SF (1984): Quetelet index in the diagnosis of anorexia nervosa. Br Med J 288: 1800.

Macdonald FC (1986): Quetelet's index as indicator of obesity. Lancet 1: 1043.

McLaren DS (1966) A fresh look at protein-calorie malnutrition. Lancet 2: 485–488.

McLaren DS (1971): Classification of protein-energy malnutrition. Lancet 2: 1208.

McLaren DS (1987a): A fresh look at some perinatal growth and nutritional standards. Wld Rev Nutr Diet 49:87–120.

McLaren DS (1987b): Three limitations of the body mass index. Amer J Clin Nutr 46: 121.

McLaren DS (1988): A fresh look at protein-energy malnutrition in hospitalized patients. Nutrition 4:1–6.

McLaren DS, Kanawati AA (1972): A somatic quotient. Am J Clin Nutr 25: 363.

McLaren DS, Pellett PL, Read WWC (1967): A simple scoring system for classifying the severe forms of protein-calorie malnutrition in early childhood. Lancet 1:533–535.

McLaren DS, Read WWC (1972): Classification of nutritional status of early childhood. Lancet 2:146–149.

McLaren DS, Read WWC (1975): Weight/length classification of nutritional status. Lancet 2:219–221.

Morgan DB, Hill GL, Burkinshaw L (1980): The assessment of weight loss from a single measurement of body weight: The problems and limitations. Am J Clin Nutr 33:2101–2105.

Nabarro D, McNab S (1980): A simple new technique for identifying thin children. J Trop Med Hyg 83:21–33.

Rolland-Cachera MF, Sempé M, Guilloud-Bataille M (1982): Adiposity indices in children. Am J Clin Nutr 36: 178–184.
Sasanour SR, Georgieff MK, Pereira GR (1986): Mid-arm circumference and mid-arm/head circumference ratios: Standard curves for anthropometric assessment of neonatal nutritional status. J Pediatr 109:311–315.
Seoane N, Latham MC (1971): Nutritional anthropometry in the identification of malnutrition in childhood. J Trop Pediatr 17:98–104.
Shah PM, Junnarkar AR, Khare RD (1976): Communitywide surveillance of 'at risk' under-fives in need of special care. J Trop Pediatr 22:103–107.
Smedman L, Sterky G, Mellander L, Wall S (1987): Anthropometry and subsequent mortality in groups of children aged 6–59 months in Guinea-Bissau. Am J Clin Nutr 46:369–373.
Sommer A, Loewenstein MS (1975): Nutritional status and mortality: A prospective validation of the QUAC stick. Am J Clin Nutr 28:287–292.
Studley HO (1936): Percentage of weight loss, a basic indicator of surgical risk in patients with chronic peptic ulcer. JAMA 106:458–460.
Trowbridge FL, Sommer A (1981): Nutritional anthropometry and mortality risk. Am J Clin Nutr 34:2591–2592.
Waterlow JC (1972): Classification and definition of protein-calorie malnutrition. Br Med J 3:566–599.
Waterlow JC, Rutishauser IHE (1974): Malnutrition in man. In Cravioto J, Hambraeus L, Vahlquist B (eds): "Early Malnutrition Mental Development." Sweden: Almqvist and Wiksell, p 13.
WHO Working Group (1986): Use and interpretation of anthropometric indicators of nutritional status. Bull WHO 64:929–941.
Zerfas AJ (1975): The insertion tape: A new circumference for use in nutritional assessment. Am J Clin Nutr 28:782–787.
Ziman JM (1976): "The Force of Knowledge: The Scientific Dimension of Society." Cambridge: Cambridge University Press, p 291.

Anthropometric Assessment
of Nutritional Status, pages 287–299

17
Growth Monitoring and Promotion

MICHAEL C. LATHAM
Division of Nutritional Sciences, Cornell University, Ithaca, New York 14853

INTRODUCTION

The regular weighing of infants and children to assess their growth has been carried out for a long time. Sometimes periodic measurements other than weight, including especially length or height, arm circumference, and skinfold thickness measures, are also used either to determine development or assess nutritional status (Latham, 1979). Such periodic secular determinations are strictly speaking anthropometric growth monitoring. The term *monitoring* means literally "to keep watch over" or "to check systematically."

In current parlance, and in medical and nutritional literature, the term *growth monitoring* now usually refers to the periodic weighing of children, the plotting of each measurement on a "growth chart" or child health card, and the use of the information on the card to influence actions by the health worker making the measurements and the mother or guardian who brings the child to be measured.

This rather simple procedure with its quite straightforward objectives is now mired in an international debate (Anon, 1985); it has strong proponents and opponents; and the literature on growth monitoring has mushroomed in the last decade (Gopalan and Chatterjee, 1985). This is probably at least in part because UNICEF has included growth monitoring as the first of its four-pronged GOBI strategy to influence child survival in developing countries (Grant, 1984). The *G* stands for growth monitoring, the *O* for oral rehydration therapy for diarrhea, the *B* for breast-feeding promotion, and the *I* for immunization. UNICEF believes that the wide adoption of these four strategies will greatly reduce infant and child mortality, and improve nutritional status in developing countries.

The recording of a child's weight on a growth chart in itself serves no useful purpose, unless accompanied by some action (Latham, 1984). This has long been recognised, but in many growth monitoring programs this is about all that is done. Under these circumstances the potential benefits of growth monitoring are not, and cannot be, realised. We now prefer to use the term *growth monitoring and promotion*, and UNICEF now uses this term for the *G* of GOBI (Hendrata, 1988). This is potentially important because the "promotion of good growth" is clearly the main objective of regular weighing.

If a growth monitoring program at a village, district, or national level concentrates on weighing and charting, but ignores or does not attempt to use the chart in a coherent positive manner, then it clearly is an exercise in futility. This is assuming that growth monitoring is being used, as it usually is, to influence growth in the individual child. Growth monitoring could be used simply to generate data for purposes of nutritional surveillance, or program evaluation. That is a different matter, and is not the subject of discussion here.

The use of growth charts and growth monitoring is not a new concept. Growth measurements have been used as a means of judging the growth and health of children for many years. In several industrialized countries well-baby clinics included child weighing as a means to judge proper development. In the 1960s Morley et al. (1968), on the basis of work in Nigeria, advocated the use of growth charts in developing countries, and this can be regarded as the birth of the growth monitoring movement. It was suggested that the chart tried out at Ilesha in Nigeria could be used for early detection of malnutrition and for identification of children at high risk (Morley, 1968). The author stated that "maintaining an adequate rate of growth" was replacing "prevention of malnutrition" as the goal towards which the clinic at Ilesha and other clinics modeled on this now direct their work (Anon, 1968). Morley stressed the use of the chart to promote growth and not to cure malnutrition; he was an advocate for the mother, rather than the clinic, holding possession of the chart; and he later stressed that the health worker and the mother should be more interested in growth velocity than in the child's position on the chart. The term *Road to Health Chart* became widely accepted (Morley, 1973).

Now there are many different weight charts in use around the world. They usually have lines which indicate "normal" or standard weight gains by age. These then are based on "reference standards," and unless accepted national standards exist, it is recommended by WHO and others that NCHS standards be used. These differ little from the Harvard, Denver, and other standards previously used (Stephenson et al., 1983). A model chart produced by the World Health Organization is shown as Figure 1.

MAIN FEATURES OF GROWTH MONITORING

Although growth monitoring could involve, for example, the use of arm circumference measurements rather than weight for age, and it could be used for nutritional surveillance or evaluation, thus involving data on groups of children, nevertheless UNICEF and most government programs use the term growth monitoring and promotion more narrowly. In general it includes sequential weighing and it is used to help caretakers maintain good growth in

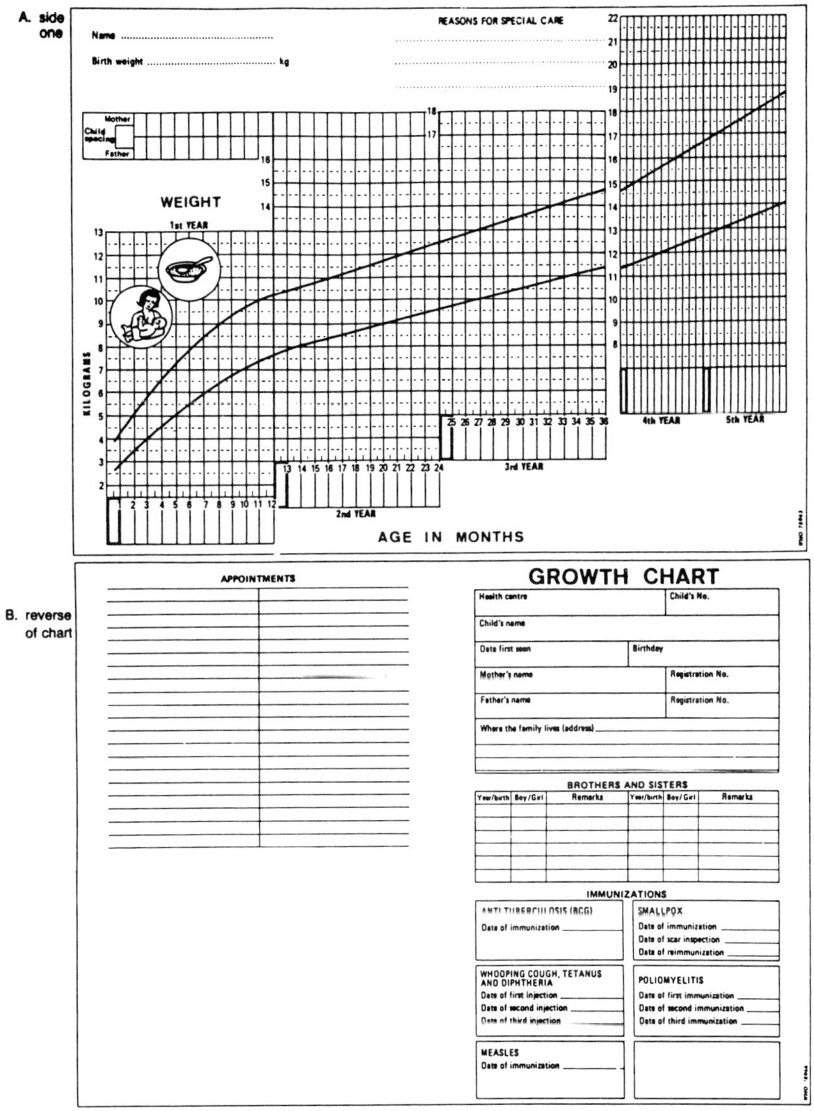

Fig. 1. World Health Organization growth chart.

the individual child. A useful definition adopted by the Indian Integrated Child Development Service is:

> Growth Monitoring and Promotion can be defined as an operational strategy of enabling mothers to visualize growth or lack of growth and to receive specific, relevant and practical guidance in ways in which she, her family and community can act to assure health and continued regular growth in her child.
>
> GM/P implies a regular and sequential measurement of growth, recognizing it to be the result of overall health, nutrition, environment, psychosocial and development factors in the child. GM/P is based on a strategy aimed at behavioural change and adoption of improved self-help actions within the family and the community in order to promote optimal health. In short, GM/P is a communication strategy for making health and nutrition education more individualized, more convincing and more effective.

Hendrata (1988) has stressed that it should be a preventive, promotive, and preemptive strategy aimed at action before malnutrition or serious growth faltering occurs; it is a strategy to cause behavioral change mainly following effective communication to achieve good growth based on home action; and it deals with the broad environment of the growing child encompassing not only nutrition, but also his or her health, psychological development, intellectual stimulation, and physical environment.

It is the view of the author that GM and P should where possible be closely integrated into primary health care (PHC) activities, and not usually be a separate program. It should concentrate on maintaining good growth in infants and children, and not as is often the case be used mainly for rehabilitating children whose growth is poor. If the former is to be the focus, then it is essential that infants enter the program soon after birth, because in general infants 0–5 months of age who are breast-fed have satisfactory growth. GM and P is then a preventive not a curative strategy, and it is designed mainly to promote good growth and health, not to deal with malnutrition and ill health. Growth promotion then includes a strategy to maintain and reinforce desirable practices, and workers in the program do not concentrate their actions on mothers whose children are doing poorly. Workers should be obtaining information on how mothers and families are managing to achieve good growth rather than mainly finding the reasons for growth failure. Praise and reinforcement should be an important feature of the program. While the major emphasis is on maintenance of good growth, which can be viewed as a preemptive strategy, nevertheless the program should include a strategy for dealing with those hopefully few cases where the program has failed, and where children are not doing well, and need some special attention. This will usually involve some special advice involving behavioral change aimed to achieve rehabilitation and in some cases will necessitate treatment or referral. Where possible praise for what the mother is doing right should be included. Scolding, including public scolding, should not be a part of the program.

Growth monitoring, then, is a strategy to empower mothers to maintain good nutritional status in their children and to prevent growth retardation. Much of the action should consist of positive reinforcement rather than corrective action. As a diagnostic exercise it should be as much to find out what mothers are doing right as what is going wrong. Of course it is also to detect early growth faltering, to find the likely reasons for this, and to suggest to mothers corrective actions which are realistic and which they might try. It is likely to be relatively unsuccessful if used mainly to try to "correct" the growth of older children who are moderately or severely stunted, especially if these children are not wasted.

In all cases meaningful involvement of mothers should be the heart of a growth monitoring and promotion program. It is a participatory exercise; it involves dialogue and discussion, not lecturing and scolding; and mothers should help in decision making, for example, about the location, the hours, and the organization of GM sessions. Mothers need also to be consulted about such matters as the need for privacy and confidentiality, whether it is appropriate in their culture to weigh children nude or clothed.

These views of growth monitoring and promotion present the concept of the author and others of what it should be, rather than what it usually is in practice in countries in Africa, Asia, and Latin America in 1988. This author continues to see growth monitoring in action which ignores these principles. Too often growth monitoring is used mainly as a weighing exercise, advice is given only to mothers whose children are doing badly (this often consists of public scolding), and advice is frequently impractical and does not recognise what is practical and useful. In some parts of the world GM is regarded by health workers mainly as a tool for diagnosis of malnutrition. In other places it is extended to be a part of a system for delivery of certain other interventions, for example, selecting children to receive free or subsidised weaning foods, or as a means of getting children to attend for immunization. These can indeed be a component of a good GM and P program, but the full potential benefits will not be realised without the level of communication, dialogue, and empowerment of mothers and communities described above. At worst growth monitoring consists of the routine exercise of weighing and weight charting with no advice given, and with no use made of the chart. Those organizing new GM efforts must also keep in mind that in some societies there may be cultural prejudices against the weighing of young children. Sensitive efforts to overcome these may be needed.

OPERATIONAL CONSIDERATIONS

Rohde (1984) has pointed out the differences between growth monitoring on the one hand and nutritional surveillance on the other. Nutritional assessment using growth data for surveillance may, for example, require only small subsamples of the population of the communities involved; rather large numbers of children can be quite quickly weighed per day because diagnosis and communication is not an important feature; and surveillance may require rather precise, accurate measurements done by a highly trained worker with the measurements repeated at rather long intervals. In contrast, GM and P programs hope to enroll all children under a particular age; the groups of children at a weighing session should be relatively small because diagnosis and dialogue are important; the measurements made need not be as precise and can be performed by a person with less education and training (sometimes even by mothers themselves); and it is very important that the children come for weighing and growth promotion sessions at rather short intervals.

Although the term diagnosis is used, this means an assessment of the child's current situation and the factors influencing either good or less than optimal growth. It is not itself a curative service, and the diagnosis is not mainly to detect disease or malnutrition so that medicine or food supplements can be provided. It is to allow reinforcement and empowerment for mothers to maintain good growth and health in their young children. The data collected in a good growth monitoring program could be used for purposes of nutritional surveillance. The point being made is that if the main objective of a program is nutritional surveillance and not growth monitoring, then the program should be different.

An important operational rule of GM and P, then, is that infants be enrolled as soon after birth as possible. Children seen for the first time in their second or third year of life often will already have evidence of growth failure, and GM and P can at this stage do relatively little to improve the situation, especially in stunted older children. Infants under 6 months of age where breast-feeding is the normal feeding practice usually show good growth. This, therefore, is a period when dialogue is most useful. GM and P can provide positive reinforcement, but it can also be a time when a dialogue becomes established for the months ahead, during the nutritional danger period, which is usually between 6 and 18 months of age. A mother can tell the health worker about what she plans to do, when she intends to introduce other foods, how long she expects to breast-feed, whether she wants to get the infant immunized, and how she will deal with illnesses such as diarrhea and respiratory infections. The worker at the GM and P session can now cautiously guide the mother and discuss with her a strategy for maintaining good growth and health in her infant during the danger period.

If this is to be the heart of the program, then it is important that the health worker have a good understanding of existing child-raising practices, and the local cultural, social, and dietary environment of the community. Without this the messages may not be relevant, practical, or feasible for mothers to implement, and may not even be credible to them. The health worker must also have a minimum knowledge of the factors most likely to lead to growth faltering. For example, he or she should understand that after about 6 months of age breast-feeding alone often provides inadequate nutrition and needs to be supplemented; that too much supplementation may reduce suckling and lead to insufficient milk; that certain foods are bulky and have low energy density but that there are ways to increase energy density; that as breast-feeding becomes less important rather frequent feeding with other foods is important; that infections may themselves lead to growth faltering, but that starvation as a treatment for diarrhea and other infections contributes to this; and that advice should be given to provide breast milk and other foods during most illnesses.

A second operational rule then is that the health worker requires adequate time to talk to each mother (at least 5–15 minutes) and needs to have a certain basic knowledge and reasonable communication skills. It is important that he or she knows how to listen and to elicit information from the mother and how to provide positive feedback and encouragement plus appropriate advice. This takes some skill, and some of these skills can be imparted in training. But obviously some individuals are better listeners and communicators than are others.

A third operational rule which follows is that GM and P be integrated into primary health care. Many of the messages and advice suggested are an integral part of PHC. Mothers should in general not have to attend separate sessions on a different day to have their children immunized, to receive vitamin A or anthelmintics, to get advice about oral rehydration, or to attend a prenatal examination or get family planning advice. In fact it should be the duty of the GM and P staff to ensure that all children attending have been immunized against the six diseases covered in the Expanded Program of Immunization and that mothers know how to use oral rehydration therapy, etc. Growth monitoring and promotion can be a part of PHC, or alternatively, it can encompass PHC activities. Hendrata has stated that "GM and P can help to shift the emphasis from professionals to parents, from clinics to homes, from dependence to empowerment. And in so doing it can help to build a genuine primary health care system." GM and P can serve as an activity which at frequent intervals brings the child into contact with the health services.

A fourth operational principle is that the advice given and the nutrition and health education be rather specific, aimed at the particular circumstances of each child; somehow this needs to be part of a dialogue which gives the mother the feeling that she herself is developing a realistic, achievable strategy to maintain the good growth and health of her child, and that she sees the benefits of the time that she has invested in the exercise. The content of the messages should be simple, and must take account of the child in a family situation. The chart, then, is used to get mothers to understand that healthy growth is feasible, and that they can follow it themselves. Increasingly with the new TALC scale described below, mothers are encouraged to weigh their own babies.

Finally, GM and P should be conducted as near as possible to peoples' homes, at a time convenient to parents, in small enough groups to allow adequate individualized dialogue and short waiting periods, and be conducted in a way mainly to suit parents, not health workers. For example, in an urban setting where mothers work away from home, the sessions could be on a Sunday, and the health workers could have Monday off. Unless some means are provided for combining GM and P with simple therapy and other preventive services, attendance may be poor. This might include, for example, deworming, administration of vitamin A, provision of ORT packets, availability of antimalarial drugs, and possibly also simple treatment for common illnesses. In all cases, and especially when the latter is not possible, the rural GM and P based in a small village must be linked with and have backup from a health centre, dispensary, or clinic. Rohde (1984) and others feel that food supplements should not be provided at GM and P sessions even if the child is faltering. Rohde feels that supplements have negative consequences for the program. Food supplements, he believes, should be reserved for a different time and place, and should be seen by all mothers as a therapeutic response to the child's persistent lack of normal growth. This view is not shared by all those involved in GM and P. In some programs GM is used as a means to identify children who are to get supplements. Several voluntary agencies use this strategy. There is now an increasing belief that where free food supplements are provided, they should be targeted to the most needy children, and this targeting may be based on weight charts and GM programs.

Under some circumstances growth monitoring and promotion may be conducted not at a health centre, but in people's homes. This will often be popular with mothers, and it will result in a wider coverage, especially of the most neglected famlies. But home visits will usually be more expensive, because one field worker can cover fewer children per day. Although GM and P can act as a catalyst in the strengthening of primary health care activities, it is also true that it is much easier to have successful GM and P in a well-functioning PHC system. So efforts to strengthen and improve primary health care will also make successful GM and P a more feasible possibility.

As stated, the nutritional danger period in most poor communities is from ages 6 to 24 months. But GM and P should if possible begin soon after birth. So it is recommended that attendance for weighing and growth promotion be monthly from 0 to 24 months, and if feasible at 3-month intervals from 24 to 48 months, but only if this will not limit what can be done in the critical first 24 months of life. The purists would suggest that when a new GM and P begins, it should only enroll newly born infants, so that the program would not be fully operational for 24 months, when all children under 2 years would be in the program. This ideal may not be feasible in practice because of the demands made. But whatever is decided, it should be realised that infants enrolled for the first time at, say, 12 or 18 months of age have entered the program too late for it to be really effective for them.

One cannot generalise about a universal growth chart suitable for all parts of the world (Morley, 1973). Many local considerations need to be taken into account. It is widely agreed that where possible the card should be kept by the mother or guardian. It should be something she values and can maintain safely, so it needs to be attractive to her and can often best be kept in a plastic pouch. It must be designed to be as easily understood as possible. There is no agreement as to whether a series of curves or a road to health is desirable and where these should be drawn. If these are desired, then they should be based on NCHS or established local standards. Often multiple lines are included, and these can be useful; different colors can be used for each channel. The design is important: It should be decided locally, and it is desirable to involve communication experts, social scientists, pediatricians, nutritionists, and others in the design. The chart should be pretested before it is widely disseminated. An experienced outside consultant and UNICEF and WHO advice may be helpful for countries lacking their own experts. A local modification of the WHO growth chart shown in Figure 1 may be considered.

In the past a variety of scales, both spring scales, such as the Salter scale, and balance scales, some made locally, such as one in the Philippines, have been used. Now UNICEF is recommending the new scale made by TALC in London called the direct recording scale, which still needs careful evaluation (Fig. 2). It allows the chart to be attached to the scale and thus a direct placing of the child's weight on the chart (Morley, 1988). This circumvents the step of placing a dot or a bubble where the weight as recorded on one axis intersects with the month of weighing (or age) on the other axis. This seemingly simple exercise has been found to be difficult and is a major cause of error in weighing programs in many countries. A new scale is now being tested which is electronic; it in fact first weighs the mother. She then holds her baby, and the scale displays the weight of the child by automatically providing the difference between the combined weight of mother and child from that of the mother alone (O'Malley-Burns and Rohde, 1988). This then saves time and reduces the often somewhat difficult task of suspending a struggling child from a hanging scale. Mother, infant, and field worker are all happier. This may be the GM tool of the future. Its wide adoption depends on its reliability and its cost. Unless the price of the scale is competitive, it will not be widely used.

Although growth monitoring is simple in concept, and is a low-cost technology for helping to reduce the extent of malnutrition, it is not easy to do it well. It takes good organisation, adequate resources, an appropriate existing infrastructure, and careful training and proper supervision of workers. In some geographic locations, it may involve overcoming cultural barriers.

CONCLUSIONS

Growth monitoring (and less frequently, growth monitoring and promotion) is being widely practiced; with the blessing and financial assistance of UNICEF, the numbers of children included in GM programs are likely to increase. UNICEF as an advocate reports many successes of growth monitoring in developing countries around the world (Grant, 1987).

All now agree that weighing of children and plotting the weight on a chart cannot itself improve the nutrition and health of children. The success or failure of GM depends on how the information and the chart are used. The weigh-

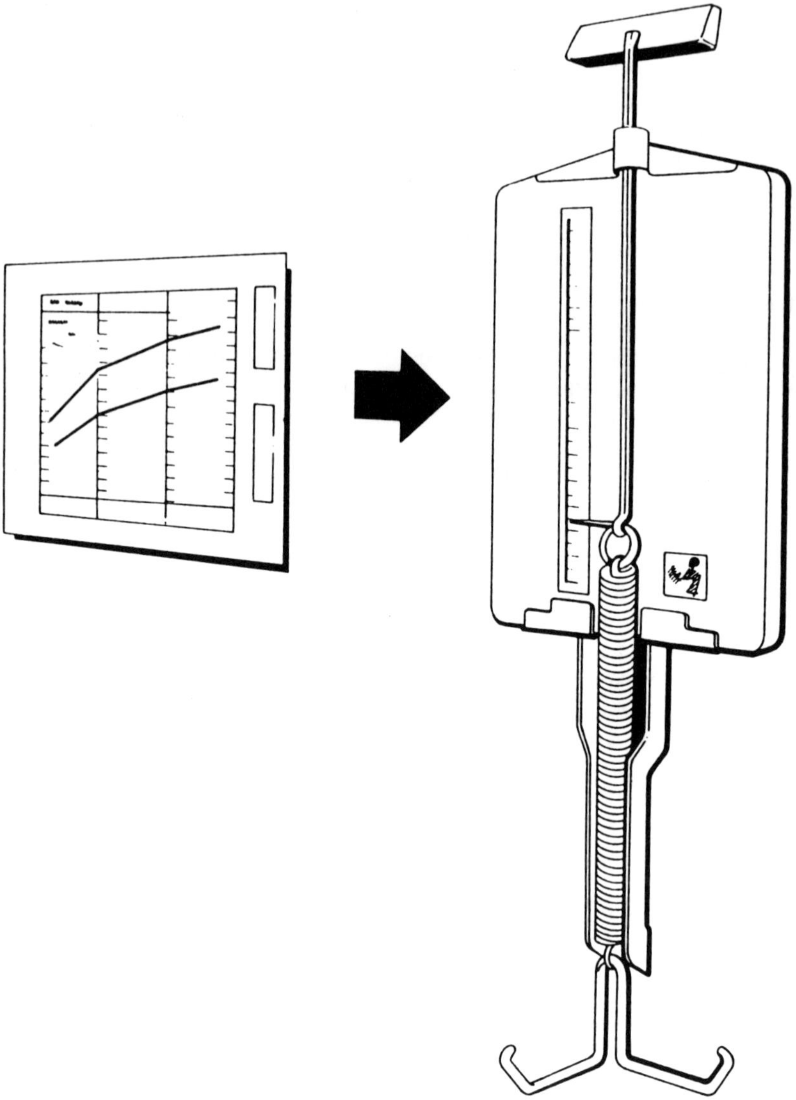

Fig. 2. TALC scales using the road to health chart for under fives. (Reproduced from Goodwin et al., 1988, with permission of the publisher.)

ing and the plotting have to result in action if there is to be a benefit. Those taking action in general are likely to be either the health worker or the mother (or parents or guardian) of the child. GM is likely to be successful if the actions are appropriate and feasible, and if they are implemented. Growth monitoring is one among several means of achieving the desired goal of healthy growth. It can only by successful, then, first, if it consists of growth monitoring and promotion, and second, if it is implemented in the right context, including those primary health care components that can assist the GM technology.

EVALUATION OF GROWTH MONITORING

The general body of opinion in applied nutrition circles is that growth monitoring and promotion is a strategy worth pursuing (Rohde, 1988). Austin et al. (1978) estimated that between 31% and 74% of nutrition projects in the nonindustrialized countries include the use of growth charts. There are also serious critics of growth monitoring who state that its value has not been demonstrated and that it is too costly a project for poor countries considering the very limited financial resources available for health and nutrition services. Another set of critics argues that the very concept of a graph and of its being understood so that it influences action by an illiterate mother is highly unlikely.

The unfortunate fact is that there have been very few scientific attempts to evaluate growth monitoring, and most of these have flaws in their design. There are studies which suggest that illiterate women can be taught to understand growth charts (Pielmeier, 1985). In some studies where growth monitoring appeared to be of value in terms of improved health or nutrition, it was not possible to separate benefits from the growth chart per se from benefits resulting from the other interventions introduced as part of the growth monitoring program, activities such as immunizations, oral rehydration therapy, supplementary feeding, treatment of disease, and others (Morley, 1973).

Growth monitoring has been widely practiced in India and in Indonesia. A detailed review of GM in India suggests major problems and a few successes, but illustrates that no well-conducted evaluation has been conducted (Gopalan and Chatterjee, 1985). In the case of Indonesia both the World Bank–funded project covering 225,000 people designed to examine the impact of community-based GM, and also the ever-expanding UPGK program using volunteers (Kaders) covering a large population, have been described at length (Griffiths, 1985). In the former project it is claimed that based on 600 program households and 400 comparison households, there was a significant improvement in mothers' nutritional knowledge and nutritional practices, and in the nutritional status of the children. Unfortunately there were many differences between the two groups, and it is not possible to judge how much improvement was due to the major efforts of nutrition communication and behavior change, and what exact role was played by the growth chart as a part of GM.

Other studies in Jamaica, Lesotho, and elsewhere also have problems and produce results that are unconvincing. The book-length publication *Use of*

Growth Charts for Promoting Child Nutrition—A Review of Global Experience by C. Gopalan and M. Chatterjee (1985) concludes that the effectiveness of GM has not been proven, but also suggests that good evaluation studies have not been undertaken. Rohde (1985) has stated that the statistical proof of the efficiency of growth monitoring has still not been demonstrated.

Currently there are attempts being made to fill this void. In the K. V. Kuppam Block near Vellore in Southern India a project is underway where GM and P has been introduced in six villages, and six villages are serving as controls with no GM. Unlike most other studies, an identical set of other health interventions are being used in both the GM and non-GM villages. And as an editorial in the Lancet (1988) suggests, any system "is only as good as the workers who operate it." Unlike oral rehydration, GM is not a curative approach with quick results, and unlike immunization, it is not a magic bullet requiring little behavioral change. Rather it is a means by which a simple technology can help people help their children. It can empower mothers, but only if properly used.

ACKNOWLEDGMENTS

This chapter expresses the views of the author. My thinking about growth monitoring has been greatly influenced by the writings of Drs. David Morley, John Rohde, Lukas Hendrata, and C. Gopalan. I have learnt and borrowed from them. I am grateful for their wisdom. I am indebted to Sabu George, whose influence and knowledge of GM has led me to be involved with him in a project to evaluate growth monitoring in India. This is being conducted in collaboration with the Christian Medical College in Vellore, with Dr. R. Abel as our Co-Principal Investigator, and with support from UNICEF and the Thrasher Research Fund.

REFERENCES

Anon (1968): The Ilesha health and weight chart. Nutr Rev 26:267–269.

Anon (1985): Growth monitoring: Intermediate technology or expensive luxury. Lancet 2:1337–1338. Editorial.

Austin J, Makin M, Pyle D, Zeitlin M (1978): "Annotated Directory of Nutrition Programs in Developing Countries." Cambridge, Mass: Harvard Institute for International Development.

Goodwin RM, Armstrong A, Bertram J, Stewart B (1988): Springtime in Ayrshire: Home weighing of neonates with a new direct recording scale. Public Health 102:335–347.

Gopalan C, Chatterjee M (1985): "Use of Growth Charts for Promotion of Child Nutrition." New Delhi: Nutrition Foundation of India, pp 1–120.

Grant J (1984): "State of the World's Children 1984." Oxford: Oxford University Press, pp 1–60.

Grant J (1987): "State of the World's Children 1987." Oxford: Oxford University Press, pp 64–79.

Griffiths M (1985): "Growth Monitoring of Preschool Children." Geneva: World Federation of Public Health Association.

Hendrata L (1988): "Growth Monitoring and Promotion." New York: UNICEF. (in press.)

Latham MC (1979): "Human Nutrition in Tropical Africa." Rome: Food and Agricultural Organization of the United Nations, pp 25–30.
Latham MC (1984): Strategies for the control of malnutrition and the influence of the nutritional sciences. Food Nutr 10:5–31.
Morley D (1968): Prevention of protein-calorie deficiency syndrome. Trans R Soc Trop Med Hyg 62:200–208.
Morley D (1973): "Paediatric Priorities in the Developing World." London: Butterworths, pp 1–250.
Morley D (1988): Personal communication.
Morley D, Bicknell J, Woodland M (1968): Factors influencing the growth and nutritional status of infants and young children in a Nigerian village. Trans Roy Soc Trop Med Hyg 62:164–195.
O'Malley-Burns J, Rohde JE (1988): Weighing scales: design and choices. Indian J Pediatr 55 (suppl)S31–S37.
Pielmeier NR (1985): Mother's knowledge related to child health and nutrition in Ghana and Lesotho. J Trop Pediatr 31:131–139.
Rohde JE (1984): Growth monitoring. World Health, May 1984, pp 17–19.
Rohde JE (1985): Community-based nutrition programs. In Waiver M, Huffman S (eds): "Health and Family Planning in Community-Based Distribution Programs:" Boulder: Waterview Press, pp 82–93.
Rohde JE (1988): Symposium: Growth monitoring and promotion: an international perspective. Indian J Pediatr 55 (suppl):S1–S123.
Stephenson LS, Latham MC, Jansen AAJ (1983): "A Comparison of Growth Standards: Similarities Between NCHS, Harvard, Denver and Privileged African Children and Differences with Kenyan Rural Children." Ithaca, NY: Cornell University International Nutrition Monograph Ser. No. 12, pp 1–95.
World Health Organization (1978): A growth chart for international use and child health care: Guidelines for primary health care personnel. Geneva: WHO.

Anthropometric Assessment
of Nutritional Status, pages 301–318
Published 1991 by Wiley-Liss, Inc.

18
Nutritional Surveillance in Developed Countries Using Anthropometry

ROBERTO J. RONA
Department of Community Medicine, The United Medical and Dental Schools of Guy's and St. Thomas's Hospitals, St. Thomas's Campus, London SE1 7EH, England

INTRODUCTION

"A child's growth rate reflects, better than any other single index, his state of health and nutrition; and often indeed his psychological situation also. Similarly, the average value of children's height and weights reflect accurately the state of a nation's public health and the average nutritional status of its citizens ... Thus a well-designed growth study is a powerful tool with which to monitor the health of a population, or to pinpoint subgroups of a population whose share in economic and social benefits is less than it might be" (Eveleth and Tanner, 1976). This quote summarizes the purposes of a surveillance system in which growth is the chosen measure of public health. If a system is to be fully effective, close links need to be developed with government agencies, as these are ultimately responsible for the organisation of and the resources allocated to a system. Furthermore, fluctuations in growth, which reflect changes in public health, should prompt remedial public health policy. If collaboration between government agencies and auxologists is not evident, growth studies tend to become academic exercises.

Tanner (1976, 1986) has repeatedly made the point that it is essential to distinguish between surveillance of individuals and surveillance of populations. For the assessment of an individual child, comparison with standards of growth provides the basis on which to decide whether a child is small, underweight, or overweight. For the assessment of a population, it is the comparison between different groups within a country or between countries that provides the basis for recommendations. A review of nutritional surveillance of populations using growth as the index is the main aim of this paper.

Few developed countries operate a nutritional surveillance based on growth. With this in mind five issues will be covered: firstly, the theoretical basis for growth surveillance from a social and biological viewpoint; secondly, the design of a growth surveillance system suitable for developed countries;

thirdly, the sort of alarm system that should be developed in relation to growth surveillance systems; fourthly, the requirements of surveillance studies; and fifthly, supplementary uses that growth surveillance data can be put to. In this paper mainly, but not only, issues related to height will be examined.

THEORETICAL BASIS FOR THE SURVEILLANCE OF GROWTH

There are two reasons for basing the nutritional surveillance of populations on anthropometry. Firstly, anthropometric measurements can give an idea of the level of nutrition and health in a community, and secondly, anthropometric assessment provides a proxy measure of the social fabric of a community because stature and growth pattern are usually related to social and economic indicators of welfare (Dowler et al., 1982).

Nutritional surveillance in developing countries often shows an overt link between anthropometric assessment and ill health. For example, Chen et al. (1980) could relate levels of poor weight for age and weight for height to mortality in preschool children in Bangladesh. This relation is no longer evident in developed counties, as nutritional levels are now too high to have an effect on infancy and childhood mortality. This gives a different role to nutritional surveillance in developed countries compared with developing countries. For example, the value of weight, a useful indicator of nutritional status for severe malnutrition, is diminished in a country where the level of nutrition is generally high. In such countries height serves as a superior indicator of malnutrition (Habicht, 1980). However, nutritional status in developed countries is still a predictor of future ill health. It has been reported that short stature in adults is related to increased mortality from cardiovascular disease (Paffenbarger and Wing, 1969; Waaler, 1984) and an increased risk of obstetric complications in women (Butler and Alberman, 1969); and that distribution of body fat, for example, the waist/hip girth ratio, is correlated with mortality for cardiovascular disease (Lapidus et al., 1984).

Social Factors and Growth

Cross-sectional comparisons between subgroups in a country or between countries have provided information about the association between growth and social circumstances. Between-country comparisons have shown that differences in growth are minimal for countries of a similar level of development, regardless of ethnic origin, while growth differences are striking between countries of a dissimilar level of development (Habicht et al., 1974). Cross-sectional analyses within developed countries have shown differences in growth according to the number of children in a family, and the father's social class and employment status (Goldstein, 1971; Rona et al., 1978). In general, however, the variation due to biological factors such as parent's height (Rona et al., 1978), ethnic origin (Rona and Chinn, 1986), and birth weight (Goldstein, 1971; Rona et al., 1978) is greater than that attributable to social factors in developed countries, although it should be recognised that these so-called biological factors may reflect not only genetic, but also environmental, influences.

Reports from Sweden indicate that differences in height between social classes have disappeared (Lindgren, 1976) or are disappearing (Peck and Vagero, 1987). The extrapolation of the findings to other European countries is limited, for although some factors are given the same name, they do in fact have different definitions. If social factors were defined in the same way for all countries, the decline of an association between height and a set of social factors in one country and their persistence in another of a similar level of development would provide sound argument for proposing in-depth assessment of remedial action in the latter. Cross-sectional studies are of limited value if the aim is to assess the possible effects of changes in the living standard in the growth of the community. For this purpose, the findings from a series of surveys on growth are more relevant than a one-off cross-sectional study. In general, information on secular trends in growth has been obtained from records kept over long periods of time for a specific group, e.g., conscripts or school children (Tanner, 1981). The great majority of studies show an increase in stature over the last 150 years in all age groups, but this has been more evident in children than in adults. Most of these studies, as is to be expected, have changed their design over time in terms of sampling frame, selection of individuals in the study, and sample size (e.g. Cameron, 1979), and it is only for the last 25 years that any degree of uniformity over time has been seen. Thus the calculation of trends between surveys is more appropriate (Roede and van Wieringen, 1985; Chinn and Rona, 1984), although the repeated finding from secular trend studies of increase in stature over time in the last century in developed countries makes it unlikely that this phenomenon is an artefact. Improvements in social circumstances and nutritional factors provide the most plausible explanation, although other factors have also been put forward (Tanner, 1962; Meredith, 1976).

An understanding of the factors governing the secular trend in growth in developed countries is central to the purpose of growth surveillance. The information to be derived from looking at secular trends of growth over long and short periods of time will be described, and the lesson for nutritional surveillance systems based on growth discussed.

Long-Term Secular Trends in Growth

The studies of Floud and Wachter (1982) and van Wieringen (1979) have been selected to illustrate the long-term trend in growth.

Floud and Wachter (1982) do not consider that prices and wages on their own give a true picture of the standard of living in a community. Other factors, such as the working conditions and the level of household overcrowding, are relevant to an analysis of the standard of living. They postulate that growth during childhood and adolescence can give an index of the standard of living in the community. This was certainly true in the 18th and 19th centuries in Britain when there was a large child-working population (Tanner, 1981).

Floud and Wachter (1982) analysed information on the age, occupation history, and heights of 50,000 very poor children who were recruited by the Marine Society between 1770 and 1860. The quantile bend estimator was used to adjust for the exclusion of the shorter children as the society changed its minimum height requirement for admission over time (Wachter and Trussell, 1982). In Figure 1 the growth curves for 13- to 16-year-old children are shown for this period. The most important features of these curves are low stature up to 1800, a deterioration of height during the Napoleonic wars, and a substantial increase in the stature after 1815. As pointed out by the authors, there are inconsistencies in these data, but the magnitude of the height changes suggests they are real changes related to socioeconomic factors. However, accepting the data's validity complicates the interpretation of the sharp positive secular trend in growth following the Napoleonic war. The collapse of food prices after the war was associated with large-scale unemployment, which was further aggravated by the 0.3 million men coming back from the war (Checkland, 1983). The recovery from this unemployment was almost complete by the early 1820s. Thus the early increase in height may have been due to a great extent simply to a recovery of height to prewar levels. An alternative explanation may be that with high unemployment levels, the Marine Society could afford to select only the better-nourished applicants. Height of British recruits for the same period would facilitate the choice between the two explanations.

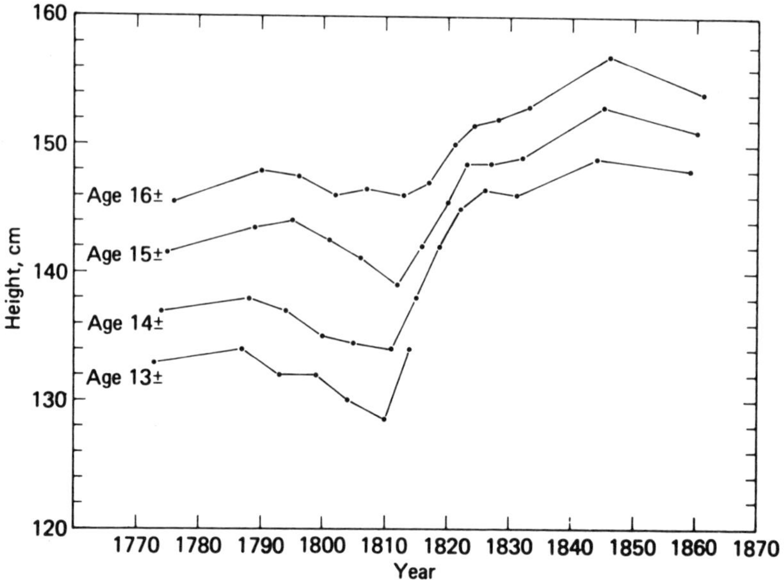

Fig. 1. Height of Marine Society recruits from 1770 to 1860. (Reproduced from Floud and Wachter, 1982, with permission of the publisher.)

Height data for Dutch conscripts have been reported annually since 1851 (with exception of the 1939–1945 period), and uncensored socioeconomic, demographic, and cultural statistics from the Central Bureau of Statistics are available and allow an ecological analysis of the relations between environmental factors and growth (van Wieringen, 1979). Figure 2 shows the distribution of heights during the period. The general trend over this period is one of substantial increase in height, albeit interrupted by short periods in which the positive secular trend of growth ceased. These periods coincide with the cholera epidemic of 1866–1867 and the agrarian crisis between 1888 and 1896. In contrast, the First World War and the depression in the thirties did not greatly inhibit the secular trend in growth for Dutch conscripts. The Second World War may have affected the growth of the 1948–1951 drafts who were between 10 and 14 years old at the height of the Dutch famine in 1944.

Short-Term Secular Trend in Growth

One means of gauging how useful growth surveillance is to public health is to examine growth changes over short periods of time, say 10 years. This will be done for the economic depression of the thirties and the period between 1965 and 1985, as the first may show growth response to economic depression and the second represents a period of unprecedented advance in data handling of large data sets.

The depression in the 1930s. In Oslo, Norway, the height and weights of school children have been monitored since 1918 (Brundtland et al., 1980). Fig-

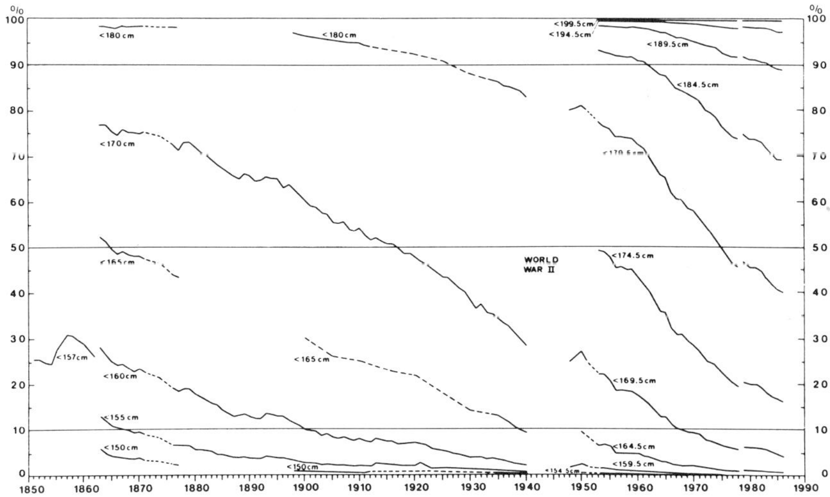

Fig. 2. Cumulative frequency, in percentages, of the heights of Dutch conscripts from 1851 to 1986. (Reproduced from van Wieringin, 1978, with permission of the publisher.)

ure 3 shows the mean height of boys for the period 1920–1975. There was a clear negative secular trend during the Second World War (1939–1945), but for all age groups the 1930s is characterised by a very marked increase in height. Brundtland et al. (1980) attributed this to the milder economic crisis experienced by Norway compared with other countries and to the general introduction of school lunches in the period 1925–1934. The Dutch (Fig. 2) and Norwegian data are compatible for the period 1920–1940 in so far that during the economic depression there was a positive secular trend of growth.

In London there was a secular trend of between 1.55 and 1.88 cm/decade over the period 1905–1938 in children between the ages of 5.0 and 13.9 years (Cameron, 1979). Thus it is very unlikely that during the economic depression the secular trend was arrested. In the Rhonda Valley, Wales, a mining area that suffered greatly during the economic depression of the 1930s, height records of 8- and 9-year-old children show no fall off in the secular trend in growth during the period (Baker et al., 1977). This is perhaps surprising given that when unemployment peaked at 2.6 million, unemployment payments were cut by 10%, contributions to inland revenue were increased, and salaries in the public sector were reduced (Checkland, 1983). Explanation for why the depression did not check the secular trend in growth are complex but can be summarised as follows: in comparison with the preceding period, the standard of living did not deteriorate in most social groups in Europe in spite of high unemployment, and governments introduced palliative measures, such as insurance cover for some unemployed groups to protect the most vulnerable groups in the society (Thane, 1982). In addition, fertility greatly diminished so that the total period fertility rate that was 2.39 in 1921–1925 reached 1.78 in 1931–1935, a figure similar to the period 1976–1980 (OPCS, 1980); family size was thus reduced.

From 1965 to 1985. The secular trend in growth for the past 20 years is examined for Holland (Roede and van Wieringen, 1985) and Britain (Rona and Chinn, 1984; Chinn and Rona, 1984), where cross-sectional studies have been undertaken of similar design.

The Dutch data show a negative secular trend in growth in children under the age of 2 years, and a substantial increase in height for older age groups. The trend in those under 2 years old is curious and will be discussed below. The Dutch survey illustrates that a negative secular trend in growth does not necessarily accompany a period of socioeconomic crisis and that even in highly developed countries the positive trend in growth continues. Furthermore, this increase in height is observed for the whole distribution and not only for the low-stature individuals.

In England and Scotland, increase of approximately 1 cm has been recorded for primary school children of both sexes for the period 1972–1980 (Chinn and Rona 1984). The National Study of Health and Growth (NSHG) includes the collection of data on social factors for children whose measurements are taken. For example, duriing the period of analysis, the number of children in a family decreased sharply. Adjusting for this diminishes the trend

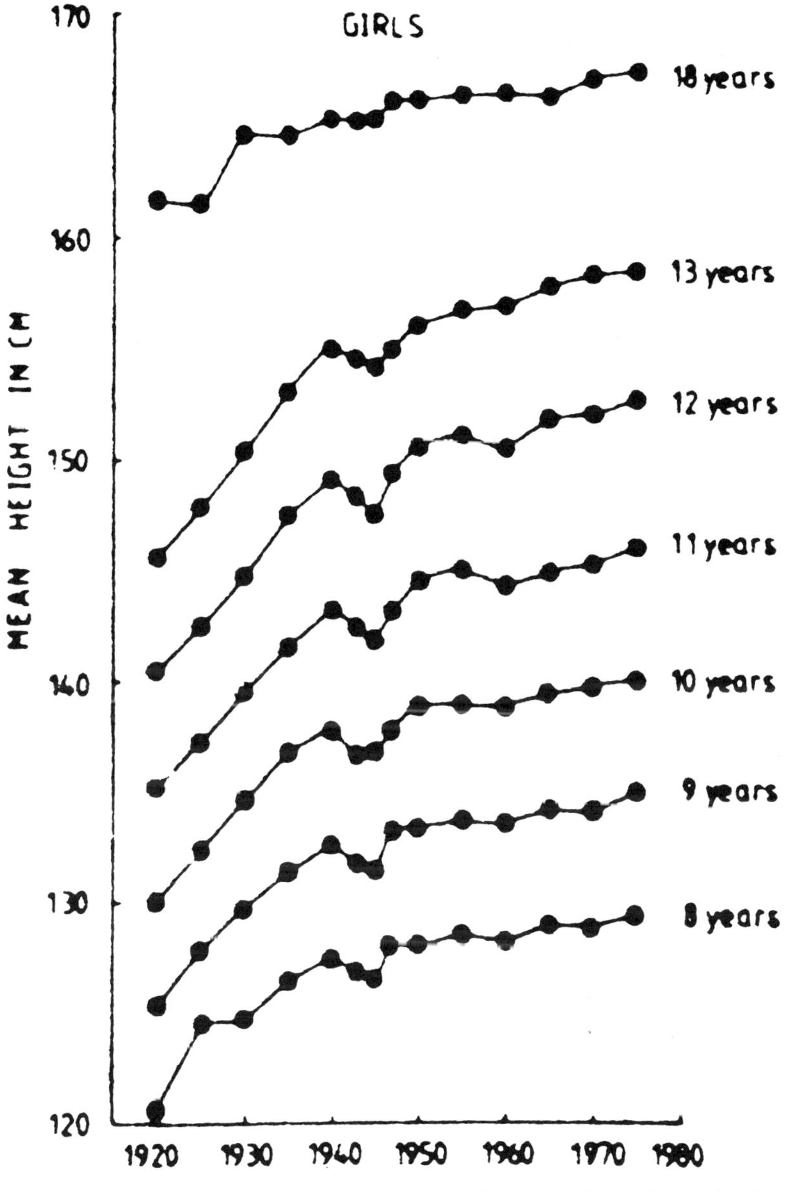

Fig. 3. Height of Oslo children from 1920 to 1980. (Reproduced from Brundtland et al., 1980, with permission of the publisher.)

in height. However, other factors must have also contributed, because a significant difference ($P < 0.05$) in boys and an insignificant difference in English girls remained after adjustment for family size (Rona and Chinn, 1984).

In the 20th century, growth deteriorated during the war years but not during major economic depressions. A series of mechanisms related to family structure and welfare policy may have acted as buffers during such periods. As family size appears to be declining and as the generosity of welfare policies may have peaked, it would be interesting to ascertain how long the secular trend in growth continues, if at all.

Biological Factors and Growth

Any assessment of the impact of socioeconomic factors and welfare policy on growth should be done in the context of biological characteristics, e.g., age and maturation. It is well documented that the secular trend in growth is greatest during adolescence, intermediate in childhood, and least in young adults (Eveleth and Tanner, 1976). There are two components to this positive secular trend in growth: Firstly, there has been a tendency towards earlier maturation over time, and secondly, there has been an absolute increase in adult height. The trend towards an earlier maturation between 1840 and 1960 has been shown for a series of European countries by assessing age of menarche (Tanner and Eveleth, 1975). Many of the factors associated with the secular trend in growth are similarly related to age of menarche (van Wieringen, 1978). However, exceptions to this have been documented. For example, Roberts et al. (1986) could find no association between social class and age of menarche. Dann and Roberts (1973) suggested that the secular trend in the age of menarche may have petered out in Britain, whereas the trend in growth continues (Chinn and Rona, 1984). More recent data seem to confirm this plateau in the age of menarche in the last 20 years in Britain (Cameron, 1979) and in Norway (Bruntland et al., 1979). However, in Holland the trend to earlier maturation continues, as the age of menarche was 1.4 months earlier in 1980 than in 1965 and most secondary sex characteristics develop at an earlier age than hitherto (Roede and van Wieringen, 1985). It can be tentatively concluded that the secular trend in growth and the secular trend towards an earlier age of maturation in the last 25 years show many interrelations, and this should be considered in any interpretation of secular change in height in age groups in a community.

Less well established is the negative secular trend in growth for the first two years of life (Roede and van Wieringen, 1985). Figure 4 shows the height of Dutch boys up to the age of 4. Boys in the 1980 survey overtake their counterparts in the 1985 survey at age 2.5. In girls the pattern is similar. In Britain the 1981–1982 survey of growth in preschool children reported that boys and girls at age 1 were on average shorter than the 50th percentile of the British standards of height based on 1959 measurements, but by age 2, their heights were similar to the British standards (personal communication). In Britain and Holland up to 1980, all other age groups had a positive trend in growth. Two explanations are offered for the observation: a change in the pattern of food intake in the very young; and a demographic change in the number of children

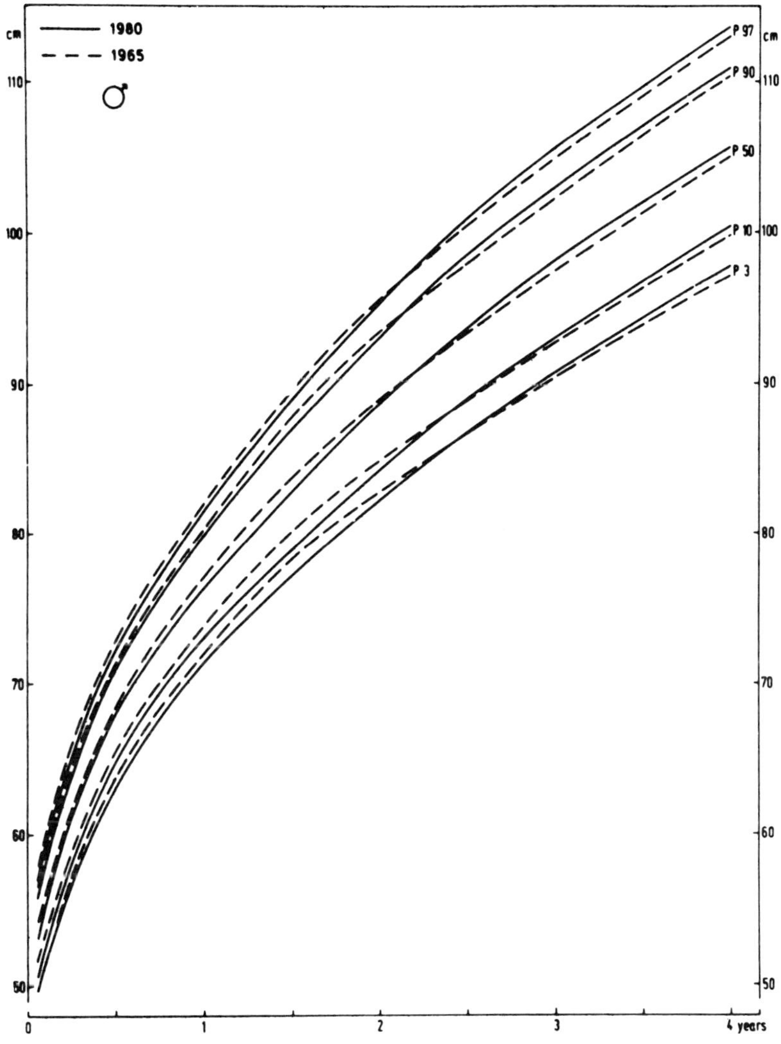

Fig. 4. Attained length (height) of 0–3-year-old boys. (Reproduced from Roede and van Wieringin, 1985, with permission of the publisher.)

in the family. The second explanation can account for both the negative secular trend in the first two years of life, and the positive secular trend in older age groups. In families, the proportion of firstborns to total births has increased, and as the firstborn generally has a lower birthweight than his siblings (Chamberlain et al., 1975), one could expect to see a negative secular trend in growth for the first two years. For older age groups, the firstborn and children from smaller families tend to be taller (Goldstein, 1971; Rona et al., 1978), and thus the trend towards smaller families may partly explain the positive secular trend of growth. Dramatic differences in the secular trend for growth between age groups demand caution in the interpretation of results based on narrow age range.

Changes in the genetic endowment of the population under observation should also be appreciated. Many European countries experienced an inflow of immigrants during the economic boom following the Second World War. In Britain the newcomers came mainly from the West Indies and from the Indian Subcontinent. These groups not only modified the gene pool of the host population but also had different socioeconomic and cultural characteristics. In terms of growth, the difference between ethnic groups are very large and are unexplained by biological and socioeconomic factors (Rona and Chinn, 1986). For example, children from Afro-Caribbean origin were between 2 and 3 cm taller than Caucasian children in spite of a lower average standard of living (Fig. 5). For children originally from the Indian Subcontinent, heterogeneity is even observed between groups according to the language spoken at home (Rona and Chinn, 1986). Children whose parents speak Punjabi are almost as tall as Caucasian children, while children from Gujarati families are nearer to the 25th centile of height of British standards. Ethnic minorities tend to oc-

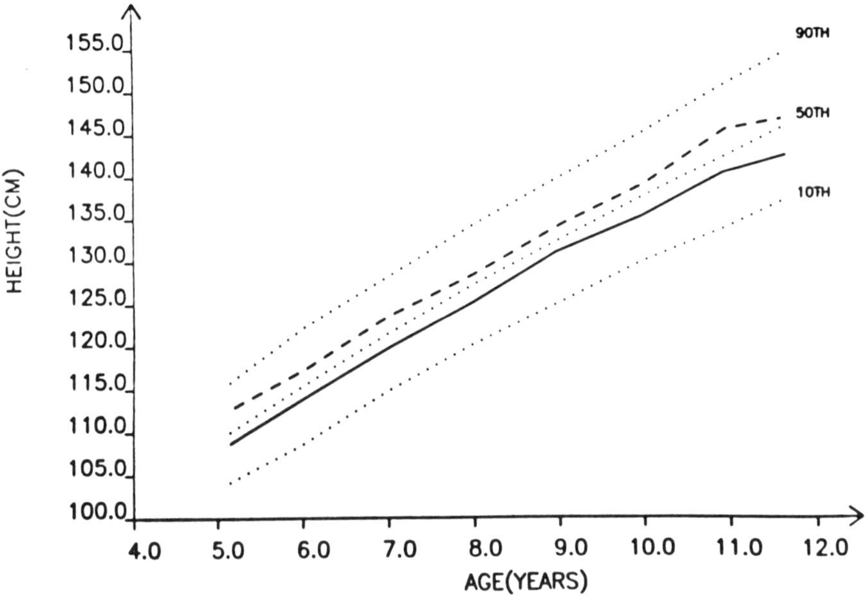

Fig. 5. Height of Caucasian (————) and Afro-Caribbean (– – – –) boys against the NSHG representative sample in 1972.

cupy the lowest socioeconomic positions in their country of adoption, and are, therefore, an important inclusion in a surveillance system.

In conclusion, the interpretation of changes, or the lack of them, in growth over time requires careful consideration. The pace of maturation, the age group selected for surveillance, new additions to the gene pool, and social characteristics of a community are relevant to the assessment of growth changes documented by a surveillance system.

DESIGN FOR A GROWTH SURVEILLANCE SYSTEM

With the realisation that the number of children to be measured is small in comparison to the population of interest, two strategies are available. An independent random sample can be drawn each time measurements are taken, or an initial selection from a sampling frame can define all future samples. An example of the second approach is the British cohort study (Butler and Alberman, 1969) that selected children on the basis of date of birth. If it is decided that surveillance will be of growth at more than one age, the design becomes mixed longitudinal, unless ages at measurement and frequency of surveys are chosen such that no child is remeasured. If such a design is adopted, then for the purposes of surveillance all children within the chosen dates of birth who can be identified should be measured, including any who have migrated and have not been measured at previous surveys.

Selection according to other criteria can also give mixed-longitudinal data. The NSHG (Irwig, 1976), which was designed primarily as a surveillance study, selected schools within specific areas, and these have been retained as far as possible in the study.

Growth surveillance based on independent random samples, although simplest in terms of data analysis, is likely to present difficulties associated with maintaining a consistent sampling frame and response rate. It has not been attempted in the United Kingdom. Apart from simplicity in estimation of trends, pure cross-sectional data has little to recommend it. Estimation of trends in rate of growth are not precluded, but precision is low (Tanner, 1951). Use of the data to relate rate of growth to individual characteristics of the child is lost. Chinn and Rona (1987) showed that the cross-sectional design had little advantage compared with mixed-longitudinal designs in precision of estimation of trends in height and weight.

The frequency of surveys will depend on how sensitive to changes in trend the system is designed to be. However, unless just one age group is observed, the precision of the estimate will depend not only on the frequency of surveys, but also on the number of age groups over which the trend is averaged, the correlation between measurements on the same child, and the proportion of children measured at each survey (Chinn and Rona, 1987). Regardless of whether a cross-sectional or mixed-longitudinal design is chosen, its precision depends primarily on the between-child variance and the number of children measured at each occasion. However, no general rules can be given to aid the choice of study design, and it is necessary to carry out the appropriate calculations to choose between potential designs.

ALARM SYSTEMS

A surveillance of growth should respond promptly to undesirable changes in the growth pattern of the population. Action should either control the ill effect of the environment on growth or initiate more detailed investigations about the possible causes of any deterioration in height or increase in obesity. In the area of growth surveillance little work has been done on developing alarm systems from anthropometric measurements, but the value of incorporating such systems can be seen from the surveillance system of malformations. In the surveillance of malformations in operation in Britain, two mechanisms are primed to respond to teratogens such as thalidomide. The first requires the calculation of the expected number of malformations for a given group, which is then compared with the observed number for the group. A difference greater than three standard deviations between observed and expected triggers an alarm response for the group investigated (Weatherall and Haskey, 1976). The second test relies on the cumulative sum (cusum) technique, which aims to detect quickly any shift in the mean level of a series of data measurements. The cusum technique adds the values of a time series and substracts the reference value. Once the cusum exceeds a critical value, called *decision boundary,* the mean level is said to have changed (Weatherall and Haskey, 1976). The critical value in the system described has been arbitrarily set so that on average 500 months pass before a false alarm is given, and, on average, only three months will be needed before a true increase is detected.

A nutritional surveillance involves the measurement of changes in level of disease (malnutrition) or population at risk in the community. Habicht (1980) pointed out that true prevalence can only be assessed if the *sensitivity* (proportion correctly identified with the disease of the total with the disease) and *specificity* (proportion correctly identified as healthy of the total healthy group) of a test to assess malnutrition is greater than one. In developed countries this can be applied to obesity, for which the prevalence is reasonably high depending on the cutoff point chosen and the age or sex group. However, the prevalence of malnutrition at a clinical level is so low that its assessment would be meaningless. In essence, a developed country requires an alarm system that detects negative changes in the secular trend for height and positive changes in the secular trend for obesity. Perhaps for the assessment of change in the prevalence of obesity in the community an equivalent to the cusum technique could be developed and tested.

Terrenato and Ulizzi (1983) attempted to assess improvement in nutritional status using continuous height data. They investigated the stature distribution curves from 1874 to 1960 in Italian military recruits, and suggested that a decrease in skewness and hyperkurtosis was compatible with a progressive improvement in living conditions. This may be a valid interpretation for studies in adults over the past 85 years. However, in their study symmetry in the distribution of height and lack of hyperkurtosis were reached by 1938, and consequently, in developed countries the examination of the third and fourth moments of the normal distribution would not be very helpful.

There are many unresolved questions which make it difficult to suggest clear-cut operational methods to establish an alarm system for nutritional status. Firstly, why have marked differences in the secular trend of growth been seen between affluent countries? In Norway, that there was no change in height of military conscripts between 1965 and 1975 (Brundtland et al., 1980) contrasts with an increase of almost 3 cm in Holland (van Wieringen, 1978). Secondly, why have different age groups experienced different secular trends, e.g., a negative secular trend in growth in the children under 2 years old and a positive secular trend in older children? Thirdly, what adjustments should be made for changes in social class structure, family size, and employment status in any comparison of groups over time? For example, in Britain, children whose fathers were unemployed in 1972 were shorter than their peers in 1981. However, the unemployed in 1981 were on average better off than in 1972, as in 1972 most unemployed were in the unskilled manual group while in 1981 a large proportion of the unemployed belonged to other social classes (Rona and Chinn, 1984). Fourthly, what adjustment should be made for inflows of new groups into the community?

The following suggestions should be considered in the establishment of an alarm system of growth surveillance: international awareness of trends, i.e., how do the results from one country compare with countries who are in the same league of socioeconomic development. A countrywide system should include four age groups of concern: preschool children, preadolescent school children, adolescent school children, and young adults, as changes in trends of growth may differ in these age groups due to changes in parity and age of maturation. Concern over changes in growth needs to focus not only on the mean but also, according to the size of the samples, on the 10th or 3rd centiles of the distribution. This suggestion is difficult to fulfill for subsets of the sample because the precision of the estimates of the low centiles of the distribution will be poor (unless the total population instead of a sample is being measured). Algorithms based on central measures (mean and median) should be developed for warning systems and these should be fully tested.

In conclusion, the development of alarm systems for surveillance of nutrition has been neglected. The positive secular trend in growth in most age groups has not demanded searching questions into the nutritional status of the population. However, it is a matter of urgency that alarm systems are developed if we are to maximise the value of a surveillance system.

REQUIREMENTS FOR ESTABLISHING A GROWTH SURVEILLANCE SYSTEM

Any surveillance system should comply with certain characteristics, each of which seems deceptively easy to fulfil. The sample should be representative of the population about which health decisions will be made. The measurements undertaken should be simple, accurate, repeatable, and acceptable if comparability over time is to be ensured. Only essential personal information about individuals in the sample should be obtained. The most important results of the surveillance process and recommendations should be released to the supporting agencies shortly after data collection so that these agencies can make informed decisions. The amount of work the project will entail should be carefully estimated when making bids for resources. Nowadays, when cost-cutting exercises are so fashionable, it is appropriate to keep in mind that long-term projects are very difficult to maintain with limited resources.

It is beyond the aim of this paper to give a recipe for the successful implementation of a surveillance system of growth. However, an element that needs consideration is the makeup of the team in charge of the surveillance system and the network of collaborators. The team needs to have expertise in biomedical and epidemiological aspects of growth, statistics, data handling, and administration. A sound administration is crucial for coordinating the study and communicating with the units. In a long-term project collaborators change, their enthusiasm dwindles, and local resource constraints become more apparent. In practice these problems can be handled provided release of reports on important results is timely and discussion of local problems in conducting the study are promptly sorted out. It is likely that parts of the sample will need to be replaced because of either local unwillingness to continue or decrease in birth rate. A clear procedure should be specified for replacing children and an assessment of whether the replacement affects the overall trend is advisable.

Another issue that needs to be addressed in the design of a nutritional surveillance in developed countries is how to ensure that the number of children in each relevant subgroup in the community is sufficient for useful analysis. This is not an easy matter to resolve, because in a developed country the "at risk" groups are also minority groups which will be small in a representative sample of the country. In the NSHG we have tackled this problem by following two samples, one a representative sample of the country, and the other selected to include children from inner-city areas and ethnic minorities (Rona and Chinn, 1986).

In a surveillance study, reports of the results should be supplied soon after data collection and, to be effective, need to be understood by a wide range of people with no particular expertise in the field. In the NSHG the style has been to produce annual reports with routine results of growth surveillance and more sophisticated analysis for publication in scientific journals. For example, using data from the three surveys in the NSHG, we reported a positive secular trend of height in the first 10 years of surveillance. The results from the routine system were confirmed in a more sophisticated longitudinal analysis (Chinn and Rona, 1984).

SUPPLEMENTARY USES OF GROWTH SURVEILLANCE DATA

A nutritional surveillance system is a wealth of data for use in research, with important implications for public health. Two examples from the NSHG will illustrate this.

The NSHG has contributed to the understanding of the influence of changes in the British food policy with regard to the availability of school meals and milk during the 1970s on the growth pattern of primary school children (Cook et al., 1979, Rona et al., 1983). It was concluded that given the standard of living at the time of the survey, the provision of free school milk did not increase the growth of 6- and 7-year-old children, and that school meals did not increase the rate of growth of primary school children in any social stratum. This assessment should be repeated over time, as socioeconomic circumstances in the community can deteriorate to a level in which welfare policy related to food could affect the growth of children.

In the NSHG, several topics of significant public interest, e.g., parents' perception of food intolerance in their children (Rona and Chinn, 1987) have been explored. A strong association between the mother's level of education and the child being perceived as food intolerant was found. A possible explanation of this finding would be that mothers with higher levels of education are more perceptive than other mothers to issues given high profile by the media or voluntary organisations. More recently it has been demonstrated that the children perceived as food intolerant were significantly shorter than children with no history of food intolerance (Price et al., 1988), and it is concluded that, regardless of the underlying aetiology, this finding indicates that parents' complaints of food intolerance in their children need to be taken seriously by doctors.

CONCLUDING REMARKS

In even the wealthiest societies there are disadvantaged groups, and socioeconomic circumstances are not immune to fluctuation. Therefore a system to assess changes in the nutritional status of the community is advisable. Only a continuous surveillance system of growth stands a chance of detecting unforeseen effects that these changes can have on the nutritional status of children. However, a surveillance study is only an observational study, and therefore, in common with all observational studies, a cause and effect relationship is difficult to infer unlike for a randomised controlled trial. Furthermore, the design of surveillance systems may not be the most efficient for every type of issue that arises, and surveillance studies are appreciated as difficult to modify once established. In practical terms it should be clear that surveillance of growth needs to be undertaken by researchers with expertise in growth epidemiology, and social policy related to child welfare.

Tanner (1986) has emphasised how important it is to distinguish between the use of auxological data to monitor the health of individuals and the health of populations. In this paper I have concentrated on surveillance of populations. Continuous and systematic assessments of growth over short periods of time in the community are uncommon in developed countries. Advances in data handling make it feasible for most developed countries to set up such a system. At the very least this type of surveillance can detect any deterioration in nutritional status in terms of height and an increase in obesity. Both of these problems can prompt intervention strategies from the appropriate agencies. In addition these projects contribute to knowledge on a variety of issues that are highly relevant to social policy. The possibility of incorporating additional measurements into the system to evaluate the health of the community may increase the efficiency of the system. On the other hand there are several aspects that need to be further explored. These are namely: the sensitivity of growth to changes in the socioeconomic circumstances of populations in developed countries and methodological issues to decide the appropriate threshold for an alarm system.

REFERENCES

Baker IA, Cochrane AL, Elwood PC (1977): Growth surveillance. (Letters to the Editor.) Int J Epidemiol 6: 293.

Brundtland GH, Liestol K, Walloe L (1980): Height, weight and menarcheal age of Oslo school children during the last 60 years. Ann Hum Biol 7: 307–322.

Butler NR, Alberman ED (1969): "Perinatal Problems. The Second Report of the 1958 British Perinatal Morality Survey." Edinburgh: Churchill Livingstone.

Cameron N (1979): The growth of London school children 1904–1966: An analysis of secular trend and inter-county variation. Ann Hum Biol 6: 505–525.

Chamberlain R, Chamberlain G, Howlett B, Claireaux A (1975): "British Births 1970, 1: The First Week of Life." London: William Heinemann.

Checkland S (1983): "British Public Policy 1776–1939. An Economic, Social and Political Perspective." Cambridge: Cambridge University Press.

Chen LC, Chowdhury AKMA, Huffman S (1980): Anthropometric assessment of energy-protein malnutrition and subsequent risk of mortality among pre-school children. Am J Clin Nutr 33: 1836–1844.

Chinn S, Rona RJ (1984): The secular trend in the height of primary school children in England and Scotland from 1972–1980. Ann Hum Biol 11: 1–16.

Chinn S, Rona RJ (1987): National Study of Health and Growth: Effect of change in design with reference to efficiency of mixed longitudinal studies for measuring trends. J R Soc Med 80: 544–546.

Cook J, Irwig LM, Chinn S, Altman DG, Florey CduV (1979): The influence of availability of free school milk on the height of children in England and Scotland. J Epidemiol Community Health 33: 171–176.

Dann TC, Roberts DF (1973): End of a trend? A 12-year study of age of menarche. Br Med J 3: 265–267.

Dowler EA, Payne PR, Seo YO, Thompson AM, Wheeler EF (1982): Nutritional status indicator: Interpretation and policy making role. Food Policy 7: 99–112.

Eveleth PB, Tanner JM (1976): "Worldwide Variation in Human Growth." Cambridge: Cambridge University Press.

Floud R, Wachter KW (1982): Poverty and physical stature. Evidence on the standard of living of London boys 1770–1870. Soc Sci Hist 6: 422–451.

Goldstein H (1971): Factors influencing the height of seven year old children. Hum Biol 43: 92–111.

Habicht J-P (1980): Some characteristic of indicators of nutritional status for use in screening and surveillance. Am J Clin Nutr 33: 531–535.

Habicht J-P, Martorell R, Yarbrough C, Malina RM, Klein RE (1974): Height and weight standards for pre-school children. How relevant are ethnic differences in growth potential? Lancet 1: 611–615.

Irwig LM (1976): Surveillance in developed countries with particular reference to child growth. Int J Epidemiol 5: 57–61.
Lapidus L, Bengtsson C, Larsson B, Pennert K, Rybo E, Sjostrom L (1984): Distribution of adipose tissue and risk of cardiovascular disease and death: A 12 year follow-up of participants in the population study of women in Gothenburg, Sweden. Br Med J 282: 1400–1404.
Lindgren G (1976): Height, weight and menarche in Swedish school children in relation to socio-economic and regional factors. Ann Hum Biol 3: 501–528.
Melia RJW, Florey CduV, Altman DG, Swan AV (1977): Association between gas cooking and respiratory disease in children. Br Med J 1: 149–152.
Meredith HV (1976): Findings from Asia, Australia, Europe and North America on secular change in mean height of children, youths and young adults. Am J Phys Anthropol 44: 315–326.
OPCS (1980): "Birth Statistics. Review of the Registrar General on Births and Patterns of Family Building in England and Wales, 1980." Ser. FM1 No. 7. London: Her Majesty's Stationery Office.
Paffenbarger RS, Wing Al (1969): Chronic diease in former college students, X: The effects of single and multiple characteristics on risk of fatal coronary diease. Am J Epidemiol 90: 527–535.
Peck AMN, Vagero DH (1987): Adult body height and childhood socioeconomic group. J Epidemiol Community Health 41: 333–337.
Price CE, Rona RJ, Chinn S (1988): The height of primary school children and parents' perceptions of food intolerance. Br Med J 296:1696–1699.
Roberts DF, Wood W, Chinn S (1986): Menarcheal age in Cumbria. Ann Hum Biol 13: 161–170.
Roede MJ, van Wieringen JC (1985): Growth diagrams 1980. Netherlands third nationwide survey. Tijdschr Noor Soc Gezandheiszorg 63 (suppl): 1–34.
Rona RJ, Chinn S (1984): The National Study of Health and Growth: Nutritional surveillance of primary school children from 1972 to 1981 with special reference to unemployment and social class. Ann Hum Biol 11: 17–28.
Rona RJ, Chinn S (1986): National Study of Health and Growth: Social and biological factors associated with height of children from ethnic groups living in England. Ann Hum Biol 5: 453–471.
Rona RJ, Chinn S (1987): Food intolerance in primary school children. The parents' perceptions. Br Med J 294: 863–866.
Rona RJ, Chinn S, Smith AM (1983): School meals and the rate of growth of primary school children. J Epidemiol Community Health 37: 8–15.
Rona RJ, Swan AV, Altman DG (1978): Social factors and height of primary school children in England and Scotland. J Epidemiol Community Health 32: 147–154.
Tanner JM (1951): Some motes on the reporting of growth data. Hum Biol 23: 93–159.
Tanner JM (1962): "Growth at Adolescence." 2nd ed. Oxford: Blackwell Scientific.
Tanner JM (1976): Growth as a monitor of nutritional status. Proc Nutr Soc 35:315–322.
Tanner JM (1981): "A History of the Study of Human Growth." Cambridge:Cambridge University Press.
Tanner JM (1986): Physical development. Br Med Bull 42: 131–138.
Tanner JM, Eveleth PB (1975); Variability between populations in growth and development at puberty. In Berenberg SR (ed): "Puberty, Biologic and Psychosocial Components." Leiden: Kroese, pp 256–273.
Terrenato C, Ulizzi L (1983): Genotype-environment relationships: An analysis of stature distribution curves during the last century in Italy. Ann Hum Biol 4: 335–346.

Thane P (1982): "The Foundation of the Welfare State." London: Longman.
van Wieringen JC (1978): Secular growth changes. In Falkner F, Tanner JM (eds): "Human Growth. Vol 2, Postnatal Growth." London: Bailliere Tindall, pp 445–473.
van Wieringen JC (1979): Secular growth and environment. An analysis of development in the Netherlands, 1850–1978. Coll Anthropol 3: 35–47.
Waaler HT (1984): Height, weight and mortality. The Norwegian experience. Acta Med Scand (suppl) 679:1–55.
Wachter KW, Trussell J (1982): Estimating historical heights. J Am Stat Assoc 77: 279–303.
Weatherall JAC, Haskey JC (1976): Surveillance of malformations. Br J Med Bull 32: 39–44.

Anthropometric Assessment
of Nutritional Status, pages 319–335

19
National Nutritional Surveys Assessing Anthropometric Status

ROBERT J. KUCZMARSKI AND CLIFFORD JOHNSON
Division of Health Examination Statistics, National Center for Health Statistics, Hyattsville, Maryland 20782

INTRODUCTION

The components of nutritional status assessment may be broadly classified under the following categories: anthropometric, biochemical, clinical, dietary, and socioeconomic. A variety of surveys conducted at university, clinic, state, regional, and national levels may gather population-based data in one or more of these assessment categories. The various settings represent levels of data collection that may or may not be statistically representative of the population being sampled. This, of course, depends upon the sophistication of the sampling design that is incorporated in the survey and the intended purposes of the survey. At the national level in the United States, there are several surveys that collect self-reported data on body size, but there is only one national survey program that actually measures body dimensions of examined persons.

Most notable among the U.S. surveys that collect nationally representative questionnaire data on heights and weights are the National Health Interview Survey (NHIS) conducted by the National Center for Health Statistics (NCHS) and the Nationwide Food Consumption Survey (NFCS) sponsored by the United States Department of Agriculture (USDA). The NHIS is conducted annually and the NFCS approximately every 10 years. The questionnaire data in these surveys provide information on a self-report of height and weight for the sample persons. The validity of such data has been discussed by others and will not be dealt with further in this chapter (Pirie et al., 1981; Stewart et al., 1987).

In addition to national surveys that provide an overall description of the nutritional status of a population at a given time, there are also surveillance programs that collect anthropometric data. Although not national in scope, the Centers for Disease Control (CDC) sponsors the Behavioral Risk Factor Surveillance System (BRFSS) and the Pediatric Nutrition Surveillance System (PedNSS). The BRFSS obtains self-reported height and weight data from telephone interviews that have allowed further estimates of overweight to be made in the United States (Forman et al., 1986). The PedNSS also collects height and weight data from clinics in 36 states on low-income, high-risk children from birth to 17 years (USDHHS, 1987). These data are from convenience samples in many different clinics that do not use standardized procedures, technicians, or equipment, and are not intended to be used as nationally representative reference data.

BACKGROUND ON HEALTH AND NUTRITION EXAMINATION SURVEYS

The only national survey program that actually measures selected body dimensions of sample persons is the Health and Nutrition Examination Survey (HANES). The HANES program consists of a series of surveys that measure and monitor selected aspects of the health and nutritional status of the U.S. population. Each survey has the capability of gathering information that is uniquely obtained by direct medical examinations and clinical tests and measurements, including anthropometric assessments.

Historically, six of these surveys have been conducted, beginning with three National Health Examination Surveys (NHES I, NHES II, and NHES III) from 1960–1970 (Table 1). Subsequently, dietary, hematological, biochemical, and clinical measures were added to assess the nutritional status of the population. The name of the survey was correspondingly changed to reflect this broader purpose, and two National Health and Nutrition Examination Surveys were conducted (NHANES I 1971–1975 and NHANES II 1976–1980).

In these national surveys, because some minority groups were sampled at a rate proportional to their density in the population, the number of minority persons in the sample was not large enough to evaluate their health and nutritional status. Therefore, in the period 1982–84, the Hispanic Health and Nutrition Examination Survey (HHANES) was conducted to evaluate the health and nutritional status of the three largest Hispanic subgroups in the United States. These three groups consisted of persons of Mexican descent residing in selected households in the five southwest states of Texas, Colorado, New Mexico, Arizona, and California; Puerto Ricans from selected counties of New

TABLE 1. NCHS Health Examination Surveys

Year	Survey	Ages covered (years)
1960–62	National Health Examination Survey I	18–79
1963–65	NHES II	6–11
1966–70	NHES III	12–17
1971–74	National Health and Nutrition Examination Survey I	1–74
1974–75	NHANES I Augmentation	25–74
1976–80	NHANES II	0.5–74
1982–84	Hispanic HANES	0.5–74
1988–94	NHANES III	2 mo.+

York, New Jersey, and Connecticut; and Cubans in Miami, Florida. The third NHANES began in October 1988 and will continue until 1994. Body measurements will be included as a vital component in the assessment of nutritional status in this survey.

SURVEY DESIGN

In the past, the NHES and the NHANES have been limited to the geographically accessible, civilian, noninstitutionalized population of the United States, excluding Native Americans residing on reservation lands and persons residing on military reservations. All surveys have used complex, multistage, stratified, cluster samples of defined population groups. For the NHES and the NHANES I, the target populations were based on a probability sample of persons in the coterminous United States. With the NHANES II, Alaska and Hawaii were, for the first time, eligible for inclusion in the sample. The HHANES was restricted to counties and neighborhoods in three areas of the country that had a sufficient proportion of Hispanics to render it economically feasible to visit households and operate an examination center for a period of four to seven weeks. In past surveys, there were upper and lower age limits. Thus, infants aged less than 6 months and adults aged more than 74 or 79 years were not included.

There are a number of common factors in each of the HANES surveys. Each consists of two major components: 1) household interviews and 2) physical examinations and interviews conducted in mobile examination centers. The household interviews are conducted prior to the examinations and are used to obtain selected demographic and socioeconomic data on the family and specific medical history information for each sample person. The body measurements are part of a series of tests and procedures performed in the mobile examination centers. These exam centers consist of several sets of specially equipped trailers that are moved from one geographic location to another. Detailed descriptions of each of the HANES surveys and the health and nutritional assessments made in each study have been published (NCHS 1973, NCHS 1977, NCHS 1981, NCHS 1985).

DATA USES

In all of the national surveys, weight, heights, skinfolds, circumferences, and breadths were included. However, in the earlier NHES surveys there was a broader array of measures reflecting the interests of the persons designing the survey and those of their consultants. These included many body dimensions that tended to be more useful in the discipline of human engineering. The diverse range of measurements that have been taken over the years are shown in Table 2. With the inception of the NHANES program in 1971, the list of measures was narrowed to focus on those that were believed to be most closely associated with health or nutritional status. Having mentioned the NHES in its historical context as the predecessor to the NHANES, the following discussion will now focus only on the HANES program.

TABLE 2. Body Measurements in the HES and Hanes Surveys

	Survey					
Body measurements	HES I 1960–62	HES II 1963–65	HES III 1966–70	NHANES I 1971–75	NHANES II 1976–80	HHANES 1982–84
Skinfolds						
Triceps	18–79 yrs	6–11 yrs	12–17 yrs	1–74 yrs rt and lft	6 mo–74 yrs rt and lft	6 mo–74 yrs rt and lft
Subscapular	18–79 yrs	6–11 yrs	12–17 yrs	1–74 yrs rt and lft	6 mo–74 yrs rt and lft	6 mo–74 yrs rt and lft
Iliac crest	X	X	X	X	X	6 mo–74 yrs rt and lft
Medial calf	X	X	12–17 yrs	X	X	6 mo–74 yrs rt and lft
Lateral chest (midaxillary)	X	6–11 yrs	12–17 yrs	X	X	X
Suprailiac	X	X	12–17 yrs	X	X	X
Circumferences and girths						
Upper arm girth	18–79 yrs	6–11 yrs rt and lft	12–17 yrs	1–74 yrs rt and lft	6 mo–74 yrs rt and lft	6 mo–74 yrs rt and lft
Medial calf circumference	X	6–11 yrs	12–17 yrs	X	X	6 mo–74 yrs rt and lft
Chest circumference						
Erect						
Full expiration	X	X	X	25–74 (Detail)	X	X
Full inspiration	X	X	X	25–74 (Detail)	X	X
Mid respiration	18–79 yrs	6–11 yrs	12–17 yrs	1–7 (Nutrition)	2–7 yrs	2–7 yrs
Supine						
Mid respiration	X	X	X	X	6 mo–3 yrs	6 mo–3 yrs

Head circumference	X	X	X	1–7 (Nutrition)	6 mo–7 yrs	6 mo–7 yrs
Forearm girth	X	X	12–17 yrs	X	X	X
Waist girth	18–79 yrs	6–11 yrs	12–17 yrs	X	X	X
Hip girth	X	6–11 yrs	12–17 yrs	X	X	X
Lengths, stature, and weight						
Sitting height	18–79 yrs	6–11 yrs	12–17 yrs	2–74 yrs	2–74 yrs	2–74 yrs
Standing height erect	18–79 yrs	6–11 yrs	12–17 yrs	2–74 yrs	2–74 yrs	2–74 yrs
normal	18–79 yrs					
Recumbent length	X	X	X	1–2 yrs	6 mo–3 yrs	6 mo–3 yrs
Crown–rump length	X	X	X	X	6 mo–3 yrs	6 mo–3 yrs
Weight	18–79 yrs	6–11 yrs	12–17 yrs	1–74 yrs	6 mo–74 yrs	6 mo–74 yrs
Cervical height	X	X	12–17 yrs	X	X	X
Acromion to olecranon	X	6–11 yrs	X	X	X	X
Acromial height	X	X	12–17 yrs	X	X	X
Foot length	X	6–11 yrs	12–17 yrs	X	X	X
Radial height	X	X	12–17 yrs	X	X	X
Buttock–knee length	18–79 yrs	X	X	X	X	X
Stylion height	X	X	12–17 yrs	X	X	X
Knee height	18–79 yrs	6–11 yrs	X	X	X	X
Iliac crest height	X	X	12–17 yrs	X	X	X
Buttock–popliteal length	18–79 yrs	X	X	X	X	X
Trochanter height	X	X	12–17 yrs	X	X	X
Popliteal height	18–79 yrs	6–11 yrs	X	X	X	X
Tibial height	X	X	12–17 yrs	X	X	X
Elbow rest height	18–79 yrs	X	X	X	X	X
Thigh clearance	18–79 yrs	6–11 yrs	12–17 yrs	X	X	X
Sphyrion height	X	X	12–17 yrs	X	X	X

(Continued)

TABLE 2. Body Measurements in the HES and Hanes Surveys (*Continued*)

	Survey					
Body measurements	HES I 1960–62	HES II 1963–65	HES III 1966–70	NHANES I 1971–75	NHANES II 1976–80	HHANES 1982–84
Skeletal widths and breadths						
Biacromial breadth	X	X	12–17 yrs	X	X	6–74 yrs
Biacromial diameter	18–79 yrs	X	X	X	X	X
Biiliac crest breadth	X	X	X	X	X	6 mo–74 yrs
Bitrochanteric breadth	X	X	12–17 yrs	1–74 yrs	6 mo–74 yrs	6 mo–74 yrs
Elbow breadth	X	X	12–17 yrs	1–74 yrs rt and lft	6 mo–74 yrs rt and lft	6 mo–74 yrs rt and lft
Foot breadth	X	6–11 yrs	12–17 yrs	X	X	X
Ankle breadth	X	X	12–17 yrs	X	X	X
Knee breadth	X	X	12–17 yrs	X	X	X
Wrist breadth	X	X	12–17 yrs	X	X	X
Bizygomatic breadth	X	X	12–17 yrs	X	X	X
Bigonial breadth	X	X	12–74 yrs	X	X	X
Elbow–elbow breadth	18–79 yrs	6–11 yrs	12–17 yrs	X	X	X
Seat breadth	18–79 yrs	6–11 yrs	12–17 yrs	X	X	X
Bicristal breadth	X	X	12–17 yrs	X	X	X
Bicristal diameter	X	6–11 yrs	X	X	X	X
Chest breadth (4th ICS)	X	6–11 yrs	X	X	X	X
Chest debth (4th ICS)	X	6–11 yrs	X	X	X	X
Bicondylar diameter	X	6–11 yrs	X	X	X	X
Handedness	X	X	X	1–74 yrs (20%)	6 mo–74 yrs	6 mo–74 yrs
First toe relative to second toe	X	X	12–17 yrs	X	X	X
Second (index) finger relative to 4th (ring) finger	X	X	12–17 yrs	X	X	X

Because the HANES has evolved into a multipurpose health survey with numerous components that must serve the needs of many, anthropometric measures that are indicators or predictors of health outcomes drive the selection of the limited number of measures that can be included in the survey. Thus, despite the fact that there continues to be an immense amount of interest in nationally representative data for a whole host of body dimensions, expressed notably by various manufacturing industries, the HANES is regrettably unable to accommodate all of these numerous requests.

The major intended uses of the HANES anthropometric data include but are certainly not limited to providing the following:

1. Normative reference data distributions by various demographic characteristics including age, race, sex, and poverty status (NCHS, 1987a).
2. Age-, race-, sex-specific distribution cut points that can be used by others to classify persons in subpopulation surveys or clinical studies (Trowbridge et al., 1987).
3. National prevalence estimates for various conditions such as stunting, wasting, overweight, and obesity (van Itallie, 1985).
4. Baseline and follow-up data for the national nutritional monitoring system and for setting and evaluating health objectives for the nation (USDHHS, 1986).
5. Analytical data that can be controlled as explanatory variables in the interpretation and prediction of morbidity and mortality (Stanton et al., 1982; NCHS, 1987b).
6. Data to create and revise the height, weight, and head circumference growth charts for children and adolescents that are used both in the United States and internationally (Hamill et al., 1979).

QUALITY OF MEASURES

In the HANES a great deal of effort has been put forth to ensure that measures are taken with standardized procedures, in a standardized setting, and using standardized equipment to minimize differences in findings among sample locations. Toward this goal, the examination component is conducted in mobile examination centers that have been specially designed and constructed for this survey, as previously mentioned. Further standardization is apparent in that examinees are required to wear only a disposable paper gown, pants, and slippers of a known weight. The health technicians on the full-time examination teams travel from one location to the next within the United States. They are specially trained to follow specific measurement protocols and are periodically evaluated by the NCHS staff and outside consultants who have expertise in anthropometry. During the course of a survey, all equipment is calibrated and checked for accuracy at regular intervals.

From the nutritional monitoring perspective, the quality of anthropometric measures included in the HANES is crucial. Because the HANES program consists of multiple surveys in a series, it is possible to monitor trends over time.

This can be accomplished with varying degrees of confidence, depending upon the measure of interest. For example, standing height data can be directly compared across all surveys because the method, equipment, and technician training were highly stable over the years.

The body weight procedure was also standardized with respect to equipment and technician training; however, in the NHES surveys, persons were weighed with light indoor clothing as oppposed to gowns. Thus, when comparisons are made between the NHES and the NHANES, or when trends over time are being investigated, adjustments should be made for clothing weight. An average clothing weight adjustment of 2.0 pounds has been used for the NHES.

A more problematic procedure has been the skinfold measurement. For skinfolds, unlike weight, it is more difficult to make adjustments for differences that may have occurred over time in equipment, training, and intratechnician or intertechnician measurement variation. With multiple sources or error possible, it is difficult to determine whether changes over time are artifactual and attributable to methodological approaches or individual observer bias or whether they represent actual biological differences or secular trends.

NHANES ANTHROPOMETRIC MEASUREMENTS

Height and Weight

The anthropometric data can be used for both cross-sectional and longitudinal applications in all age groups. The NHANES height and weight data can be used in pediatric clinics and public health screening or surveillance programs to follow an individual child's growth over time in relation to growth charts based on observation in a representative sample of the population (Hamill et al., 1979; Moore and Roche, 1982; Chumlea, 1986; CDC, 1987). Similarly, when cases of stunting or wasting are identified, growth charts may be used to monitor the progress or remedial intervention. At the other end of the spectrum, children and adolescents who are overweight for their height, age, and sex can have their values plotted and monitored on the growth charts.

These percentile distributions are also used for surveillance of populations. For example, the previously mentioned PedNSS of the CDC receives anthropometric data from 36 states, the District of Columbia, and Puerto Rico on low-income children who participate in publicly funded health, nutrition, and food assistance programs. With smoothed percentile distributions of data from the NCHS surveys, the CDC uses the following criteria to identify individuals with low or high values (CDC, 1985):

1. Low height-for-age: Height-for-age less than the 5th percentile for children of the same sex and age in the reference population.
2. Low weight-for-height: Weight-for-height less than the 5th percentile for children of the same sex and height in the reference population. This indicator describes thinness.

3. High weight-for-height: Weight-for-height greater than the 95th percentile for children of the same sex and height in the reference population. This indicator describes overweight.

For adults, the height, weight, and skinfold data have been used to identify persons who were overweight or obese (Cronk and Roche, 1982). The height and weight data, when used to create a new variable that yields an index of body mass, have been especially useful in establishing the prevalence of overweight and severe overweight. To achieve this, weight in kilograms is divided by height in meters squared (kg/m^2). This particular index is known as the body mass index (BMI) or the Quetelet index and is derived from data on persons aged 20–29 years. The rationale for using persons aged 20–29 years as the reference population was that most young adults are relatively lean; the increase in body weight that usually occurs as men and women age is assumed to be due almost entirely to fat accumulation (Najjar and Rowland, 1987.) The percentiles beyond which overweight and severe overweight are characterized have been (somewhat arbitrarily) set by the NCHS at the 85th and 95th percentiles respectively. For the most recent national survey (NHANES II, 1976–1980) the 85th and 95th percentile cutpoint values for males and females are shown in Table 3.

Using these criteria, current estimates indicate that approximately 34 million U.S. adults (15 million men, 19 million women) are overweight, and among these, approximately 13 million adults (5 million men, 8 million women) are severely overweight. As Table 4 indicates, the prevalence is markedly higher among black women compared with white women.

Body weight and standing height are considered as essential in any nutritional assessment for adults and most youths. For children who are unable to

TABLE 3. BMI Percentile Cut Points for Defining Overweight and Severe Overweight: NHANES II, 1976–1980[a]

	Percentile	
	85th	95th
Males	27.8	31.1
Females	27.3	32.3

[a]Excludes pregnant women. Overweight and severe overweight are defined as a sex-specific body mass index (kg/m^2) equal to or greater than the 85th and 95th percentile, respectively, for examinees aged 20–29 years.

TABLE 4. Prevalence of Overweight and Severely Overweight Persons Aged 20–74 Years by Race, Sex, and Age: United States 1976–1980

	Overweight (%)			Severely overweight (%)		
	All races	White	Black	All races	White	Black
Both sexes	25.7	24.8	35.7	9.4	8.9	15.2
Male	24.2	24.4	25.7	8.0	7.8	10.2
Female	27.1	25.1	43.8	10.8	9.8	19.3

stand erect independently, a recumbent length is taken. The crown—rump length has been recorded in past HANES surveys, but since it is apparently seldom used, it is a candidate for elimination from future surveys in favor of other measures that are in higher demand. However, sitting height will continue to be included. Analyses have shown distinct ethnic group differences for this measure in adults (NCHS, unpublished data). In addition, when subtracted from standing height, a new variable, leg length, can be created. Ethnic differences have also been observed for this measure when group medians are examined, with longer legs in blacks, shorter legs in Hispanics, and intermediate length legs in persons of European origin who reside in households in the United States (NCHS, unpublished data).

Skinfolds

Skinfold measurements are used to assess the thickness of subcutaneous fat at various body sites and have been included in each of the HANES surveys. They have been incorporated in other studies for a number of years in prediction equations to estimate the amount of excess body fatness or obesity. For example, the well-known Durnin-Womersley equations that use the sum of four skinfolds to indicate obesity have received wide application (Durnin and Womersley, 1974). However, such equations do have problems in that they tend to be specific to the sample populations from which they were derived and are not generalizable to other samples (Norgan and Ferro-Luzzi, 1985).

Using the NHANES I data, the sum of the triceps and subscapular skinfolds was used to characterize obesity and generate distributions of obesity for adults in the U.S. population (NCHS, 1983). A potential limitation is that it assumes that subcutaneous fat is evenly distributed throughout the body and that these two sites are highly correlated with overall body fatness. These assumptions may be true for small sample studies where body types are fairly homogeneous, but may not hold in national surveys where all body types are encountered with varying amounts and distributions of internal and subcutaneous fat. The underlying difficulty in validating skinfold data as markers of obesity in national surveys is the lack of a dependent variable that quantifies body composition and parcels out body fat. Nevertheless, as for other anthropometric measures, percentile distributions for each skinfold site provide useful reference standards by age, race, and sex groups (NCHS, 1987a), tend to be confirmatory of the overweight data (Abraham, 1983), and are variables that can be controlled in other data analyses to assess their influence on health outcomes (Stallones et al., 1982). With the current interest in fat patterning, researchers have analyzed the HANES skinfolds from the trunk and limb to assess central versus peripheral fat distributions (Frisancho and Flegal 1982, Blair et al., 1984).

Breadths

Skeletal breadth measurements have limited utility in nutritional assessment. At best, selected breadths may be used to categorize the overall skeletal frame size. This categorization is potentially important in determining an acceptable weight for a given height. That is, persons with larger frames should be permitted to carry more soft tissue as skeletal muscle along with a proportional amount of additional body fat. It can be hypothesized that together with a standing height measurement, the biacromial, biiliac, and bitrochanteric breadths should adequately describe frame size (Katch and Freedson, 1982; Katch et al., 1982). Among these measures, the most problematic is the bitrochanteric breadth because of the difficulty encountered in compressing the fat pads at this site. Others have used the bony chest breadth (Garn et al., 1983), although Katch and Freedson (1982) have observed that the chest and biiliac widths may also be subject to considerable measurement error. The elbow breadth from the NHANES II has been used in the publication of the 1983 Metropolitan height–weight tables as an indicator of frame size although the appropriateness of this particular application remains questionable (Rosenberg and Sitrin, 1983; Knapp, 1983). Others have found that the ankle or wrist breadths may give a better prediction of frame size than does the elbow breadth (Himes and Bouchard, 1985). However, these predictions remain equivocal because there are insufficient data in the literature that have explored an appropriate dependent variable to describe and predict skeletal frame size.

Circumferences

Various circumferences have been included in all of the previous national surveys, although until recently their predictive value for selected chronic conditions had not been fully recognized. Most notably, the waist and hip (buttocks) circumferences, when taken as a ratio, appear to indicate upper and lower body fat stores, with a high waist-to-hip ratio being associated with an increased risk for a number of conditions of public health importance (Ohlson et al., 1985; Bjorntorp, 1987; Gillum, 1987; VanGaal et al., 1988,). Unfortunately, the importance of these two measures was not fully appreciated when the earlier surveys were being planned and, therefore, were not included in the NHANES.

The upper arm circumference is a measure that is commonly made in population surveys. It is a relatively simple measure and may be indicative of either undernutrition or overnutrition. Given that certain assumptions are made, when the mid-upper arm circumference is put into formulas with the triceps skinfold, the cross-sectional arm muscle and fat areas can be estimated (Wright et al., 1984). Thus, this measure may be particularly useful in some groups of elderly adults as well as in young children who may be particularly vulnerable to loss of body energy reserves.

Head circumference as a screening tool is not a sensitive index of undernutrition because the brain is spared in starvation (Davidson et al., 1979). In developed countries, other indicators such as standing height or recumbent length and weight would more readily and appropriately identify potential cases of wasting. The head circumference standards are only of occasional value in assessing the relatively rare genetic disorders causing microcephaly or macrocephaly. Thus, head circumference, together with other clinical observations, may identify hydrocephalus, Tay-Sachs disease, Down syndrome, or similar conditions (Nellhaus 1968). However, although head circumference growth charts have been published (Roche et al., 1987), head circumference should not be considered the method of choice in a cross-sectional assessment of current nutritional status.

NHANES III PLANS

The protocol for the NHANES III, which began in October 1988 and will continue for six years, includes an array of anthropometric measures in each of the above-mentioned categories that have been referenced (Woteki et al., 1988). Among these, the measures that are new to the survey are knee height, midthigh skinfold, wrist breadth, and waist, buttocks, and midthigh circumferences. The knee height is included for persons aged 60 years or more to gather nationally representative data that can be used to refine predictive equations for standing height. Such equations could then be used in certain clinical cases where it is not possible to obtain a standing height or recumbent length on nonambulatory elderly persons (Chumlea et al., 1985; Muncie et al., 1987). The midthigh measurements are important predictors of body fatness, especially in overweight persons (Fanelli and Kuczmarski, 1984; Fanelli and Kuczmarski, 1988). The thigh area is known to be a major fat depot in both females and obese individuals. The importance of the waist and buttocks circumferences and the wrist breadth have already been mentioned. Where applicable, all anthropometric measurements will be taken on the right side of the body. Only one measure, buttocks circumference, will be taken over the paper garment; all others are done where the measuring instruments make direct contact with the examinee's skin.

A bioelectrical impedance analyzer will be used to record resistance and reactance values for persons aged 12 years or older. With the appropriate equations that are currently being developed and validated, it is anticipated that these values can eventually be used to yield total body water, and lean and fat body masses (Lukaski et al., 1985; Pasco and Rutishauser, 1985; Kushner and Schoeller, 1986; Lukaski et al., 1986).

The NHANES III will be somewhat unique among the national surveys in that both the lower and upper age ranges will be expanded beyond those in the past. Exams will begin at 2 months of age for infants, and there will be no upper age limit criterion for inclusion of adults in the survey.

AVAILABILITY OF THE DATA

In addition to the growth charts made available gratis by some proprietary firms, the anthropometric data from the national nutritional surveys are available primarily through three major channels. First, data analysts can access the data directly via the public use data tapes that are released by the NCHS through the National Technical Information Service (NTIS). Second, the NCHS publishes a variety of reports that provide population distributions as well as background and technical information for analysis of the data. A list of these documents that are available through the U.S. Government Printing Office may be obtained from the Scientific and Technical Information Branch at the NCHS. Third, the data appear in articles in scientific and medical journals and in chapters of books. The NCHS encourages authors to use the appropriate survey acronym in the title and abstract of journal articles so that others may more easily find these anthropometric data analyses through automated retrieval systems.

ANALYTICAL CONSIDERATIONS

The HANES, like all surveys, is subject to various types of biases and errors. A concerted effort has been made to eliminate or reduce the effects of these biases and errors through standardization of methodological approaches and the implementation of numerous quality control procedures (NCHS, 1981; NCHS, 1985). However, despite these procedures, problems do arise, and the data need to be carefully analyzed to identify sources of error that might affect the interpretation of the data.

Two possible sources of bias in survey data are nonresponse bias and measurement bias. If the sample persons who did not participate in the survey are different from those who did participate, the results of the survey will not truly represent the population being studied. There are many sources of nonresponse in a survey such as the HANES, and researchers need to evaluate the potential for nonresponse bias before proceeding with any analysis of the data. In addition, the possibility of measurement bias must be considered. If some systematic change in procedure or methodology occurs, the impact on analysis and interpretation of the data can be considerable. This type of evaluation is especially important when comparing results from different surveys or the same survey at different points in time.

The HANES surveys are subject to an additional analytic consideration because of the nature of their design. Since these are large, complex, sample surveys, the analysis of the data is not a straightforward task, and the use of common statistical software packages that assume simple random sampling is usually not appropriate.

Each person in the sample represents a large number of people in the U.S. population. If each sample person represented the same number of people in the population, the data could be used without weights to study relationships. Because they do not, the sample weights, which incorporate the selection probabilities, a nonresponse adjustment, and poststratification, must be used to produce correct population estimates (NCHS, 1982; NCHS, 1985; Yetley and Johnson, 1987).

The clustering that is done in the complex sample survey design often produces variance estimates that are larger than would have been obtained if the survey had been based on a simple random sample. These variances become important when confidence intervals are computed and when testing for statistical significance. There are some computer software programs available that will compute complex sample variances, although they may not be readily available or familiar to data users (NCHS, 1982). An alternative approach is to adjust the results obtained based on the assumption of simple random sampling through the use of "design effects" (Kovar and Johnson, 1987). The *design effect* is defined as the variance from the complex sample divided by the variance of a simple random sample of the same size. If the design effect is near unity, the complex sample design has little effect on the variances, and one could consider assuming simple random sampling for the analysis. More detailed discussions on the appropriate analysis of the HANES data have been published (NCHS, 1982; Kovar and Johnson, 1987; NCHS, 1987a).

In any analysis of anthropometric data, including that of the HANES, the choice of criterion or "cutoff" values is critical to the interpretation of the findings. They should be selected with a survey's design and methodologies as well as the researcher's study objectives in mind. A recent report has discussed the limitations of cutoff points in assessing nutritional and health status (USDHHS and USDA, 1986).

The above analytical considerations have been presented relative to the HANES surveys. However, any survey, whether national, regional, state, or clinical in scope, is subject to most of the same issues. The correct use of anthropometric data from national nutritional surveys can tremendously increase our scientific knowledge. Inappropriate use of the data, whether intentional or unintentional, is a major concern. Responsible and informed use of these national data by all users, especially scientific researchers, is the ultimate objective.

REFERENCES

Bjorntorp P (1987): Classification of obese patients and complications related to the distribution of surplus fat. Am J Clin Nutr 45:1120–1125.

Blair D, Habicht JP, Sims EA, Sylvester D, Abraham S (1984): Evidence for an increased risk for hypertension with centrally located body fat and the effect of race and sex on this risk. Am J Epidemiol 119:526–540.

Centers for Disease Control (1985): Nutrition Surveillance 1983, issued August 1985. DHHS Publ. No. (CDC) 85-8295.
Centers for Disease Control (1987): Nutritional status of minority children—United States, 1986. Morbidity and Mortality Weekly Report 36:366–369.
Chumlea WC (1986): Clinical methods of assessing obesity in children. Perspect Lipid Disord 3:14–19.
Chumlea WC, Roche AF, Steinbaugh ML (1985): Estimating stature from knee height for persons 60 to 90 years of age. J Am Geriatr Soc 33:116–120.
Cronk CE, Roche AF (1982): Race- and sex-specific reference data for triceps and subscapular skinfolds and weight/stature. Am J Clin Nutr 35:347–354.
Davidson S, Passmore R, Brock JF, Truswell AS (1979): "Human Nutrition and Dietetics." New York: Churchill Livingstone.
Durnin JV, Womersley J (1974): Body fat assessed from total body density and its estimation from skinfold thickness: Measurements on 481 men and women aged from 16 to 72 years. Br J Nutr 32:77–97.
Fanelli MT, Kuczmarski RJ (1984): Ultrasound as an approach to assessing body composition. Am J Clin Nutr 39:703–709.
Fanelli MT, Kuczmarski RJ (1988): Estimation of body fat from ultrasound measures of subcutaneous fat and circumferences in obese women. Int J Obes 12:125–132.
Forman MR, Trowbridge FL, Gentry EM, Marks JS, Hogelin GC (1986): Overweight adults in the United States: The behavioral risk factor surveys. Am J Clin Nutr 44:410–416.
Frisancho AR, Flegal PN (1982): Advanced maturation associated with centripetal fat pattern. Hum Biol 54:717–727.
Garn SM, Pesick SD, Hawthorne VM (1983): The bony chest breadth as a frame size standard in nutritional assessment. Am J Clin Nutr 37:315–318.
Gillum Rf (1987): The association of the ratio of waist to hip girth with blood pressure, serum cholesterol, and serum uric acid in children and youths aged 6–17 years. J Chron Dis 40:413–420.
Hamill PV, Drizd TA, Johnson CL, Reed RB, Roche AF, Moore WM (1979): Physical growth: National Center for Health Statistics percentiles. Am J Clin Nutr 32:607–629.
Himes JH, Bouchard C (1985): Do the new Metropolitan Life Insurance weight–height tables correctly assess body frame and body fat relationships. Am J Public Health 75:1076–1079.
Katch VL, Freedson PS (1982): Body size and shape: Derivation of the "HAT" frame size model. Am J Clin Nutr 36:669–675.
Katch VL, Freedson PS, Katch FI, Smith L (1982): Body frame size: Validity of self-appraisal. Am J Clin Nutr 36:676–679.
Knapp TR (1983): A methodological critique of the "ideal weight" concept. JAMA 250:506–510.
Kovar MG, Johnson C (1987): Design effects from the Mexican portion of the Hispanic Health and Nutrition Examination Survey: A strategy for analysts. 1986 Proceedings of the Section on Survey Research of the American Statistical Association 1987. Alexandria, Va: Statistical Association.
Kushner RF, Schoeller DA (1986): Estimation of total body water by bioelectrical impedance analysis. Am J Clin Nutr 44:417–424.
Lukaski HC, Bolonchuk WW, Hall CB, Siders WA (1986): Validation of tetrapolar bioelectrical impedance method to assess human body composition. J Appl Physiol 60:1327–1332.

Lukaski HC, Johnson PE, Bolonchuk WW, Lykken GI (1985): Assessment of fat-free mass using bioelectrical impedance measurements of the human body. Am J Clin Nutr 41:810–817.

Moore WM, Roche AF (1982): "Pediatric Anthropometry." Columbus, Ohio: Ross Laboratories.

Muncie HL, Sobal J, Hoopes JM, Tenney JH, Warren JW (1987): A practical method of estimating stature of bedridden female nursing home patients. J Am Geriatr Soc 35:285–289.

National Center for Health Statistics, Miller HW (NCHS) (Feb. 1973): Plan and operation of the Health and Nutrition Examination Survey, United States, 1971–73. Vital and Health Statistics Ser. 1, No. 10a—Development, Plan, and Operation. DHEW Publ. No. (PHS) 79-1310. U.S. Public Health Service. Washington, DC: GPO.

National Center for Health Statistics (NCHS) (Jan. 1977): Plan and operation of the Health and Nutrition Examination Survey. Vital and Health Statistics Ser. 1, No. 10b—Data Collection Forms of the Survey. DHEW Publ. No. (HRA) 77-1310. U.S. Public Health Service. Washington, DC: GPO.

National Center for Health Statistics, McDowell A, Engel A, Massey JT, Maurer K (NCHS) (July 1981): Plan and operation of the Second National Health and Nutrition Examination Survey, 1976–80. Vital and Health Statistics Ser. 1, No. 15. DHHS Publ. No. (PHS) 81-1317. U.S. Public Health Service. Washington, DC: GPO.

National Center for Health Statistics, Landis J, Lepkowski J, Eklund S, Stehouwer S (NCHS) (Sept. 1982): A statistical methodology for analyzing data from a complex survey, the first National Health and Nutrition Examination Survey. Vital and Health Statistics. Ser. 2, No. 92. DHHS Publ. No. 82-1366. U.S. Public Health Service. Washington, DC: GPO.

National Center for Health Statistics, (NCHS) Abraham S (Jan. 1983): Obese and overweight adults in the United States. Vital and Health Statistics. Ser. 11, No. 230. DHHS Publ. No. 83-1680. U.S. Public Health Service. Washington, DC: GPO.

National Center for Health Statistics (NCHS) (Sept. 1985): Plan and operation of the Hispanic Health and Nutrition Examination Survey, 1982–84. Vital and Health Statistics Ser. 1, No. 19. DHHS Publ. No. (PHS) 85-1321. U.S. Public Health Service. Washington, DC: GPO.

National Center for Health Statistics, Najjar MF, Rowland M (NCHS) (Oct. 1987a): Anthropometric reference data and prevalence of overweight, United States, 1976–80. Vital and Health Statistics. Ser. 11, No. 238. DHHS Publ. No. (PHS) 87-1688. U.S. Public Health Service. Washington, DC: GPO.

National Center for Health Statistics, Hadden WC, Harris MI (NCHS) (Feb. 1987b): Prevalence of diagnosed diabetes, undiagnosed diabetes, and impaired glucose tolerance in adults 20–74 years of age, United States, 1976–80. Vital and Health Statistics Ser. 11, No. 237. DHHS Pub. No. (PHS) 87-1687. U.S. Public Health Service. Washington, DC: GPO.

Nellhaus G (1968): Head circumference from birth to eighteen years: Practical composite international and interracial graphs. Pediatrics 41:106–114.

Norgan NG, Ferro-Luzzi A (1985): The estimation of body density in men: Are general equations general? Ann Hum Biol 12:1–15.

Ohlson LO, Larsson B, Svardsudd K, Welin L, Eriksson H, Wilhelmsen L, Bjorntorp P, Tibblin G (1985): The influence of body fat distribution on the incidence of diabetes mellitus. Diabetes 34:1055–1058.

Pasco Ja, Rutishauser HE (1985): Body fat estimated from anthropometric and electrical impedance measurements. Hum Nutr: Clin Nutr 39c:365–369.
Pirie P, Jacobs D, Jeffery R, Hannan P (1981): Distortion in self-reported height and weight data. J Am Diet Assoc 78:601–606.
Roche AF, Mukherjee D, Guo S, Moore WM (1987): Head circumference reference data: Birth to 18 years. Pediatrics 79:706–712.
Rosenberg IH, Sitrin MD (1983): The role of body weight in nutritional evaluation. Clin Consultations 3:1–2.
Stallones L, Mueller WH, Christensen BL (1982): Blood pressure, fatness, and fat patterning among USA adolescents from two ethnic groups. Hypertension 4:483–486.
Stanton JL, Braitman LE, Riley AM, Khoo CS, Smith JL (1982): Demographic, dietary, life style, and anthropometric correlates of blood pressure. Hypertension 4(suppl 3):135–142.
Stewart AW, Jackson RT, Ford MA, Beaglehole R (1987): Underestimation of relative weight by use of self-reported height and weight. Am J Epidemiol 125:122–126.
Trowbridge FL, Marks JS, deRoma GL, Madrid S, Boutton TW, Klein PD (1987): Body composition of Peruvian children with short stature and high weight-for-height, II: Implications for the interpretation for weight-for-height as an indicator of nutritional status. Am J Clin Nutr 46:411–418.
U.S. Department of Health and Human Services and U.S. Department of Agriculture (USDHHS and USDA) (July 1986): Nutrition monitoring in the United States—A report from the Joint Nutrition Monitoring Evaluation Committee. DHHS Publ. No. (PHS) 85-1255. U.S. Public Health Service. Washington, DC: GPO.
U.S. Department of Health and Human Services (USDHHS) (1987): Nutritional status of minority children—United States, 1986. Morbidity and Mortality Weekly Report. HHS Publ. No. (CDC) 87-8017. 36:366–369.
Van Gaal L, Rillaerts E, Creten W, De Leeuw I (1988): Relationship of body fat distribution pattern to atherogenic risk factors in NIDDM. Diabetes Care 11:103–106.
van Itallie, TB (1985): Health implications of overweight and obesity in the United States. Ann Intern Med 103:983–988.
Woteki CE, Briefel RR, Kuczmarski R (1988): Contributions of the National Center for Health Statistics. Am J Clin Nutr 47:320–328.
Wright RA, Heymsfield S, McManus CB (eds) (1984): Nutritional assessment. St. Louis: Blackwell Scientific.
Yetley E, Johnson C (1987): Nutritional applications of the health and nutrition examination surveys (HANES). Annu Rev Nutr 7:441–463.

Anthropometric Assessment
of Nutritional Status, pages 337–346

20
Choosing Appropriate Reference Data for the Anthropometric Assessment of Nutritional Status

FRANCIS E. JOHNSTON AND ZHEN OUYANG
Department of Anthropology, University of Pennsylvania, Philadelphia, Pennsylvania 19104-6398 (F.E.J); School of Public Health, Harbin Medical University, Harbin, People's Republic of China (Z.O.)

INTRODUCTION

The basis of any evaluation is comparison. Without some criterion against which observations may be compared, there is no foundation for any judgment of adequacy or success. And, unless the criterion employed is grounded both on a sound theoretical premise and a solid empirical base, there will be no sense of either reliability or validity, whatever conclusions are reached. For these reasons, the anthropometric assessment of nutritional status will be no better than the criterion selected for comparison.

The criteria utilized in assessing nutritional status are frequently called "standards," or "reference standards." If we accept the Webster's dictionary definition of a *standard* as something established as a rule or basis of comparison, then the term is a simple and useful. However, for reasons discussed below, the word has all too often been used to indicate a norm for attainment and, as a result, many workers in the area prefer to refer to the comparative criterion simply as "reference data."

There is no shortage of descriptive data which have been proposed for reference use in nutritional evaluation. As a result, the problem becomes, not finding data, but sifting through the available mass to find those that fit the criterion of appropriateness:

1. Anthropometric reference data must be based on a sound theoretical base.
2. Anthropometric reference data must be based on an adequate empirical set of observations.
3. Anthropometric reference data must be valid for the specific purpose of the evaluation being conducted.

In this chapter, these issues will be discussed within the context of the anthropometric evaluation of nutritional status.

REFERENCE DATA AND THE CONCEPT OF NORMAL

Reference data serve as criteria against which to compare the measurements either of an individual or of a sample. However, they have been interpreted operationally in two different ways, based upon one's concept of the term "normal." Since not only the interpretation, but also the choice, of reference data will be dictated to a significant degree by our understanding of the term normal, it is necessary to contrast here the two concepts which exist in the minds of anyone making evaluations (see Johnston, 1977, for a more detailed consideration).

There are those who see normal as an ideal, from which any deviation is significant. King (1944) notes that "... normality ... has nothing whatsoever to do with the average ... nor is it related to variations of different individuals from this average." Normal is seen as "that which functions in accordance with its inherent design." At the same time, others argue that, because of the wide range of variability which exists among apparently healthy individuals, the criterion of normal must be seen in a statistical sense, embodied in the idea of an acceptable range of variation. With this approach no single state of nature is seen as normal except the central tendency (Simonson, 1966).

While no one would be likely to disagree with the first concept of normal, virtually all who have used anthropometric data have rejected its application to the evaluation of nutritional status. The determinants of anthropometric variability are many and include genetic and environmental factors, as well as their interaction. As a result, it is improper to hold up as a "gold standard" any population of individuals as a norm of attainment for all others (Goldstein and Tanner, 1980; Cameron, 1986; Johnston, 1986).

Reference data, therefore, are yardsticks, constructed so as to provide us with accurate statistical distributions of anthropometric indicators in a well-defined and well-nourished population. Using appropriate techniques, individuals or populations may be related to those distributions in a precise way, e.g., expressing measurements as percentiles of the reference population. The reference data thus provide a measure of position relative to the reference population. The interpretation of the nutritional significance of that position is another matter altogether and requires information on the relationship between anthropometric variation and nutriture.

The separation of anthropometric reference data from the evaluation of abnormality is an important conceptual step in the assessment of nutritional status. First of all, it recognizes the multiplicity of factors which determine anthropometric dimensions and therefore the complexity of the process of evaluation. Second, it emphasizes the importance of reference data which are reliable statistically and which are relevant to the particular component of nutriture being assessed.

REFERENCE DATA VERSUS DESCRIPTIVE DATA

From the preceding, it is apparent that reference data become the standard for relating a body of anthropometric variables to a more useful framework, one which may then be interpreted within the context of nutriture. The selection of reference data therefore becomes a critical step since, in a very real sense, the raw measurements will be converted into values relative to the reference set. This leads us to consider just what reference data are.

Tanner (1986) distinguishes between standards, reference populations, and samples for population comparison. *Standards* refer to individuals, used either to screen out those individuals suspected of some abnormality or to assess the effects of treatment or other intervention. *Reference populations* are distributions of variables from appropriate populations which are widely accepted as reference data for evaluations at the population level. *Samples for comparison* are sets of sample data taken from the literature, generally close genetically and/or geographically to the group under study, which provide descriptive information on similarity or difference.

Unfortunately, many investigators have promoted data they collect from the samples they study as reference data, i.e., data which can serve in the assessment of the nutritional status of a population. In the same vein, other investigators have uncritically used such samples in their own studies, treating those samples as if they were reference data. This is not to say that comparisons between samples should not be made, for comparison is the basis of scientific investigation. However, it is important to stress that most samples reported in the literature are not appropriate for reference use. Subjects are usually not enrolled with regards to established sampling procedures. For a variety of reasons, often as not legitimate, individuals are enlisted opportunistically, with little consideration of their representativeness in the population under study, and frequently using procedures which introduce a bias into the research. Genetic (or environmental) factors may be distorted by incorporating whole families into a sample or, in the case of longitudinal studies of children, by including the same individual in more than one age group and reporting the data as cross-sectional. Practices such as this result in an overrepresentation and an underrepresentation of particular sources of variation in the sample.

Other strategies may further vitiate the appropriateness of such samples as reference data. Some studies may be undertaken to test rather specific hypotheses and hence employ a correct, but highly constrained, sampling protocol. Many others are carried out on a much smaller scope and do not include a large enough number of subjects to allow the characterization of the distributions of the variables measured. Bias introduced by sampling strategy or sample size are not so important if the focus is upon the mean or the median. However, as is usually the case in nutritional assessment, the investigator is more concerned with the tails of the distribution, and so great care must be taken to ensure the accuracy of the data and hence the representativeness of the sample throughout its range of variation.

None of the above concerns should be seen as criticisms of such studies. On the other hand, they do point specifically to the inappropriateness of the vast majority of data sets available from around the world for use as reference data. They may be highly useful for comparisons, but they should not be employed for the nutritional assessment of populations, for the monitoring of a population over time, nor for the evaluations of individuals.

CHARACTERISTICS OF REFERENCE DATA

Waterlow et al. (1977) presented a minimal set of criteria which must be satisfied in order for anthropometric data to serve as reference data. These criteria, listed in Table 1, speak to three primary concerns for anyone seeking to find appropriate data to use. First, the population should be well nourished. While there will be variability among individuals in the degree to which their nutritional requirements have been satisfied, there must not be a large amount of significant nutritional deficiency or excess. This implies that a sample composed of only the elite members of a population might not be appropriate since intake may exceed requirements.

Second, careful sampling procedures must be followed, and they must be stated explicitly. Each socioeconomic and genetic component should be included in the sample in proportion to its representation in the population. Age/sex groups should be large enough to ensure that the extreme percentiles, at least to the 5th and 95th, can be calculated with sufficient confidence. And each individual should be represented only once in the sample.

Third, the anthropometric data used for reference purposes in nutritional assessment should be presented in a usable way. The extremes of the distribution must be available, especially when the purpose is to evaluate individuals at risk of malnutrition. In addition to percentiles, standard deviations should be published, though care must be exercised in the event of skewed distributions. Finally, since reference distributions are likely to have been smoothed, the techniques used must be available to those who use such data.

The criteria given in Table 1 rule out the overwhelming majority of descriptive data sets for use as reference data. In fact, if followed scrupulously, they may rule out virtually every data set available. For example, the reference data of the U.S. National Center for Health Statistics (NCHS) (Hamill et al., 1977) are widely used throughout the world and recommended by most interna-

TABLE 1. Minimal Criteria for Anthropometric Reference Data in Nutritional Evaluation[a]

1. The population should be well-nourished.
2. Each age/sex group of the sample should contain at least 200 individuals.
3. The sample should be cross-sectional.
4. Sampling procedures should be defined and reproducible.
5. Measuring procedures should be optimal.
6. Measurements should include all variables to be used in nutritional evaluation.
7. Raw data and smoothing procedures should be available.

[a]From Waterlow et al., 1977.

tional bodies as the best currently available. Yet 20%–30% of subjects examined between 6 and 11 years of age were reexamined between 12 and 17.

TYPES OF REFERENCE DATA

There are several issues of significance in the selection of appropriate reference data for nutritional evaluation, even when the criteria of Table 1 have been sufficiently satisfied. These issues revolve primarily around the "type" of reference population which is most useful for specific purposes. This section will be devoted to a consideration of those types with particular reference to the issues involved.

International Versus Local Reference Data

Many investigators have discussed the issue of a single, international reference data set for nutritional evaluation. For example, Johnston (1986) argues for the advisability of a single standard on a number of grounds. First of all, reference data simply provide a criterion against which samples can be compared. Since the meaning of any observed deviation is a separate matter, the issue is primarily one of selection of one or more appropriate populations to provide the reference data. Second, a single reference standard provides international comparability analogous to some unit of measurement, for example, the meter. Third, the criteria of Table 1 are explicit and impose requirements which increase the cost of developing a reference population. The collection of data from a population is one thing, but the development of reference data is a completely different task, and the cost is likely to exceed the resource base available to many countries or regions. Local reference data have their place (see the following section), but an international standard of reference is necessary as a first step in a nutritional evaluation.

In their discussion of assessing the nutritional status of populations, Waterlow et al. (1977) recommend that the reference data from the United States NCHS be adopted as an international standard of reference. This opinion has been widely shared by other groups and bodies charged with developing recommendations on nutritional monitoring and has resulted in the NCHS data as being the most widely employed data in the world for that purpose (e.g., WHO, 1978). Smoothed heights and weights by age and sex are available from the Health Examination Survey (HES) and the Health and Nutritional Examination Survey (HANES) for children (Hamill, 1977) and adults (Abraham et al., 1979). Since these surveys did not include infants, the national data have been supplemented by the inclusion of young subjects from the longitudinal study conducted by the Fels Research Institute in southern Ohio. Although presented in a more obscure publication, percentiles for the triceps and subscapular skinfolds and for upper arm circumference, smoothed by cubic splining, are also available, though only for ages 2 through 18 years (Johnson et al., 1981).

Reference data from HANES I for skinfolds, upper arm circumference, and the upper arm muscle circumference have also been published for children and adults by Frisancho (1981) and Bishop (1981). For assessments of the elderly, combined HANES I and II data have been published by Frisancho (1984) for one-year age groups from 62 through 74 years, though the more extreme percentiles are not always available for the oldest groups. Neither Bishop and his colleagues nor Frisancho employed an algorithm for smoothing the data. However, by using adjustments similar to those employed by the NCHS, Bishop's data represent a true U.S. national probability sample, rather than a large sample of subjects from the United States, as in the case of Frisancho's distributions.

Local Reference Data

A number of investigators have questioned the utility of a single international reference population, arguing that the NCHS data are not applicable to the samples which they are studying. It seems clear that, when environmental factors are adequately controlled, there are significant, though relatively small, differences in stature, and possibly in weight as well (Eveleth, 1986). Garn (1974) has suggested that "appropriate size standards should now be used for boys and girls of largely-African ancestry." A similar point is made by Goldstein and Tanner (1980) when reference data are employed as growth standards in the clinical management of individuals.

Some authors question the validity of nutritional status assessments in local groups using international reference data (Richardson, 1973; Cameron, 1986; Van Loon et al., 1986). Walker and Richardson (1973) suggest that, while international standards are of "great value," it is inappropriate to "stigmatize" that proportion of a local population, perhaps from a disadvantaged economic section, that does not attain the standard.

Two central and related positions underlie this controversy. The first assumes that an international reference population such as the NCHS data, from an economically privileged nation, overestimates the prevalence of undernutrition in third world groups (e.g., Cameron, 1986). Or, at the least, there are significant differences between the local group and the international reference population that cannot be explained solely by nutritional factors (e.g., Johnston et al., 1984). The second assumption holds that local reference data from third world countries cannot be used with confidence because of the high proportion of undernourished individuals who would be included in the sample.

The majority of investigators take an intermediate position. An international reference population is important in providing maximum comparison and evaluation across a wide range of groups. However, local standards may also be utilized for more specific purposes within countries, ethnic groups, or ecological zones, *providing* these standards are derived following, as closely as possible, the guidelines presented in Table 1.

While there are countless studies of body size and composition of samples from around the world, only a small percentage of them are appropriate for use as reference data, and virtually all of these focus on children rather than adults, especially the elderly. Some notable exceptions are the large surveys of children in the United Kingdom (Rona and Altman, 1977), Cuba (Jordan, 1979), the Netherlands (van Wieringen, 1986), and India (Indian Council of Medical Research, 1972).

Reference Standards for Clinical Use: Cross-Sectional and Incremental

Tanner differentiates reference population data, used in evaluating and monitoring groups, from growth standards, used for screening individuals at risk or for managing patients clinically (Tanner, 1980, 1986; Tanner et al., 1970). In the latter case, the purpose is more specific, and longitudinal data are frequently desirable in order to permit the development of increments or velocities for the growth of children.

The two data sets most widely used for this purpose are from the Institute of Child Health, London, and the Fels Research Institute, Yellow Springs, Ohio. The British data (Tanner et al., 1966) are used throughout the world to follow the growth of individuals and to assess the response to treatment. They provide smoothed percentiles for height and weight and for velocity of growth, adjusted for use both with populations and individuals.

The Fels Longitudinal Study is a long-term, in-depth examination of individuals from southwestern Ohio. From this base, Roche and Himes (1980) and Baumgartner et al. (1986) have published sex-specific percentiles of increments over 6-month intervals, adjusted for chronological age at examination; diurnal, secular, and seasonal effects; and familial relationships.

Conditional Reference Data

The reference data discussed so far are specific only in terms of age, sex, and, in the case of local reference populations, geography. However, other limitations may be necessary in the case of more focused nutritional assessment; i.e., other characteristics must be taken into account. Tanner (1986) refers to these more limited reference data as conditional standards.

A number of conditional reference standards have been proposed though, for obvious reasons, they cannot conform to all of the criteria of Table 1. For example, in the assessment of the nutritional status of children, it may be desirable to control for the height of the parents. Tanner et al. (1970) have provided reference standards for children from 2 to 9 years of age. "Parent specific" reference data for U.S. children from birth to 18 years of age have been published by Himes et al. (1985).

Frame size has been seen as an important factor in the assessment of nutritional status, especially in the case of overnutrition and obesity. Most famous are the Metropolitan weight tables (Metropolitan Life Insurance Company, 1983), though they employ a subjective assessment of frame size. Frisancho (1984) has provided reference data from HANES I and II for the assessment of weight, skinfolds, and arm circumference in adults and the elderly, controlling for frame size by measuring the biepicondylar breadth of the elbow.

Of increasing importance has been the development of reference standards for the assessment of nutritional and health status in conjunction with pregnancy. Such assessments involve not only the assessment of the adequacy of weight gain, but also of the newborn infant, who may be at risk of intrauterine growth retardation. Recent reference data against which to assess maternal weight gain have been published by Rosso (1988), while data for the evaluation of size at birth are available from Blidner et al. (1984), Brenner et al. (1976), or Lubchenco (1963).

Secular Change

The term "secular change" refers to the modification of the patterns of growth, maturation, and morphology which a population undergoes through time (van Weieringen, 1986). This modification may be seen, e.g., in an increase in the rate of maturation, or as a greater stature or weight at a given age than was the case in the same population at some time in the past. Populations are not static units but themselves are changing dynamically across time. These changes reflect concomitant change in nutrition, in the level of health care, or in the general environment and have been widely studied in Western and non-Western populations by many investigators. (Apparent change may also result from migration, as a population gradually becomes admixed with, or even replaced by, another.)

The choice of an appropriate reference population in nutritional assessment is conditioned by the existence of a secular trend. Because of the logistics involved, current reference standards are almost always constructed from data collected some time in the past. For example, the NCHS reference data were collected in the 1960s and 1970s and the British standards of Tanner even earlier. If there have been secular changes in the population, a reference population, or any extant data set used as a local standard, might not provide a meaningful comparison for assessment. For example, Cuban teenagers attending an academically select school display significantly greater median skinfold thicknesses than are found in the Cuban reference standards (Suarez and Argülles, 1986). It is unclear whether this means greater tendency towards obesity among the study sample, or a secular trend in a rapidly modernizing country. The interpretation of the differences is important for nutritional monitoring and the implementation of public health programs.

This problem is complicated further by the fact that secular trends are certainly not always rectilinear, nor are they necessarily positive (Roche, 1979). Since, for the most part, such trends are responses to environmental changes, both quantitative and qualitative aspects of those changes will affect the existence and magnitude of secular change.

CONCLUSIONS

The selection of appropriate reference data in the anthropometric assessment of nutritional status is crucial and involves a clear understanding of many determinants of the selection process. Investigators must have a clear idea of whether they need a true reference standard, an international reference population, or local reference data. They must be sensitive to the necessity of controlling for additional factors, leading to the search for appropriate conditional standards. Most important, any potential data set must itself be evaluated as a valid reference standard. This requires the consideration of the criteria set forth in Table 1, as well as the imposition of additional ones, depending upon the specificity of the assessment being carried out. There are many descriptions of anthropometric variation in populations, but only a few of these can be considered as appropriate for reference data.

REFERENCES

Abraham S, Johnson CL, Najjar MF (1979): Weight by height and age for adults 18–74 years, United States, 1971–1974. DHEW Pub (PHS) 79–1656. Hyattsville, Md: National Center for Health Statistic.

Baumgartner RN, Roche AF, Himes JH (1986): Incremental growth tables: Supplementary to previously published charts. Am J Clin Nutr 43:711–722.

Bishop CW, Bowen PE, Ritchey SJ (1981): Norms for nutritional assessment of American adults by upper arm anthropometry. Am J Clin Nutr 34:2530–2539.

Blidner IN, McClemont S, Anderson GD, Sinclair JC (1984): Size-at-birth standards for an urban Canadian population. Can Med Assoc J 130:133–140.

Brenner WE, Edelman DA, Hendricks CH (1976) A standard of fetal growth for the United States of America. Am J Obstet Gynecol 126:555–564.

Cameron N (1986): Standards for human growth: Their construction and use. S Afr Med J 70:422–425.

Eveleth PB (1986): Population differences in growth. In Falkner F, Tanner JM (eds): "Human Growth, Vol 3," 2nd ed New York: Plenum Press, pp 221–239.

Frisancho AR (1981): New norma of upper limb fat and muscle areas for assessment of nutritional status. Am J Clin Nutr 34:2540–2545.

Frisancho AR (1984): New standards of weight and body composition by frame size and height for assessment of nutritional status of adults and the elderly. Am J Clin Nutr 40:808–819.

Garn SM (1974): The question of race differences in stature norms. Ecol Food Nutr 3:319–320.

Goldstein H, Tanner JM (1980): Ecological considerations in the creation and the use of child growth standards. Lancet 1:582–585.

Hamill PVV, Drizd T, Johnson CL, Reed RB, Roche AF (1977): "NCHS Growth Curves for Children, Birth–18 Years, United States." DHEW Pub (PHS) 78–1650. Hyattsville, Md: National Center for Health Statistics.

Himes JH, Roche AF, Thissen D, Moore WM (1985): Parent-specific adjustments for evaluation of recumbent length and stature of children. Pediatr 75:304–313.

Indian Council of Medical Research (1972): "Growth and Physical Development of Indian Infants and Children." New Delhi: Medical Enclave.

Johnson CL, Fulwood R, Abraham S, Bryner JD (1981): "Basic Data on Anthropometric Measurements and Angular Measurements of the Hip and Knee Joints For Selected Age Groups 1–74 Years of Age, United States, 1971–1975." DHHS Pub (PHS) 81–1669. Hyattsville Md: National Center for Health Statistics.

Johnston FE (1977): The problem of normative values in the evaluation of the biological state of human individuals and populations. In Wolanski N (ed): "Metody Kontroli Rozwoju Człowieka i Zmian Struktury Populacji Ludzkich." Warsaw: Ossolineum, pp 341–357.

Johnston FE (1986): Reference data for physical growth in nutritional anthropology.

In Quandt SA, Ritenbaugh C (eds): "Training Manual in Nutritional Anthropology." Washington, DC: Am Anthropol Assoc, pp 60–65.
Johnston FE, Bogin B, MacVean RB, Newman BC (1984): A comparison of international standards versus local reference data for the triceps and subscapular skinfolds of Guatemalan children and youth. Hum Biol 56:157–171.
Jordan J (1979): "Desarollo Humana en Cuba." La Habana: Editorial Scientifico-Técnica.
King CD (1944): The meaning of normal. Yale J Biol Med 17:493–501.
Lubchenco LO, Hansman C, Dressler M, Boyd E (1963): Intrauterine growth as estimated from liveborn birthweight data at 24 to 42 weeks of gestation. Pediatrics 32:793–800.
Metropolitan Life Insurance Company (1983): Metropolitan height and weight tables. Stat Bull 64:1–9.
Richardson BD (1973): Growth standards: An appraisal with special reference to growth in South African Bantu and white pre-school children. S Afr Med J 47:699–702.
Roche AF (ed) (1979): "Secular Trends in Human Growth, Maturation, and Development." Monogn Soc Res Child Dev, Vol. 44, Nos 3–4, ser 179.
Roche AF, Himes JH (1980): Incremental growth charts. Am J Clin Nutr 33:2041–2052.
Rona RJ, Altman DG (1977): National study of health and growth: Standards of attained height, weight, and triceps skinfold in English children 5 to 11 years old. Ann Hum Biol 4:501–523.
Rosso P (1988): A new chart to monitor weight gain during pregnancy. Am J Clin Nutr 41:644–652.
Simonson E (1966): The concept and definition of normality. Ann NY Acad Sci 134:541–558.
Suarez A, Argülles JM (1986): Nutritional evaluation of adolescents: Usefulness of anthropometric indicators in the diagnosis of obesity. Acta Paediatr Hung 27:303–310.
Tanner JM (1980): Growth as a monitor of nutritional status. Proc Nutr Soc:35:315–322.
Tanner JM (1986): Use and abuse of growth standards. In Falkner F, Tanner JM (eds): "Human Growth, Vol 3." New York: Plenum Press, pp 95–109.
Tanner JM, Goldstein H, Whitehouse RH (1970): Standards for children's height at ages 2 to 9 years, allowing for height of parents. Arch Dis Child 41:755–762.
Tanner JM, Whitehouse RH, Takaishi M (1966): Standards from birth to maturity for height, weight, height velocity, and weight velocity: British children, 1965. Arch Dis Child 41:454–471;613–635.
Van Loon H, Saverys V, Vuylsteke JP, Vlietinck RF, Eeckels R (1986): Local versus universal growth standards: The effect of using NCHS as universal reference. Ann Hum Biol 13:347–357.
van Wieringen JC (1971): "Growth Diagrams, 1965, Netherlands." Groningen: Wolters-Noordhoof.
van Wieringen JC (1986): Secular growth changes. In Falkner F, Tanner JM (eds): "Human Growth, Vol 3." 2nd ed. New York: Plenum Press, pp 307–331.
Walker ARP, Richardson BD (1973): International and local growth standards. Am J Clin Nutr 26:897–900.
Waterlow JC, Buzina A, Keller W, Lane JM, Nichaman MZ, Tanner JM (1977): The presentation and use of height and weight data for comparing the nutritional status of groups of children under the age of 10 years. Bull WHO 55:489–498.
World Health Organization (1978): A growth chart for international use in maternal and child care: Guidelines for primary health care personnel. Geneva: WHO.

Anthropometric Assessment
of Nutritional Status, pages 347–364

21
Measurement Issues Related to the Anthropometric Assessment of Nutritional Status

NOEL CAMERON
Department of Anatomy, Medical School, University of the Witwatersrand, Johannesburg 2193, South Africa

This chapter seeks to discuss some of the issues related to the measurement of nutritional status using anthropometry. The reader will note that many of the comments relate to developing countries and the problems in carrying out nutritional assessments in those environments. For this I make no apologies; nutritional assessment assumes major importance specifically in those countries, and those of us who, by choice, have decided to practice our skills with disadvantaged populations are faced with these issues on a daily basis. Thus these issues should not only be judged on a theoretical basis but on their practical importance in the assessment of nutritional status.

Anthropometry, in an historical context, represented a descriptive aspect of natural science involving body measurement, classification, and correlation. Washburn (1951, 1953) described a new "strategy" for physical anthropology moving from purely descriptive research to a functional, problem-oriented approach (Johnston and Lampl, 1984). This functional approach lies at the core of nutritional anthropometry, in which measurements of the body are used not only to describe a particular degree of over nutrition, or, more commonly, undernutrition but are also used for diagnostic purposes and as a means of monitoring change in the body due to treatment. Because of this alteration in the practical use of anthropometry, it is not surprising that some confusion exists as to the uses of nutritional anthropometry. In 1953 Josef Brozek stated that "the anthropologist," using anthropometry, "is concerned with the degree of under and over-nutrition, *not* with the diagnosis of malnutrition." One central issue thus facing nutritional anthropometry is whether anthropometry describes or diagnoses. For instance, can the anthropometric description of a child below an agreed cutoff point for weight for age be diagnostic and thus imply a functional association between the external dimension and the internal milieu, or is the anthropometric description simply an indicator that functional tests are required? This issue is not merely a theoretical one. In the majority of developing countries, where undernutrition is common, anthropometric measurements indicating that a child is below agreed cutoff points trigger refeeding programmes. Conversely, in a developed country, low weight for age would indicate the need for exhaustive biochemical tests of function. Practically then, description and diagnosis are dependent on the scenario in which anthropometry is used and the purpose for which it is used. If we are to understand the use of anthropometry to assess nutritional status and thus some of the measurement issues involved in that use, we must be absolutely clear about the concept of "nutritional status."

Jelliffe and Gurney (1974) called nutritional status an "abstract concept," an "expression of nutriture in a specific variable," such as weight or height. The term *nutriture* was used by Brozek (1953) in his landmark monograph, *Measuring Nutriture,* simply as an alternative to the phrase *nutritional status,* but it has been more specifically defined by McLaren (1976) as the result of the balance between the intake and expenditure of energy and nutrients by an organism. More recently Johnston and Lampl (1984) state that the "task of anthropometry is to provide indicators of nutritional status (nutriture)." *Nutriture* and *nutritional status* are thus used interchangeably in the literature, although they have essentially different meanings; *nutriture* is a functional concept involving the dynamic process of "intake" and "expenditure," whereas *nutritional status* is a description of the physical result, i.e., status, of nutriture. But we must be aware that the anthropometric assessment of nutritional status inherently involves other aspects of *physical* status. For instance, particular external dimensions, e.g., weight for age or height for age, may be used to denote the nutritional status of a child reflecting a particular nutriture. If those dimensions are to change, should we assume the nutriture has also changed, i.e., that the function we are trying to monitor has changed? There are obvious situations in which that is not so; when a child grows its external dimensions change at varying rates. During the takeoff phase of preadolescent growth the rate of change slows to, at times, imperceptible levels, and yet the functional basis of those dimensions, i.e., the nutriture, is not necessarily at risk. In this case the external dimensions are reflecting a normal growth process, controlled perhaps by a critical point of gene expression, and are not necessarily reflecting a change as a result of an alteration in nutriture. Tanner (1976) also recognised that nutritional status, as reflected by anthropometric measurement, did not always imply a threat to adequate nutriture: " ... There is good evidence that the heights of children at given ages, including adulthood, reflect, in most countries, something we may call nutritional status ... But we have to remember that the whole concept of nutrition is an abstraction from a much more complex reality, which includes parasites, maternal behavior, the distribution of family income, the energy cost of older siblings, even the happiness and security of the child." We are, therefore, not discussing simply nutrition, but "microecology," and not the monitoring of nutritional status, but of health itself (Tanner, 1976). Thus anthropometry, when used to assess nutritional status, is actually assessing the total health of the child and should be seen as part of a complex of tests carried out to investigate that phenomenon. Monitoring the total health of the child involves monitoring not just nutriture, i.e., intake and expenditure, but also the variety of factors, some of which Tanner (1976) outlined, that affect that health. It is obvious that anthropometry cannot monitor all these things but only those that find physical expression. It cannot, for instance, monitor the degree of psychological deprivation that an abused child is subjected to, but, because adverse psychological stress affects the child's growth rate, anthropometry can monitor the effect of the stress on the growth rate. In addition anthropometry can monitor the effect of the alleviation of the stress when that child's environment is altered. Thus we have to be clear about the limitations of anthropometry. If anthropometry is limited by its inability to directly monitor functional changes within the child, what is the rationale for its use to grade the effect of nutriture in the current context?

Johnston and Lampl (1984) identify two assumptions underlying the concept of nutritional anthropometry which, they suggest, provide the rationale for its use. The first assumption is that the growth of an individual is an appropriate indicator of adequacy of essential nutrients. It is, of course, not necessary to argue that a child slows down in growth if for any reason he becomes undernourished. Evidence of this has been provided by a multitude of studies in both man and animals. The point should be made here, however, that when we talk of growth "slowing down," we are implying that the rate of growth changes. To monitor this rate it is necessary to perform serial measurements which, certainly in the context of the third or developing world, are simply not done because of logistical problems and often the need for immediate intervention. The second assumption involves body composition. It is assumed that there is a normal range of variation in the relationship between the fat and the lean components of body mass, reflecting a normal intake of nutrients. Deficiencies or excesses in nutrient intake, relative to needs, will be associated with deviations in body composition from the norm. Anthropometric techniques for assessing body composition may then be used to evaluate the adequacy of body stores.

At this point it is necessary to be more definite about the *subject* of nutritional assessment. It seems reasonable, because it is the most common situation, to take the child in a developing country as the subject of our assessment. This subject is highly unlikely to be suffering from an overabundance of food. Indeed, the usual situation is for our subject to experience a chronically poor nutritional environment allowing him or her to live on the borderline between "adequate" and "less-than-adequate" nutritional levels. "Adequate" is not meant to imply "good" in the conventional sense, but rather a nutritional level just above "less-than-adequate." It is the nutritional level that those working in developing countries associate with children living in rural environments. In this situation there is usually no regular income to provide additions to the diet, the families' food supply may not be divided so that the children are favoured, and the source of food is primarily that which is grown using inadequate techniques on perhaps inadequate soil. The borderline between adequate and less-than-adequate may be crossed and recrossed several times each year as a result of fluctuations in food supply due to climatic conditions, economic conditions, and, particularly in the young child, fluctuations in the child's ability to eat as a result of infection and infestation. The majority of such children are able to stay on the adequate side of the borderline, but the minority—about 30% of children in developing countries according to weight-for-age data (Bengoa, 1970)—fall to the less-than-adequate side.

This distinction between adequate and less-than-adequate children is of major importance to the anthropometric assessment of health and nutritional status. In the simplest case the child in a less-than-adequate environment exhibits obvious signs of malnutrition. The child with marasmus or kwashiorkor is easily identifiable to the nutritional field worker, and measurement is used only to confirm the clinical impression, if it is used at all. In this situation measurement issues are of little importance in terms of diagnosis or treatment and may be of no great importance in terms of duration of treatment. The alleviation of clinical signs and symptoms reflects the success of the treatment regime. Measurement issues assume greater importance in the former situation of the child bordering on the adequate side of the nutritional borderline. The reasons for this are numerous and some, because they relate to the financial cost of improving nutritional status, may appear to be callous depending on the scenario in which the child presents.

There is little argument in the literature, or indeed amongst nutritional field workers, that measurements of height and weight are the most important. That is, in the cross-sectional measurement situation, measurements of height and weight, combined if possible with age, provide the necessary information to decide on the adequacy of the child's nutritional status; in other words, the growth of the child as reflected in his or her height and weight is adequate when compared to some accepted norm or standard. It is the acceptance of that norm or standard that is another major measurement issue.

A number of authors have drawn attention to the difficulty created in conceptual thinking by describing a growth chart as a "standard" (Tanner and Goldstein, 1980; Waterlow, 1984; Cameron, 1986). Waterlow (1984) suggests that it is best, "though very difficult," to avoid the use of the word *standard* altogether. He points out that the word has two clear and distinct meanings in the English language, and it is not surprising, therefore, that "reference standard," or simply "standard," is used in both of these ways in the literature and confuses two concepts, that of "normal," or "standard," growth and that of the target growth which one would expect a normal child to achieve. Perhaps the point should be made more clearly: The normal growth to be found in America approximates that of the National Center for Health Statistics (NCHS) charts, and, in this context, these charts represent the *standard* of growth in America. That is to say, they represent the normal pattern of growth *and* the target that one would expect a child to achieve. The same charts used in Africa or India would not reflect the normal, i.e., usual or common, pattern of growth to be found in these areas, but, if all genetic potentials for growth are the same, they would reflect a target to be aimed at. It would be better, because it is conceptually easier for the majority of field workers in this area, if the term *reference data* or *reference chart* was used instead of *standard*, as has been suggested by Waterlow (1984) and Neumann (1979).

Neumann (1979) discusses the meaning of and criteria for reference data in some detail. The major, and as yet unresolved, problem that falls within this discussion of measurement issues concerns the concept that "bigger is best," i.e., that the faster a child grows, the earlier it exhibits adolescent growth, the larger it is as an adult, then the better its chance of survival and thus the better its overall health. Yet a number of authorities argue that this is not so. Neumann (1979) argues that "health-related effects of overgrowth and undergrowth such as mental and neurological development, immunocompetence, and long-term sequelae need further elucidation." Kannel and Dawber (1972) point out that long-term sequelae of large, rapidly growing, early maturing children may be diabetes, obesity, or one in five succumbing to atherosclerosis. Malcolm (1974) found that mortality rate was highest in those toddlers who were growing most rapidly and had, presumably, greater nutritional requirements. Whilst these studies were carried out in developed countries on children with an abundant supply of food, a parallel situation has been documented in children who live in the impoverished nutritional environment of developing countries.

Garrow and Pike (1967) reported that a sample of severely malnourished children in Jamaica grew better than their peers who had not been diagnosed as malnourished following treatment and during long-term follow-up. The only longitudinal, as opposed to follow-up, study to investigate the long-term effects of malnutrition was the study on ex-kwashiorkor patients carried out by Bowie, Moodie, Mann, and Hansen (1980) in Cape Town, South Africa. Their major finding was that ex-patients, when compared to controls, showed no significant difference for weight and height 15 years after the original episode of severe malnutrition. This finding was criticised by Cameron, Jones, Moodie Mitchell, Bowie, Mann, and Hansen (1986) because the analysis had used cross-sectional methods to analyse longitudinal data. For instance, data at each age point had been analysed independently without regard to the fact that the same children may have been present in the age groups either side of the one being analysed. In addition, no allowance had been made for the subjects who had missed examinations within a series and were thus present in some but not all of the age group analyses. Cameron et al. (1986) applied longitudinal curve–fitting techniques to the longitudinal data to arrive at a more sensitive analysis. They looked specifically at the adolescent growth of those children who had been admitted to hospital suffering from kwashiorkor between the ages of 5 months and 4 years 4 months. Following treatment and release from hospital, the children were followed up for a period of 15 years. A "control" group was also followed that consisted of children from the same families, but they were not, in most cases, siblings of the ex-patients. There was no doubt, however, that their nutritional environment was in every way similar to that of the ex-patients, although, because the controls were older than each matched patient, they had perhaps experienced the deprived environment for longer than the ex-patients.

Analysis of the biological landmarks at adolescence revealed that there were no significant differences between mean heights of males or females when the ex-patient and control groups were compared throughout the growth period (Figs. 1, 2). There were some differences in the males in that ex-patients had significantly greater takeoff velocities and significantly smaller peak velocities at adolescence. In terms of weight there were no significant differences between the female groups, but male ex-patients were significantly heavier than the controls at adulthood in addition to having greater takeoff velocities and greater weights at peak velocity. The authors concluded that the findings suggested that "boys who experience this single acute insult may eventually end up heavier, and perhaps taller, than non-affected children from the same geographic and socio-economic circumstances." Females were not affected, in relation to controls, by having experienced kwashiorkor in their early years. In comparison to British reference charts both groups ended up with heights and weights not too dissimilar from the 50th centile as demonstrated in Figures 1 and 2.

Garrow and Pike (1967) interpreted their result by postulating that all children in a family experience a similar nutritional environment but not all have acute malnutrition. Affected children may have a genetic potential for greater height and weight and thus require a greater quantity or quality of food to maintain normal growth velocity and avoid clinical malnutrition. Cameron et al. (1986) extended the explanation by adding that once refed, such children

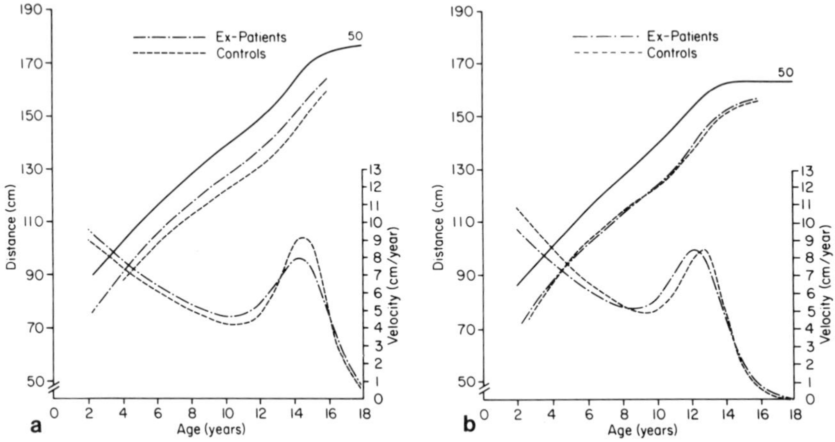

Fig. 1. Mean constant curves for height distance and velocity of male **(a)** and female **(b)** kwashiorkor ex-patients and controls compared to the British 50th centile.

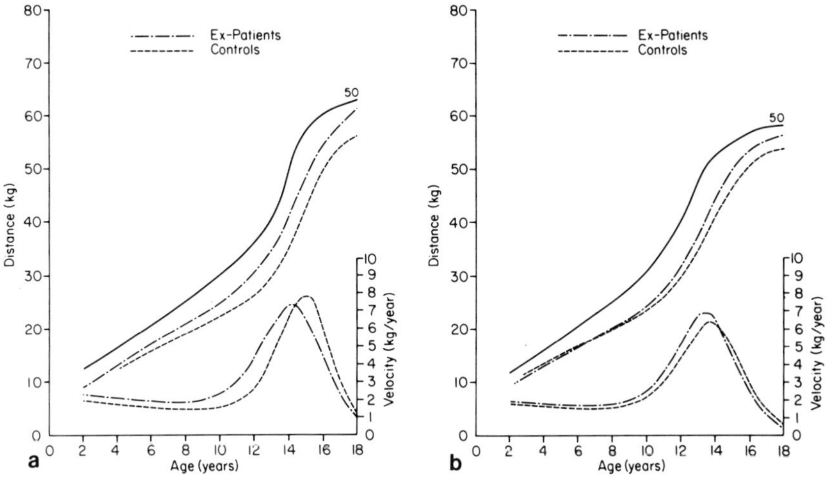

Fig. 2. Mean constant curves for weight distance and velocity of male **(a)** and female **(b)** kwashiorkor ex-patients and controls compared to the British 50th centile.

may catch up and revert to their genetically determined growth channel ending up taller and heavier than their siblings or, at least, demonstrating no long-term effect of their malnutrition. Thus, given the same impoverished nutritional environment, the child within a family that has the genetic potential for greater size will be the one most affected by that environment. A reference chart should not, therefore, necessarily be one incorporating the children who demonstrate the fastest growth velocities with early maturation, because they may be fortuitously blessed with genes for largeness.

The ideal reference data, as defined by the International Union of Nutritional Sciences (IUNS, 1972), is statistically sound but all but impossible to create in developing countries where such data is of immediate use. Neumann (1979), paraphrasing the IUNS, states that the population "must be large, representative, well described and well defined samples of 100 to 200 children per age group. Data must be periodically updated so as to be reasonably contemporary. Measurement techniques must be well described and well executed, with validation of measurement techniques ... knowledge of precise chronological age is preferable to age-independent standards, though these may become essential in lesser developed countries where age is not always known." Although the functional basis of such ideal standards is good in that they must "relate to health status and should indicate the level below which an individual or group is at risk of Protein Calorie Malnutrition (PCM) and an upper level above which an individual is at risk for overnutrition," the logistical basis to achieve such standards is simply not available in these countries because they *are* developing countries without the infrastructure necessary to succeed with these tasks. In short, the nutritional field worker, or indeed the human scientist, who attempts to document the nutritional status of the individual or community in a developing country is constantly faced with less than ideal circumstances within which he has little or no opportunity to exercise "ideal" procedures.

In the absence of surveys which could conform to these ideal criteria, should we be investigating groups of "elite" or "privileged" children and using their growth as a "standard" in developing countries? The objections against this system are, again, numerous. Elite groups may not be racially representative of the total population, although Habicht (1974) has shown that during the first two years of life growth curves of elite children in developing countries are remarkably similar to those from the United States, Scandinavia, Holland, and England. Further evidence has accumulated from India (Neumann et al., 1969); Nigeria (Janes, 1974); Ghana (Neumann et al., 1975); Ethiopia (Eksmyr, 1969); and Malaysia (McKay, 1969). One of the most oft-quoted scenarios to substantiate the equality of genetic potential between African children and those of other racial groups is that American black children demonstrate no significant differences in their height attainment to similar white children (Watson and Lowry, 1975; Wingerd et al., 1971). There is little argument in the historical literature that the majority of American blacks are descendents of slaves. Steckel (1987), in a most eloquent review of the"bio-history" of American slaves, provides evidence that such slaves were highly selected individuals—as they must have been to survive the rigours of the slave trade and remain healthy enough to warrant a good price at the slave markets! Using data from the "coastal slave trade," practiced in America until the latter part of the 19th century, Steckel showed that whilst born with relatively low birth weights and exhibiting poor growth in childhood, slave children demonstrated "remarkable" catch up in the period in which they started labouring. It was at this time that they presumably obtained far better nutrition. The fact remains, however, that the genes for largeness, or at least size equivalence to the 27th and 35th centiles of British growth charts of 1966 (Tanner et al., 1966), must have been present. To put the physical status of this slave population into perspective, Steckel compares the slaves to other contemporary samples. By 16.5 years of age, "American slave males were taller than factory workers and labouring classes in England, the poor of Italy, Habsburg military schools, the middle classes of the Carlschule, German peasants, and factory workers in Russia. As adults the American slave males also exceeded the aristocrats of the Carlschule and the Moscow middle schools, and were only 1.3 cm below the Swedish schools and 2 cm below the non-labouring classes in England. At age 17.5, American slave women exceeded Boston women of American or Irish parents, factory workers in England or Russia, and the upper class in Italy, and were only 2.7 cm below the tallest group (schools in Sweden)." In his concluding remarks Steckel adds, "High infant and child mortality rates may have eliminated individuals who adapted poorly to deprivation and those who remained may have been relatively more efficient at utilizing a given level of nutrition for growth." In addition it could be argued that largeness, which was presumably an advantage to the individual in terms of survival in this environment, must have been positively selected for with a consequent reduction in the prevalence of genes expressing smallness. Thus when the nutritional environment was good enough, these genes were allowed to express themselves. This is not to say, of course, that genes for largeness do not exist in the African continent, simply that those modern-day individuals who form the basis for arguments that *all* blacks have a genetic potential for largeness are, perhaps, not a good sample from which to make this argument because they have been selected by a controlled environment. This argument will, I believe, only be solved when we succeed in carrying out research that documents the normal growth of children from developing countries who have been given the opportunity to live with the advantages of a developed society, in terms of health and nutrition, rather than the barely adequate health and nutrition that they currently experience.

It is terribly important, also, that these studies do not simply concentrate on children under the age of 5 years. Considerable documentation exists that children from almost any country demonstrate roughly the same growth curves in their infant years as long as they are breast-fed. The "acid test" for equality of growth potential is to document growth from post-breast-feeding onwards and particularly to document the heights of young adults. In this context it is extremely important to be sure that these adults are sexually mature and not to delineate them purely on the basis of being older than 18 years. Our own research on rural children in South Africa demonstrates that true adult heights are not reached until the very late teens and early twenties and that adult height, as defined by a height velocity of less then 1 cm per year, may not be achieved until the midtwenties. If then it is not advisable to use American blacks as the norm, and it is impossible to adequately research "elite" or "privileged" children in developing countries, what do we do? I have argued (Cameron, 1986), and continue to argue, that we have to be realistic about what we mean by normal. Normal growth must be that reflected by children who live in a particular environment and demonstrate good health. In the context of a developing country "good health" is usually taken as being freedom from illness or disease as reflected in a normal growth rate, i.e., a growth rate that maintains a child's centile position relative to his peers. The fact that the distance centile resulting from this velocity may be below the NCHS centiles does not, in itself, indicate that the child is unhealthy. It does mean, however, that given the environment within which the child is living, the child is managing to maintain a normal growth rate. That is to say, a growth rate which is not causing it to fall behind its peers. Of major importance is the fact that we do not accept such a growth rate as being equivalent to the target growth which could be achieved given better nutritional and socioeconomic conditions.

Figures 3 and 4 illustrate the mean heights and weights of rural children from two areas of South Africa. Both groups are subjects in longitudinal stud-

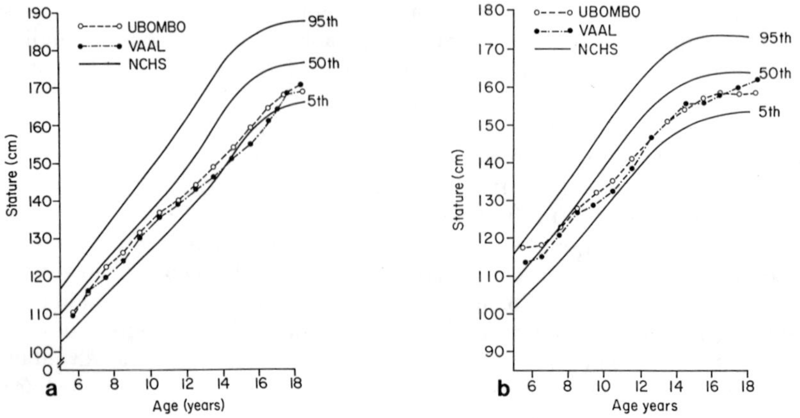

Fig. 3. Mean heights of male **(a)** and female **(b)** black rural children in South Africa compared to the NCHS reference charts. Vaal = Vaalwater sample; Ubombo = Ubombo sample.

ies. The Vaalwater (VW) group are children living and attending school on a farm owned by a paediatrician. This individual runs clinics for his staff and maintains a high level of health care compared to the usual care available to such children. The Ubombo (UB) group are children living in traditional kraals (groups of mud or brick huts) near the Mozambique border. These children

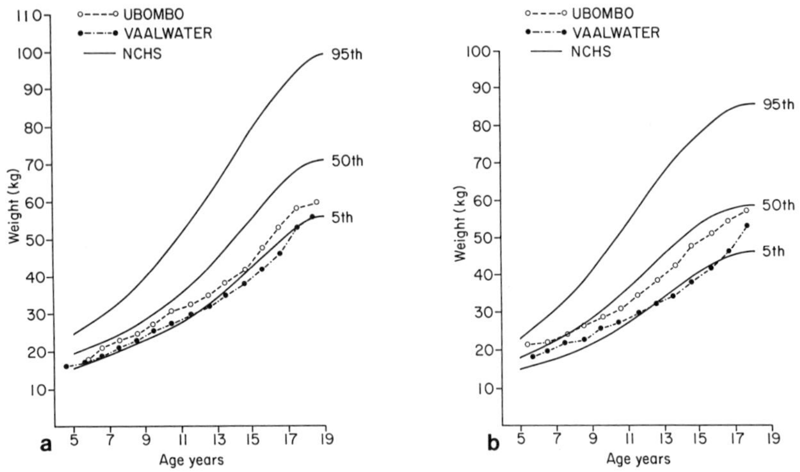

Fig. 4. Mean weights of male **(a)** and female **(b)** black rural children in South Africa compared to the NCHS reference charts. Vaal = Vaalwater sample; Ubombo = Ubombo sample.

fall under the jurisdiction of a primary health care scheme but are not monitored on the same regular basis as the VW sample. Note that the pattern of growth in height is the same for both groups and both sexes. The mean values are close to he 50th centile of NCHS charts at 5–6 years of age and then fall to the 10th centile by the early adolescent years. A relatively late adolescence brings the mean values to within close approximation of the 50th centile by late teenage/early adult ages. This pattern of growth is, I would suggest, common in developing countries and illustrates two important points. Firstly, almost 50% of these subjects were below limits of normality according to international norms at early adolescence. Yet very few of these children were unwell with any overt signs of infection, infestation, or malnutrition.

Figures 5 and 6 of the mean weight for height show the UB and VW samples to be near to the 50th centile. Thus according to criteria for malnutrition based on weight for height, these children are indeed not malnourished.

The issue of which standard of growth to compare one's anthropometric measurements to thus boils down to an awareness of actual genetic potential for growth and, in the absence of such knowledge, the normal or most common growth to be found in the community in which the child lives. It would, of course, be ideal if the growth charts recommended by most authorities—the NCHS charts—did reflect true genetic potential, but we do not, as yet, have that evidence. To work on the basis that genetic potential is equivalent without hard evidence leads to a misappropriation of funding in developing countries that simply cannot afford such misappropriation. Money that could

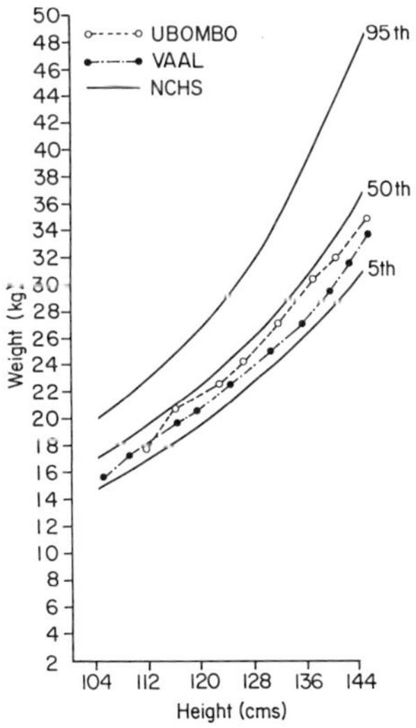

Fig. 5. Mean weight for height of black rural males in South Africa compared to the NCHS reference charts. Vaal = Vaalwater sample; Ubombo = Ubombo sample.

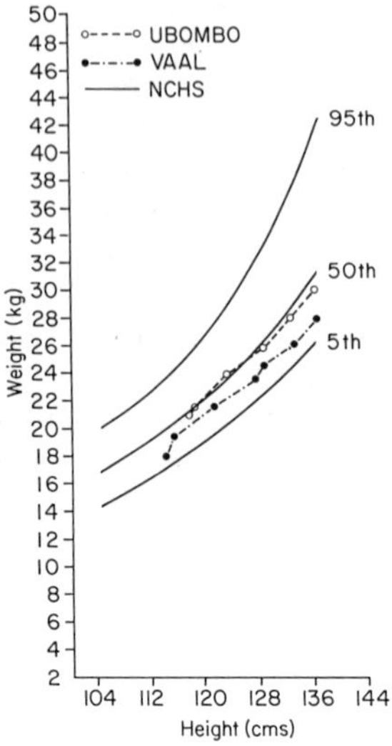

Fig. 6. Mean weight for height of black rural females in South Africa compared to the NCHS reference charts. Vaal = Vaalwater sample; Ubombo = Ubombo sample.

be spent on housing, schooling, and improved agricultural methods is instead directed towards refeeding programmes when such programmes on a large scale may not be necessary. We do not, as yet, know what the effects of this pattern of growth are on the ability of the child to learn and achieve in the conventional sense. It may be that fast growth and a short preadolescent phase of growth in some way enhance the learning ability of the child. Indeed it would seem reasonable to assume that because slow growth is an adaptation to a poor nutritional environment and that, therefore, a higher percentage of the food intake is being used for maintenance than would be the case in a good nutritional environment, that the energy available for the nonessential task of learning is going to be less. Thus learning might be impaired. The problem of obtaining evidence for this is compounded by the substandard education available in most developing countries and our inability, as yet, to be able to properly grade educational attainment in such an impoverished environment.

There are a number of other subissues that relate to the choice of reference chart, such as appropriate cutoff points and targets, but these have been discussed in detail, in other chapters of this book, by experts in the field, and the reader can do little better than to refer to these chapters (e.g., Chapters 16 and 20, this volume.)

The next issue relevant to this chapter is that of which anthropometric measurement should be used to indicate health and well-being. Again many arguments are evident in the literature, but Waterlow's classification of *wasting* and *stunting* as diagnostic results of using weight for height and height for age is difficult to better. Measurements of weight and height with, if possible, the inclusion of chronological age are, without doubt, the absolute base measurements. Of equal importance is that data collected should be collected on a longitudinal basis. We must remember that if we accept the premise that growth is the reflection of good nutriture, then growth, like nutriture, is a dynamic process. Physical status is a cross-sectional concept involving the child's position relative to others on a single occasion. "Growth" is a "longitudinal" concept involving the change in a child's physical status over a period of time. Its importance is paramount during the first few months of life when we need to know as soon as possible if a child is at risk of falling below a particular cutoff point, e.g., 80% weight for age, below which we know that mortality and morbidity assume major importance. It is, in many respects, useless to wait until the child is below the cutoff point. The problem facing most nutritional field workers in developing countries is that knowledge of chronological age is usually impossible. Children, particularly in rural African areas, simply do not know when they were born or indeed how old they are. Age, per se, is of no practical importance to such children or their families; it is not celebrated with the passing of the seasons and is usually only known if a bureaucracy has arisen out of religious or governmental need. Thus age-independent measurements assume major importance, and the search for such measurements is constantly in the mind of the nutritional or growth researcher dealing with this problem. An example of a recent attempt to develop such a measurement will illustrate the issues involved.

The basic premise involved in this search is that a "new" indicator of nutritional status must be noninvasive and have a clear biological interpretation in addition to being age independent. One of the most recently published indices of nutritional status is the width coefficient, *K*, developed by Kotze and Vivier (1986). They maintained that *K* has a biological meaning in that it estimates body width at the waist, which they put forward as an advantage over the "abstract numerical value" obtained from weight for height. Kotze and Vivier (1986) argue that *K* can be used instead of the ratio weight for height as a percentage of the reference norms for age.

Of secondary importance to this chapter, but of major importance to the moral philosophy of the nutritional field worker or human scientist working in this area, is that *K* was used by these authors to demonstrate that different ethnic groups have different allometric ratios and that, therefore, ethnicity must be considered in the anthropometric assessment of nutritional status. In addition, a follow-up paper by Kotze, Williams, MacIntyre, de Hoop, and Vivier (1986) uses *K* to show that accepted indices of nutritional status *overestimate* the incidence of PCM in South African Indian, black, and so-called coloured children. *K* was developed by scientists from the South African Departments of Health and Welfare and Constitutional Development and Planning. Cameron and Levy (1988) maintained that it seems reasonable to expect *K* to be used by these departments in their assessment of nutritional status of children in South Africa and thus in the provision of national resources such as health care and nutrition. Cameron and Levy (1988) further stated that it is of major importance that estimates of the incidence of malnutrition are reliable and that when a new index alters the previously accepted incidence, it must be carefully and critically examined. The political importance of using an apparently scientifically derived measure to show that particular sections of a country's population do not have genetic potentials equivalent to other sections should not be underestimated. In particular in a developing country it is encumbent on all scientists to constantly monitor statistics developed by the government, especially if they purport to show biological differences between racial groups.

K is purported to have biological meaning in that it represents body width at the waist. It is calculated according to the following formula:

$$K = 2\sqrt{(\text{Weight (g)} / \pi \times \text{Height (cm)})}$$

The formula incorporates weight and height and is based on two assumptions: 1) that the body may be viewed as a cylinder with its inherent geometrical properties and 2) that the density of the body is 1.0 g/ml. There is no doubt that because *K* uses height and weight it is easily measured, thus its validity as a new indicator of nutritional status rests on its age independence, relative to other more conventional parameters, and the truth of its biological meaning. The biological meaning of *K* rests on the truth of the assumption that the body can be viewed as a cylinder and the accuracy of the assumption that body density is 1.0 g/ml. Cameron and Levy (1988) tested the former assumption on a group of rural black children. They found significant differences between waist breadth and depth both within age groups and for their total sample of 150 children. Thus the assumption that the body is a cylinder is empirically incorrect. In addition *K* was significantly different from estimates of waist diameter derived from waist circumference, waist breadth, waist depth, and the average of waist breadth and depth, although it was significantly correlated with waist breadth with an $r = 0.703$. With regard to a body density of 1.0 g/ml, Cameron and Levy (1988) argued that because this value was based on the Grande and Keys (1980) "reference body" derived from three adult male cadavers, its application to children was extremely doubtful. The acceptance of this value would also require an acceptance of an age- and sex-independent value of body density, and considerable evidence exists that body composition changes during growth causing a sexually dimorphic increase in body density. In addition, and of major importance in the assessment of nutritional status, is that body composition shows major changes in conditions of malnutrition (Friis-Hansen, 1961).

K was found to be age dependent to a similar magnitude as weight for height. Correlations between age and weight for height and *K* were 0.378 and

TABLE 1. Subjects Identified as Malnourished According to the Criteria of Different Investigators

	Reference										
	Gomez et al. (1956)			Waterlow & Rutishauser (1974)		McLaren & Read (1972, 1975)			Kotze & Vivier (1986)		
	Weight for age			Wt/Ht	Ht/Age	Weight for height			*K*		
	90%	75%	60%	80%	90%	90%	85%	75%	90%	85%	75%
Females (N = 78)	36	11	0	0	7	8	1	0	9	2	0
Common to *K*	9	8			5	5	1				
Males (N = 72)	34	10	0	0	11	9	1	0	12	0	0
Common to *K*	12	10			8	3	1				
Total	70	21	0	0	18	17	2	0	21	2	0
Total common to *K*	21	18			13	8	2				
Percent common	30	85.7			72.2	47.1	100				

0.403 respectively. Thus *K* could not be said to be age independent relative to other indices.

The final point concerned the interrelationship of different assessment methods of nutritional status. This interrelationship is vital to the current discussion because of the variety of anthropometric nutritional status cutoff points that are available to the observer. Gomez, Ramos-Galvan, Frenk, Cravioto, Chavez, and Vasquez (1956) delineated mild, moderate, and severe malnutrition by 90%, 75%, and 60% weight-for-age barriers respectively. Waterlow and Rutishauser (1974) used 80% weight-for-height and 90% height-for-age cutoff points, and McLaren and Read (1972, 1975) advocated 90%, 85%, and 75% weight-for-height cutoff points. These three criteria—the Gomez, Waterlow, and McLaren criteria—are probably the most widely used criteria for nutritional assessment.

Table 1 indicates the number of children identified as malnourished according to the different classification systems including 90%, 85%, and 75% of *K* as suggested by Kotze and Vivier (1986). Of major importance is the number of individuals identified both by standard criteria and *K*. *K* performs best at identifying almost 86% of children "moderately" malnourished according to the Gomez system of 75% weight for age. It also performs reasonably well against the Waterlow criteria for stunting but poorly against McLaren's cutoff of 90% weight-for-height identifying less than 50% of such children. The importance of investigating subjects common to a new indicator and other methods of indicating malnutrition is shown by the fact that whilst similar numbers of children were identified by *K* and McLaren's criteria of 90% weight for height, only 47% of such children were identified by both systems. Thus over 50% of children identified as malnourished according to *K* were adequately nourished according to weight for height. If the new index was a better estimator of malnutrition, one would expect all those identified by *K* to be within the malnourished group according to weight for height. *K* does, however, have some merit in that it identified 70% of children mildly malnourished according to the weight-for-age criteria of Gomez. It is important that this was achieved in the absence of an age determination.

This discussion highlights the problems of deriving a new indicator of nutritional status. Ease of use and application have to be balanced against whether the indicator is biologically valid and has internal validity, in that it actually measures nutritional status. The further one moves away from the actual physical expression of nutriture, the less sensitive is the power of the measurement to identify nutritional status.

ACKNOWLEDGMENTS

The author gratefully acknowledges the financial assistance of the South African Medical Research Council, the Council for Scientific and Industrial Research—Foundation for Research Development, and the Senate Research Committee of the University of the Witwatersrand.

REFERENCES

Bengoa JM (1970): Recent trends in the public health aspects of protein-calorie malnutrition. WHO Chron 24:552–561.

Bowie MD, Moodie AD, Mann MD, Hansen JDL (1980): A prospective 15-year follow-up study of kwashiorkor patients, I: Physical growth and development. S Afr Med J 58:674–676.

Brozek J (1953): Measuring nutriture. Am J Phys Anthropol 11:147–180.

Cameron N (1986): Standards for human growth—their construction and use. S Afr Med J 70:422–425.

Cameron N, Jones PRM, Moodie A, Mitchell J, Bowie MD, Mann MD, Hansen JDL (1986): Timing and magnitude of adolescent growth in height and weight in Cape Coloured children after kwashiorkor. J Pediatr 109:548–555.

Cameron N, Levy M (1988): A critical assessment of the width coefficient, K, as an indicator of nutritional status. S Afr Med J 73:603–606.

Eksmyr R (1969): The upper arm circumference in privileged Ethiopian children. J Trop Pediatr 15:195.

Friis-Hansen B (1961): Body water compartments in children. Paediatrics 58:169–181.

Garrow JS, Pike MC (1967): The long-term prognosis of severe infantile malnutrition. Lancet 1:1–4.

Gomez F, Ramos-Galvan R, Frenk S, Cravioto JM, Chavez R, Vasquez J (1956): Mortality in third-degree malnutrition. J Trop Paediatr 2:77–83.

Grande F, Keys A (1980): Body weight, body composition and caloric status. In Goodhart RS, Shils ME (eds): "Modern Nutrition in Health and Disease." Philadelphia: Lea & Febiger.

Habicht JP (1974): Height and weight standards for preschool children: How relevant are ethnic differences in growth potential? Lancet 2:611–614.

International Union of Nutritional Sciences (1972): The creation of growth standards, a committee report. Am J Clin Nutr 25:218–220.

Janes MD (1974): Physical growth of Nigerian Yoruba children. Trop Geogr Med 26:389–398.

Jelliffe EFP, Gurney M (1974): Definition of the problem. *In* Roche AF, Falkner F (eds): "Nutrition and Malnutrition." London : Churchill-Livingstone.

Johnston FE, Lampl M (1984): Anthropometry in studies of malnutrition and behaviour. In Brozek J, Schurch B (eds): "Malnutrition and Behaviour: Critical Assessment and Key Issues." Lausanne: Nestle Foundation.

Kannel WB, Dawber TR (1972): Atherosclerosis: A pediatric problem. J Pediatr 80:544–554.

Kotze JP, Vivier FL (1986): The width coefficient *K:* A new parameter of nutritional status compared to other allometric relationships. S Afr J Sci 82:327–329.

Kotze JP, Williams WN, MacIntyre U, de Hoop ME, Vivier FL (1986): Anthropometric and dental data on different population groups in South African primary schools. S Afr J Sci 82:329–334.

McKay DA (1969): Experience with the mid-arm circumference as a nutritional indicator in field surveys in Malaysia. J Trop Pediatr 15:213–216.

McLaren DS (1976): Protein energy malnutrition (PEM). In McLaren DS, Burman D (eds): "Textbook of Paediatric Nutrition." London: Churchill-Livingstone.

McLaren DS, Read WWC (1972): Classification of nutritional status in early childhood. Lancet 2:146–149.

McLaren DS, Read WWC (1975): Weight/length classification of nutritional status. Lancet 2:219–221.

Malcolm LA (1974): Ecological factors relating to child growth and nutritional status. In Roche AF, Falkner F (eds): "Nutrition and Malnutrition." New York: Plenum Press.

Neumann CG (1979): Reference data. In Jelliffe DB, Jelliffe EFP (eds): "Nutrition and Growth." New York: Plenum Press.

Neumann CG, Lawlor GJ, Stiehm ER, Swendseid M, Newton C, Amman A, Jacob M (1975): Immunological responses in malnourished children. Am J Clin Nutr 28:89–104.

Neumann CG, Shanker H, Uberoi IS (1969): Nutritional and anthropometric profile of young rural Punjabi children. Indian J Med Res 57:1122–1149.

Steckel RH (1987): Growth depression and recovery: The remarkable case of American slaves. Ann Hum Biol 14:111–132.

Tanner JM (1976): Growth as a monitor of nutritional status. Proc Nutr Soc 35:315–321.

Tanner JM, Goldstein H (1980): Ecological considerations in the creation and use of child growth standards. Lancet 1:582–587.

Tanner JM, Whitehouse RH, Takaishi M (1966): Standards for birth to maturity for heights, weight, height velocity and weight velocity: British children in 1965. Arch Dis Child 41:454–571, 613–635.

Washburn S (1951): The new physical anthropology. Trans NY Acad Sci 13:298–304.

Washburn S (1953): The strategy of physical anthropology. In Kroeber AL (ed): "Anthropology Today." Chicago: Chicago University Press.

Waterlow JC (1984): Current issues in nutritional assessment by anthropometry. In Brozek J, Schurch B (eds): "Malnutrition and Behaviour: Critical Assessment of Key Issues." Lausanne: Nestle Foundation.

Waterlow JC, Rutishauser IHE (1974): Malnutrition in man. In Cravioto J, Hambrens L, Vahlquist B (eds): "Early Malnutrition and Mental Development." Stockholm: Almqvist and Wiksell.

Watson EH, Lowry GH (1975): "Growth and Development of Children." Chicago: Yearbook.

Wingerd J, Schoen EJ, Solomon JL (1971): Growth standards in the first two years of life based on measurements of White and Black children in a prepaid health care program. Pediatrics 47:818–825.

Anthropometric Assessment
of Nutritional Status, pages 365–381

22
Anthropometric Assessment of Nutritional Status in Hospitalized Patients

MOLLY McMAHON AND BRUCE R. BISTRIAN
Division of Endocrinology, Metabolism and Internal Medicine, Mayo Medical School, Rochester, MN 55905 (M.M), New England Deaconess Hospital, Boston, Massachusetts 02215, Harvard Medical School, Cambridge, Massachusetts 02138 (B.R.B.)

INTRODUCTION

The value of the nutritional assessment of the hospitalized patient may be attributed to its ability to first detect the presence of and second to define the type of malnutrition. Such an assessment permits the identification of patients who require prompt nutritional support, prediction of the risk of complications related to protein-calorie malnutrition (PCM), definition of energy, protein, micronutrient and macronutrient requirements, and an evaluation of the response to nutritional therapy (Bistrian, 1984). Although the body's response to injury/inflammation is stereotyped, its expression is modulated by the energy stores of the individual. It is the balance between the severity of stress and the body's endogenous energy reserves that determines whether malnutrition will present as uncomplicated semistarvation (marasmus) or as hypoalbuminemic malnutrition (kwashiorkor). An understanding of the body's adaptation and response to both semistarvation and illness/injury will allow an appreciation of how these two forms of PCM can be differentiated by a complete nutritional assessment (Table 1).

MARASMUS: ADAPTATION TO SEMISTARVATION

Semistarvation results if the caloric intake is insufficient for the body's requirements. Since protein is vital for the maintenance of body structure, muscle function, and enzymatically regulated pathways, the body attempts to limit breakdown of visceral proteins by taking advantage of fat (100,000–150,000 kcal) and skeletal muscle (40,000 kcal) stores (Cahill et al., 1966; Shafrir, 1987). Although carbohydrate is quantitatively a limited energy reserve (1,200 kcal), it serves as an obligate energy source for the brain, hematopoietic system, and renal medulla under normal conditions. The ability of amino acids to be converted to glucose explains why the requirement for glucose as a fuel source may hasten the depletion of body protein stores in starvation.

TABLE 1. Comparison of Marasmus and Hypoalbuminemic Malnutrition (Kwashiorkor)

	Marasmus	Hypoalbuminemic malnutrition
Cause	Insufficient energy intake	Metabolic response to injury
Hormonal and metabolic alterations	Depression in metabolic rate Hypoinsulinemia	↑ Counterregulatory hormones ↑ Aldosterone ↑ Antidiuretic hormone ↑ Insulin resistance ↑ Monokine response
Visceral protein stores	Normal serum albumin No acute phase protein response Liver and gut diminished	Low serum albumin Acute phase protein response Liver increased but gut diminished
Immune function	Intact, unless current/ideal body weight < 85%	Impaired, if injury response prolonged
Clinical presentation and anthropometrics	Weight loss Low AMC	Markers of stress: fever, leukocytosis with elevation in band forms, hypoalbuminemia and elevated catabolic index Normal/low AMC
Anticipated response to appropriate nutritional therapy	Restoration of lean tissue Positive nitrogen balance	Restoration of lean tissue may or may not occur Persistent hypoalbuminemia Return of immunocompetence
Prototypic disease states	Starvation Anorexia nervosa Cardiac cachexia Malabsorption Esophageal cancer	Sepsis Head injury Burns Multiple trauma Selected cancers

The decrease in energy intake is quickly followed by a decline in basal energy expenditure. This protective reduction in the basal metabolic rate is primarily regulated by a decrease in thyroid and sympathetic nervous system activity. Although the serum total thyroxine (T4) level is maintained in the normal range during semistarvation (Vagenakis et al., 1977), most studies have shown a decrease in the concentration of total triiodothyronine (T3) (Portnay et al., 1974), the biologically active form of the hormone. It is primarily the fall in serum insulin that permits the mobilization of fat to meet energy requirements, the catabolism of skeletal muscle amino acids to promote visceral organ protein synthesis, and the ketosis to supply the brain with fuel, thus lessening the requirement for carbohydrate as a fuel source and pari passu the sparing of muscle breakdown (Cahill et al., 1966). The weight loss of marasmus is accompanied by a steady decline in the reserves of body fat and fat-free mass (FFM); in men, at 50% below the ideal body weight, only 10% of fat stores and 50%–60% of FFM remain (Grant, 1983). Protein must then serve as the main fuel source. The resultant increase in urinary nitrogen, a marker of protein breakdown, termed the "premortal rise in N excretion," (Lusk, 1976; Peret and Jacquot, 1972) signals a shortened survival. Weight loss exceeding 40% is generally incompatible with survival (Keys et al., 1950).

HYPOALBUMINEMIC MALNUTRITION: METABOLIC RESPONSE TO ILLINESS/INJURY

By contrast, hypoalbuminemic malnutrition evolves as a result of the body's response to injury/infection. The response, mediated by neuroendocrine- and monokine-induced alterations, is typified by a low serum albumin concentration. It is the balance between the synthesis and catabolism of albumin and its equilibrium between the intravascular and extravascular compartment that determines the plasma level of albumin. The daily hepatic synthetic rate averages 120–270 mg/kg (Gersovitz et al., 1968), or 15 g for a 70 kg person. After synthesis, the albumin molecule enters the circulation to distribute in the intravascular and extravascular space. Approximately 10% of the pool is catabolized daily in the inestinal tract and the vascular endothelium (Rothschild et al., 1971). In semistarvation, decreases in the rates of both synthesis and catabolism (James and Hay, 1968), coupled with an intravascular shift of the protein (James and Hays, 1968), maintain the serum albumin in the normal range. It is the increase in the catabolism of albumin (Rothschild et al., 1971) combined with the decrease in its synthesis that contributes to the hypoalbuminemia of injury. The liver, in response to illness, produces acute phase proteins, rather than albumin. During injury, therefore, the serum albumin concentration should be viewed as an imperfect measure of nutritional status, but an excellent marker for the injury response.

Hormones and monokines may be viewed as key modulators of the alterations in carbohydrate, protein, and lipid metabolism which occur during illness. Responses which may be directly or indirectly mediated by stress-induced hormonal changes include an elevation in basal metabolic rate (catecholamines), an impairment of water excretion with sodium and water retention (aldosterone and antidiuretic hormone), and the maintenance of blood pressure (sympathoadrenal axis activation). In addition, stress causes a pronounced rise in serum glucagon, epinephrine, cortisol, and growth hormone. In general, the elevation of these counterregulatory hormones fosters glucose production while decreasing its utilization (fuel provision for the central nervous system, wound healing, and hematopoietic system); promotes skeletal muscle breakdown leading to a negative nitrogen balance (precursors for the synthesis of glucose and protein); and stimulates lipolysis (energy source) (Schade et al., 1983). The insulin resistance of stress is directly or indirectly mediated by the rise in counterregulatory hormones.

The other major arm of the injury response is attributed to the actions of cytokines (for reviews, Dinarello and Mier, 1986; Dinarello, 1988; Flores et al., 1988; Pomposelli et al., 1988). The combined metabolic, immunologic, and hematologic response of a host to injury has been termed the acute phase response. Designed to limit the extent of injury and to promote healing through optimization of defense mechanisms and mobilization of energy reserves, this response is in part mediated by monokines, including interleukin-1, alpha and beta (IL-1), and tumor necrosis factor alpha/cachectin (TNF). These monokines are synthesized by activated cells, primarily monocytic and phagocytic cells lining the liver and spleen, in response to injury of inflammation. In addition to promoting lymphocyte proliferation, these peptides may enter the circulation to regulate physiologic responses in other tissues. IL-1 can cause fever, leukocytosis with release of immature forms from the marrow, a redistribution in plasma trace metals with a depression in serum iron and zinc and a rise in serum copper, an increase in the synthesis of hepatic acute phase proteins, and an elevation in certain complement components and procoagulants. All of these parameters may be similarly affected during illness. TNF, capable of inducing some of the same acute phase changes, is uniquely able to mimic endotoxin shock (Tracey et al., 1986; Tracey et al., 1987).

It is believed that many of the alterations in intermediary metabolism that are observed during illness may be mediated by monokines (Pomposelli et al., 1988). Recombinant cloning of monokines, while providing an opportunity to study and isolate the effects of each monokine, has also necessitated the reinterpretation of results of earlier studies in which preparations were likely contaminated with several monokines. Effects, observed during stress, that can be caused by an IL-1 infusion include an increase in the level of counterregulatory hormones (Pomposelli et al., 1987), an enhancement of the use of glucose as a fuel (Pomposelli et al., 1988), an increase in the rate of lipid oxidation (Tocco-Bradley et al., 1988), and a rise in the energy expenditure (Tocco-Bradley et al., 1988). Protein metabolism is primarily affected by TNF. TNF infusion alone (IL-1 infusion only if in combination with TNF) is capable of promoting leucine oxidation and skeletal muscle breakdown (Flores et al., 1986), which may lead to the negative nitrogen balance characteristic of injury.

ANTHROPOMETRY: BASIC ASSUMPTIONS

The clinical use of anthropometry both to estimate stores of energy and protein and to divide the body fat and FFM is a useful adjunct to the nutritional assessment. In a healthy individual, the composition of adipose tissue approximates 80% fat, 18% water, and 2% protein (Keys, 1953). FFM is composed of protein, water, glycogen, and mineral. In general, protein (19.5%), water (72.5%), and bone mineral (8%) occur in fixed proportions (Garrow, 1974). One-third to 1/2 of the protein is in skeletal muscle with the remainder divided among other lean tissues. It is the accessibility of muscle to anthropometric measuring techniques that makes muscle a useful marker of severe PCM.

Measurements of arm muscle circumference (AMC) and triceps skinfold (TSF) aim to define muscle and fat compartments in the midarm. The calculations required for the measurements assume a circular cross-section of the arm and muscle compartment, a symmetric distribution of fat around the arm, and a constant fraction of bone to muscle area (Heysmfield et al., 1984b). Although direct measurement of fat, bone, and muscle tissue by computerized axial tomography revealed that each of these approximations was in error (Heymsfield et al., 1979), in persons 60%–120% of ideal body weight anthropometric estimates of arm muscle area and fat area correspond reasonably well with the radiographic values. Estimates are closely correlated when presented in terms of percentage of standard, as the standard also contains "nonskeletal muscle" components.

The use of anthropometry in PCM is based on the assumption that the size of muscle in both the nourished and malnourished bears a constant relationship to muscle composition, specifically muscle protein, and energy content. Because histologic (Montgomery, 1962) and radiographic (Heymsfield et al., 1979) data had suggested that muscle composition was altered in PCM, this basic assumption was tested through an analysis of muscle harvested from three autopsy groups: controls (n = 11, traumatic death), early semistarvation (n = 6, acute preterminal disease), and chronic semistarvation (n = 34, severe weight loss over time) (Heymsfield et al., 1982). Early semistarvation produced no detectable change in muscle mass, protein, or total energy content. Chronic semistarvation caused muscle atrophy and a different chemical composition with all measured constituents not being reduced by the same degree. The atrophic muscle contained more water and lipid and less protein and energy when compared to muscle from the control group. As a result, anthropometry underestimated the relative reduction in muscle protein and energy in the malnourished muscle by 5%–15%. As will be discussed later, this degree of potential error is of little clinical significance.

CLINICAL APPLICATION OF ANTHROPOMETRICS

The first use of upper arm anthropometric measurements to assess PCM in hospitalized patients revealed striking incidences of malnutrition in surgical (50%) (Bistrian et al., 1974) and medical (44%) (Bistrian et al., 1976) patients. At the time of the initial survey the only available standards were those of Jelliffe (Jelliffe, 1966). As clinical experience with arm anthropometry evolved, it was recommended that a definition of PCM be restricted to an AMC either below the 5th percentile or less than 80% of standard (Bistrian, 1980). The AMC measurement correlates with both serum albumin and with percentage of weight loss (Bistrian et al., 1974; Bistrian et al., 1976; Young et al., 1979). By contrast, the use of TSF to diagnose PCM is fraught with problems. Fat is an expendable tissue, and its lack may not correlate with function (Bistrian, 1977a) or hospital morbidity or mortality (Harvey et al., 1978; Mullen et al., 1979). Very little fat reserve is sufficient for the healthy individual in nitrogen balance (as an athlete), whereas such limited fat stores in a patient in negative energy balance carries a very different prognosis. The TSF measurement is, however, required for calculation of both the AMC measurement and the prognostic nutritional index (Buzby et al., 1980), designed to predict postoperative complications in patients undergoing elective gastrointestinal surgery.

A review of other anthropometric measures commonly used in clinical medicine will precede a discussion of their importance in selected disease states. In healthy subjects, urinary creatinine excretion correlates with FFM, muscle mass, surface area, and body weight (Heymsfield et al., 1984a; Miller and Blyth, 1954). Some investigators have proposed a constant relationship between creatinine excretion and muscle mass; one gram of creatinine excreted over a 24-hour period has been estimated to be derived from 18 to 20 kg (Talbot, 1938; Forbes and Bruining, 1976) of muscle mass. An accurate interpretation of urinary creatinine excretion requires an appreciation of factors capable of affecting its measurement. Firstly, there is an intraindividual variability of 4%–8% in daily urinary creatinine excretion (Cryer and Sode, 1970). Secondly, since diet can affect daily creatinine output, the creatine-creatinine content of the diet should not be changed during the testing period. Adherence to a creatine and creatinine-free diet (meat-free protein source, casein) for six weeks has been shown to cause a significant reduction (approximately 21%) in creatinine excretion (Bleiler and Schedl, 1972). Similarly, urinary creatinine increased rapidly when subjects were switched back to a general diet. Thirdly, severe trauma (Frawley et al., 1955) and infection (Waterlow et al., 1972) may increase the urinary excretion of creatinine independently of changes in body cell mass. Fourthly, renal impairment increases the nonrenal clearance of creatinine (Jones and Burnett, 1974) so that in patients with serum creatinine levels greater than 4–6 mg/dL the correlation between creatinine excretion and FFM is poor. Finally, creatinine excretion declines with age (Tomlinson et al., 1969) reflecting the reduction in lean tissue.

In the malnourished, creatinine excretion is reduced (Ryan et al., 1957) and no longer correlates with total body weight but does correlate with body cell mass. Since height is, in general, not affected by malnutrition, a useful measure of relative muscle mass is the creatinine–height index. This index represents the ratio between the observed and expected creatinine excretion for a healthy adult of the same sex and height (Bistrian et al., 1975b; Viteri and Alvarade, 1970). The expected 24 hour creatinine excretion is calculated according to the normal creatinine excretion of healthy females (18 mg/kg/day) and males (23 mg/kg/day), using the patient's ideal weight for height. A reduction in muscle mass is assumed to produce a proportional reduction in the creatinine–height index. An index between 60% and 80% indicates moderate depletion of muscle mass, and a value below 60% suggests severe depletion (Bistrian et al., 1975b).

In clinical medicine, the energy expenditure or caloric requirement of an individual is often estimated by the Harris-Benedict equation (Harris and Benedict, 1919), which is based on the premise that basal energy needs are related to body cell mass. The variable of height, weight, age, and sex in the equation reflect the relationship between body weight and body cell mass. Relating resting energy expenditure to body weight, however, assumes a normal body composition, which is not true of the malnourished (Roza and Shizgal, 1984). Since 24-hour urinary creatinine is a reasonable marker of lean body mass even in the presence of malnutrition, an estimate of energy expenditure based on creatinine excretion, expressed as kcal/g urinary creatinine, would have value in this group (Shanbhogue et al., 1987). In summary, urinary creatinine excretion is helpful to assess lean body tissue, to confirm the completeness of a 24-hour urine collection, and to estimate renal function. In addition, estimates of energy expenditure which are related to creatinine excretion are of value in the malnourished and in those with increased total body water in whom the direct relationship between body weight and body cell mass is not maintained.

Nitrogen balance studies may be employed to estimate the degree of catabolism, to calculate the catabolic rate, and to monitor the efficacy of nutritional intervention. Nitrogen (N) balance represents the quantity of nitrogen taken in by the diet minus the quantity lost. N balance = N in − N out (urine urea nitrogen + 4 g). Since dietary protein is assumed to have an average nitrogen content of 16%, the protein can be multiplied by 0.016 or divided by 6.25 in order to be converted to nitrogen. Most nitrogen is lost in the urine and primarily as urea. Total nitrogen excretion can be estimated by adding a correction factor of 4 g to the measured urea nitrogen: 2 g/day are lost in the feces and from the skin, and an additional 2 g/day as nonurea nitrogenous losses.

Urea nitrogen excretion is a variable required for calculation of the catabolic index (CI) (Bistrian, 1979). An estimate of the degree of stress, this index separates total urea excretion into that resulting from protein intake and obligatory urea excretion from that caused by an increase in endogenous protein catabolism due to gluconeogenesis and ureagenesis. CI represents the difference between the measured and predicted urine urea nitrogen: 24-hour urine urea nitrogen excretion − (0.5 dietary nitrogen intake + 3 g). The degree to which the measured value exceeds the estimated amount may be viewed as an indicator of the degreeof stress. A CI of less than zero indicates no stress; 0–5, moderate stress; and greater than 5, severe stress (Bistrian, 1979).

NUTRITIONAL ASSESSMENT

The clinical nutritional assessment combines the history and physical examination with the laboratory tests that are needed to help confirm the clinical impressions. The history should elicit information about timing and amount of weight loss, medical illnesses, medications, and dietary habits. In general, a recent weight loss of < 10% from usual weight represents mild PCM; 10%–20%, moderate PCM; and > 20%, severe PCM taking into account the presence of excess fluid, tumor, and/or organomegaly. Knowledge of the degree of weight loss alone, however, is insufficient to define the composition of the loss. While semistarved men and women may lose 25% and 35% of total weight loss as lean tissue, respectively, following injury, this may rise to as much as 50% (Runcie and Hilditch, 1974). By contrast, obese individuals dieting with a higher protein intake (1.5 g/kg) will lose fat only (Hoffer et al., 1984). Regardless, weight loss in excess of 10% from usual weight necessitates a more complete nutritional assessment. Although in uncomplicated semistarvation mortality rates do not increase until weight loss exceeds 40%, in the presence of injury weight loss of 25% (Kinney et al., 1978) may be fatal.

While the physical examination may help both to define the cause(s) of PCM and to identify specific micronutrient deficiencies, it is only the marasmic form of PCM that is clinically obvious. Accurate recording of the patient's height and weight is important, and it is useful to express the weight as a relative value in order to compare the individual to a healthy population. As previously discussed, markers of stress and monokine activation include the presence of fever, hypoalbuminemia, leukocytosis with an increase in the release of immature forms from the bone marrow, negative nitrogen balance, and an elevated catabolic index.

INDICATIONS FOR NUTRITIONAL INTERVENTION

At this point the clinician has sufficient information to determine which patients require nutritional support. It is the magnitude of recent weight loss, the presence or absence of clinician markers of stress, and the anticipated time that the patient will be unable to eat that combine to determine the need for nutritional support. In general, in the well nourished, the metabolic response to injury is beneficial for up to two weeks. If further protracted, immune function becomes impaired. Such impairment occurs earlier if the patient is initially malnourished. Provision of energy and protein will allow the beneficial aspects of the injury response to persist until resolution of the injury. A recent unintentional weight loss of < 10% from usual weight is well tolerated. In general, if the patient is well nourished and unstressed (afebrile, normal white blood cell count and differential, and normal serum albumin) or mildly to moderately stressed and unable to meet nutritional requirements for up to 10 days, the simple provision of fluid and electrolytes will not impair clinical outcome. Prompt nutritional support should be provided if these subjects become severely stressed (head injury, major burn, multiple trauma, or severe sepsis), as this stress response will reliably persist for longer than 7–10 days and the outcome will be improved by feeding. Those who have lost 10%–20% of their usual weight should receive supplemental nutrition if moderately or severely stressed. Individuals who have lost more than 20% of body weight (e.g., anorexia nervosa) will benefit from nutritional repletion even without stress.

The report that protein-malnourished individuals were often afebrile, while septic, was one of the earliest studies linking the importance of nutrition with full expression of the injury response (Scrimshaw et al., 1968). Altered nutritional status has been shown to affect monokine production in man. The capability of mononuclear cells, in vitro, to produce IL-1 was found to be diminished in hypoalbuminemic malnutrition (Hoffman-Goetz et al., 1981; Keenan et al., 1982). Short-term (1–7 days) parenteral nutrition restored the production of IL-1. Marasmus, on the other hand, did not significantly affect the ability of blood leukocytes to produce IL-1. Cellular immune function, essential to the body's defense against infection, was also adversely affected by hypoalbuminemic malnutrition (by marasmus only if the current weight/ideal body weight $< 85\%$) (Bistrian et al., 1975a). The skin test response can be lost from nutritional deprivation within seven days and can be restored by approximately two weeks of adequate nutrition if PCM was the reason for the impairment. These studies support the need for nutritional intervention in the malnourished to optimize their metabolic response to injury and to restore immune function.

Special consideration has been focused on the indications for preoperative nutrition. The original observation that postoperative mortality rates were closely associated with preoperative weight loss dates back more than 50 years (Studley, 1936). Mortality rates were found to be increased in patients undergoing surgery for duodenal ulcer disease if the preoperative weight loss exceeded 20%. Recent prospective studies have shown that, in certain patients, five to seven days of preoperative nutrition decreases the rate of major postoperative complications and mortality (Foschi et al., 1986; Heatley et al., 1979; Moghissi et al., 1977; Muller et al., 1982; Williams et al., 1976). Therefore, we believe that patients with greater than 10% weight loss and or hypoalbuminemia should be considered as candidates for preoperative nutritional therapy.

MONITORING THE RESPONSE TO NUTRITIONAL SUPPORT

The same indices that are used in the baseline nutritional assessment can be used to monitor the response to nutritional therapy provided certain points are kept in mind (Bistrian, 1977a). In the stressed hospitalized patient receiving nutrition, day to day weight changes generally reflect shifts in fluid balance, rather than alterations in energy stores. Clinical indicators of lean tissue (AMC and urinary creatinine) are not capable of detecting the effect of nutritional support during acute care parenteral nutrition (Jeejeebhoy et al., 1982), the mean value of which is 19 days (Padberg et al., 1981). Initiation of nutritional support may actually cause a 5%–10% increase (Heymsfield et al., 1982) in muscle size, which is caused by rapid changes in muscle glycogen as a result of water-binding properties of glycogen and not by an increase in the protein content of lean tissue. In the unstressed patient with marasmus, appropriate protein and calorie intake should cause a slow weight gain and a positive nitrogen balance of 2–6 g N (60–180 g lean tissue) per day. In the hypoalbuminemic patient, no longer stressed, a similar nutritional regimen will lead to a comparable weight gain and positive nitrogen balance and to an increase in serum albumin in two to four weeks. In the stressed patient with hypoalbuminemic malnutrition, appropriate nutritional support will often not restore lean tissue but will optimize the response to stress. Although serum albumin will not normalize in the presence of stress, the associated consequences of hypoalbuminemia, an anergy and impaired monokine production, should improve with seven to ten days of nutrition. The persistence of immunoincompetence, despite nutritional support, is an ominous prognostic sign.

Recently, attention has been focused on the functional effects of PCM on the musculoskeletal system. Malnutrition has been shown to reduce ATP turnover, alter muscle energetics, cause muscle fiber atrophy and Z-band degeneration (an index of calcium-dependent proteolysis) (Jeejeebhoy, 1986). In a study of 225 patients admitted for major abdominal surgery, a reduction in muscle power (dynamometry) was found to be a better indicator of postoperative complications than was weight loss or AMC (Klidjian et al., 1980). Subsequent studies have examined muscle function and fatigue by measuring the contraction–relaxation of the adductor pollicis muscle in response to an electrical stimulus of the ulnar nerve at the wrist (Jeejeebhoy, 1986). Muscle power has been found to be affected by nutritional changes in the absence of a change in AMC (Brough et al., 1986), suggesting that reduced nutrient intake may alter function early and independently of changes in lean tissue. This is not unexpected given the importance of muscle glycogen stores for optimal muscle function. The role of these functional assessments in the hospitalized patient is unclear.

NUTRITIONAL ASSESSMENT IN SELECTED DISEASE STATES

Although body weight, the sum of total body water and of sources of protein and fat, and weight/height are the most easily obtained markers of energy reserves, their use may be misleading under certain circumstances. These include states characterized by a relative increase in total body water (hepatic, renal, and cardiac disease), by the presence of tumor or organomegaly, or by those which develop because of therapeutic measures (as fluid resuscitation postoperatively). As discussed earlier, in patients with a relative increase in total body water, there is an inability to relate either resting energy expenditure to body weight, or urinary creatinine excretion to body weight. This, combined with the inability to use serum albumin as a marker of nutritional status during injury, adds to the difficulty of properly assessing the nutritional status of such patients.

Although PCM is prevalent in patients with end-stage liver disease (ELD) (Hehir et al., 1985; O'Keefe et al., 1980), the interpretation of a nutritional assessment in these patients is difficult. A study in which 13 patients with ELD underwent nutritional assessments prior to orthotopic liver transplantation provides an illustration and discussion of the lack of sensitivity provided by individual nutritional parameters (Hehir et al., 1985). Weight, when expressed as a percentage of ideal body weight, was greater than 85% (normal lower limit) in 11 of the 13 patients. By contrast, mean TSF and AMC were 49% and 78% of standard, respectively. Mean serum albumin was 2.7 g/dL. All had depressed lymphocyte counts, and 7 of the 12 were anergic by skin testing. The relative increase in total body water (secondary hyperaldosteronism, renal dysfunction, and depressed colloid osmotic pressure of ELD) helped to maintain weight and weight/height in the normal range even in the malnourished. AMC was a more sensitive indicator of depleted energy stores than was weight, in part because the upper extremity is largely unaffected by dependent edema.

The clinical applicability of relating resting energy expenditure to the amount of urinary creatinine (vide supra) was demonstrated in a group of patients with ELD (Shanbhogue et al., 1987). Use of the Harris-Benedict equation to predict resting energy expenditure in this group of patients would lead to an overestimation of energy needs since the elevated body weight reflects a relative increase in total body water and not a relative increase in total body mass. However, when energy expenditure was related to lean tissue (urinary creatinine), patients with ELD demonstrated an increased energy expenditure compared to the control group, confirming a hypermetabolic state (Shanbhogue et al., 1987).

Nutritional depletion and continued weight loss, common among cancer patients, causes an increase in morbidity and morality (Bristrian, 1986; DeWys et al., 1980; Stein, 1978; Warren, 1932). The severe weight loss and the emaciated appearance of this group have been termed *cancer cachexia.* A consecutive survey of 54 patients (93% with metastatic disease) admitted to a major teaching hospital oncology ward assessed their nutritional status through the measurement of anthropometrics, urinary creatinine excretion, and serum albumin (Nixon et al., 1980). Of the 54 patients 88% had a creatinine height index less than 80% of standard, and 53% less than 60% of standard. Although 42% of the group had a TSF less than 80% of standard, only 23% had a midarm muscle area measurement of less than 80% of standard. Serum albumin was less than 3.5 g/dL in 31% of the patients. Creatinine–height index was clearly the most sensitive marker of PCM in this study. In the subset of patients with colon cancer, nutritional parameters were correlated with survival. Those patients who had both a creatinine-height index and a TSF measurement less than 60% of standard in addition to a plasma albumin less than 3.5 g/dL were more likely to die within 70 days of study initiation.

A study design combining anthropometric, radiographic, and biochemical methods facilitated the division of body mass into fat, FFM, and skeletal muscle and provided volume determinations of visceral organs and tumor mass (Heymsfield et al., 1985). These methods were used to evaluate body composition longitudinally in nine cancer patients during an 8–85 week follow-up period. Two control groups, 46 healthy age-, sex-, and height-matched subjects and 3 patients with weight loss due to anorexia nervosa, also underwent baseline studies. There were two estimates of fat (anthropometric total body fat and radiographic subcutaneous fat volume) and three measures of skeletal muscle (anthropometric arm muscle area, radiographic muscle volume, and 24-hour urinary creatinine excretion). Radiographic procedures estimated the size of the heart, liver, spleen, and kidney, and, in selected cases, tumor volume. All of the patients with cancer developed progression of metastatic disease; seven of the nine lost weight with an average loss of 10.5 kg. Although cachexia was a dominant clinical feature, body composition differed in the two groups. Fat and muscle depletion were similar in the two groups, but atrophy of visceral organs differed. In the subjects (note the small number) with anorexia nervosa, all measured components of FFM (muscle and visceral organs) were proportionally reduced. In the group with cancer cachexia, liver and spleen size remained unchanged or enlarged, while that of the heart and kidney remained unchanged or atrophied by 5%–30%. Relatively speaking, the patients with cancer had a larger visceral organ mass than did the patients with anorexia nervosa, supporting conclusions of earlier studies. Again, weight was not the best marker of energy stores in this subject of patients.

According to most surveys assessing the nutritional status of patients with chronic renal failure, PCM is common (Attman et al., 1980; Blumenkrantz et al., 1980; Miller et al., 1983; Schoenfeld et al., 1983). Malnutrition may be caused by the restricted protein or energy intake, increased catabolism caused by associated illnesses, nutrient loss through dialysis, and/or a hemodialysis-associated increase in catabolism (Kopple, 1988), which may in part be caused by IL-1 (Dinarello, 1988a). In a study of 43 diabetic patients (40 insulin dependent) who were on peritoneal dialysis or hemodialysis, AMC was $< 5\%$ in 44% of the group, weight was $< 85\%$ of ideal weight in 26% of the patients, while the mean serum albumin was maintained in the normal range (Miller et al., 1983). AMC was the most sensitive indicator of PCM.

Finally, injury causes an increase in the plasma concentration of antidiuretic hormone (ADH) and aldosterone (Deutsch, 1975). Postoperatively the elevation in ADH can persist for three to five days and is not suppressed by hydration (Moran et al., 1964). The impairment in sodium and water excretion may be further accentuated by administration of dextrose-containing intravenous solutions. The hyperinsulinemia which occurs as a result of hypertonic dextrose infusion leads to a decrease in sodium excretion (DeFronzo et al., 1985). This antinatriuresis can combine with the other factors to cause edema formation and a significant weight gain in patients who often have preexisting increases in total body water due to hepatic, renal, or cardiac disease. These points should be kept in mind when interpreting perioperative weight fluxes.

CONCLUSIONS

In conclusion, the nutritional assessment is invaluable for initiation and monitoring of nutritional support of the hospitalized patient. The assessment differentiates between the two forms of protein-calorie malnutrition, each of which is associated with a different requirement for nutritional therapy. An individualized nutritional assessment requires an understanding of the body's adaptation to semistarvation and response to illness as well as a knowledge of the patient's specific disease state. Timely nutritional intervention is crucial for optimization of the body's metabolic response to injury.

REFERENCES

Attman P, Ewald J, Isaksson B (1980): Body composition during long-term treatment of uremia with amino acid supplemented low-protein diet. Am J Clin Nutr 33:801–810.

Bistrian BR (1977a): Interaction of nutrition and infection in the hospital setting. Am J Clin Nutr 30:1228–1232.

Bistrian BR (1977b): Nutritional assessment and therapy of protein-calorie malnutrition in the hospital. J Am Diet Assoc 7:393–397.

Bistrian BR (1979): A simple technique to estimate severity of stress. Surg Gynecol Obstet 148:675–678.

Bistrian BR (1980): Anthropometric norms used in assessment of hospitalized patients. Am J Clin Nutr 33:2211–2214.

Bistrian BR (1984): Nutritional assessment of the hospitalized patient: A practical approach. In Wright RA, Heymsfield S, McManus CB (eds): "Nutritional Assessment." Boston: Blackwell Scientific, pp 183–205.

Bistrian B (1986): Nutritional assessment of the cancer patient. Cancer 58:1863–1866.

Bistrian BR, Blackburn GL, Hallowell E, Heddle R (1974): Protein status of general surgical patients. JAMA 230:858–860.

Bistrian BR, Blackburn GL, Scrimshaw NS, Flatt JP (1975a): Cellular immunity in semistarved states in hospitalized adults. Am J Clin Nutr 28:1148–1155.

Bistrian BR, Blackburn GL, Sherman M, Scrimshaw NS (1975b): Therapeutic index of nutritional depletion in hospitalized patients. Surg Gynecol Obstet 141:512–516.

Bistrian BR, Blackburn GL, Vitale J, Cochran D, Naylor J (1976): Prevalence of malnutrition in general medical patients. JAMA 235:1567–1570.

Bistrian BR, Sherman M, Blackburn GL, Marshall R, Shaw C (1977): Cellular immunity in adult marasmus. Arch Intern Med 137:1408–1411.

Bleiler RE, Schedl HP (1962): Creatinine excretion: Variability and relationships to diet and body size. J Lab Clin Med 59:945–955.

Blumenkrantz M, Kopple J, Gutman R (1980): Methods for assessing nutritional status of patients with renal failure. Am J Clin Nutr 33:1567–1585.

Brough W, Horne G, Blount A, Irving MH, Jeejeebhoy KN (1986): Effects of nutrient intake, surgery, sepsis, and long term administration of steroids on muscle function. Br Med J 293:983–998.

Buzby GP, Mullen JL, Matthews DC, Hobbs CL, Rosato EF (1980):Prognostic nutritional index in gastrointestinal surgery. Am J Surg 139:160–166.

Cahill CF, Herrera MG, Morgan AP, Soeldner JS, Steinke JS, Levy PL, Reichard GA, Kipnis DM (1966): Hormone–fuel interrelationships during fasting. J Clin Invest 45:1751–1769.

Cryer PE, Sode J (1970): Variation in urinary creatinine excretion and its relationships to measurement of urinary 17-hydroxy-corticosteroids. Clin Chem 16:1012–1015.

DeFronzo R, Cooke C, Andres R (1985): The effect of insulin in renal handling of sodium, potassium, calcium, and phosphate in man. J Clin Invest 55:845–855.

Deutsch S (1975): Effects of anesthetics on the kidney. Surg Clin North Am 55:775–786.

DeWys W, Begg C, Lavin P et al. (1980): Prognostic effect of weight loss prior to chemotherapy in cancer patients. Am J Med 69:491–497.

Dinarello C (1984): Interleukin-1 and the pathogenesis of the acute phase response. N Engl J Med: 311:1413–1418.
Dinarello C (1988): Biology of interleukin 1. FASEB 2:108–115.
Dinarello C, Koch K, Shaldon S (1988): Interleukin-1 and its relevance in patients treated with hemodialysis. Kidney Int 33:S21–S26.
Dinarello C, Mier J (1986): Interleukins. Annu Rev Med 37:173–178.
Edwards K, White H (1959): Creatinine excretion and body composition. Clin Sci 18:361–365.
Flores E, Drabik M, Bistrian BR (1986): The acute phase response to human recombinant mediators. Surg Forum 37:28–30.
Flores EA, Pomposelli JJ, Bistrian BR (1988): Interleukin-1. In Nadler P., Marcel Dekker (eds): "Protein and Peptides as Drugs." (in press)
Forbes GB, Bruining GJ (1976): Urinary creatinine excretion and lean body mass. Am J Clin Nutr 29:1359–1366.
Foschi D, Cavagna G, Callioni F, Morandi E, Rovati V (1986): Hyperalimentation of jaundiced patients on percutaneous transhepatic biliary drainage. Br J Surg 73:716–719.
Frawley JP, Artz CP, Howard JM (1955): Muscle metabolism and catabolism in combat casualties. Arch Surg 71:612–616.
Garrow JS (1974): Energy stores: Their composition, measurement and control. In "Energy Balance and Obesity in Man." Amsterdam, North Holland: pp 177–224.
Gersovitz M, Munro HN, Udall J, Young VR (1968): Albumin synthesis in young and elderly subjects using a new stable isotope methodology: Response to level of protein intake. J Clin Invest 47:1958–1972.
Grant JP (1983): Clinical impact of protein malnutrition on organ mass and function. In Blackburn GL, Grant JP, Young VR (eds): "Amino Acids: Metabolism and Medical Applications." Boston: John Wright, pp 347–358.
Harris JA, Benedict FG (1919): A biometric study of basal metabolism in man. Washington, DC: Carnegie Institute of Washington, Publication No. 279.
Harvey KB, Moldawer LL, Bistrian BR, Blackburn GL (1981): Biological measures for the formulation of a hospital prognostic index. Am J Clin Nutr 34:2013–2022.
Harvey KB, Ruggiero JA, Regan CS, Bistrian BR, Blackburn GL (1978): Hospital morbidity-mortality risk factors using nutritional assessment. Clin Res 26:581A.
Heatley RV, Williams RHP, Lewis MH (1979): Preoperative intravenous feeding—a controlled trial. Postgrad Med J 55:541–545.
Hehir DJ, Jenkins RL, Bistrian BR, Blackburn GL (1985): Nutrition in patients undergoing orthotopic liver transplant. J Parenter Enteral Nutr 9:695–700.
Heymsfield S, Arteaga C, McManus C, Smith J, Moffitt S (1984a): Measurement of muscle mass in humans: Validity of the 24-hour urinary creatinine method. Am J Clin Nutr 37:478–493.
Heymsfield SB, McManus CB (1985): Tissue components of weight loss in cancer patients: A new method of study and preliminary observations. Cancer 55:238–249.
Heymsfield SB, McManus CB, Seitz SB, Nixon DW, Andrews JS (1984b): Anthropometric assessment of adult protein-energy malnutrition. In Wright RA, Heymsfield SB, McManus CB (eds): "Nutritional Assessment." Boston: Blackwell Scientific, pp 27–82.
Heymsfield SB, Olafson RP, Kutner MH, Nixon DW (1979): A radiographic method of quantifying protein-calorie undernutrition. Am J Clin Nutr 32:693–702.
Heymsfield SB, Stevens V, Noel R, McManus CB, Smith J, Nixon D (1982): Biochemical composition of muscle in normal and semistarved human subjects: Relevance to anthropometric measurements. Am J Clin Nutr 36:131–142.

Hoffer LJ, Bistrian BR, Young VR, Blackburn GL, Matthews D (1984): Metabolic effects of very low calorie weight reduction diets. J Clin Invest 73:750–758.

Hoffman-Goetz L, McFarlane D, Bistrian BR, Blackburn GL (1981): Febrile and plasma iron responses of rabbits injected with endogenous pyrogen from malnourished patients. Am J Clin Nutr 34:1109–1116.

James WPT, Hay AM (1968): Albumin metabolism: Effect of the nutritional state and the dietary protein intake. J Clin Invest 47:1958–1972.

Jeejeebhoy KN (1986): Muscle function and nutrition. Gut 27:25–39.

Jeejeebhoy KN, Baker JP, Wolman SL, Wesson DE, Langer B, Harrison JE, McNeill KG (1982): Critical evaluation of the role of clinical asessment and body composition studies in patients with malnutrition and after total parenteral nutrition. Am J Clin Nutr 35:1117–1127.

Jelliffe DB (1966): "The Assessment of the Nutritional Status of the Community. " WHO Monograph 53. Geneva: WHO.

Jones JD, Burnett PC (1974): Creatinine metabolism in humans with decreased renal function: Creatinine deficit. Clin Chem 20:1204–1212.

Keenan RA, Moldawer LL, Yang RD, Kawamura I, Blackburn GL, Bistrian BR (1982): An altered response by peripheral leukocytes to synthesize or release leukocyte endogenous mediator in critically ill, protein-malnourished patients. J Lab Clin Med 100:844–857.

Keys A, Brozek J (1953): Physiol Rev 33:245–316.

Keys AJ, Brozek A, Henschel O, Michelson O, Taylor HL (1950): In "The Biology of Human Starvation." Minneapolis: University of Minnesota Press, pp 130–160.

Kinney JM, Duke JH, Long CL (1978): Tissue fuel and weight loss after injury. J Clin Pathol 4 (suppl):65–72.

Klidjian AN, Foster KJ, Kammerling RM, Cooper A, Karran SJ (1980): Relation of anthropometric and dynamometric variables to serious postoperative complication. Br Med J 281:899–901.

Kopple JD (1988): Dietary considerations in patients with advanced chronic renal failure. In Schrier RW, Gottschalk CW (eds): "Diseases of the Kidney." Boston: Little, Brown and Co, pp 3387–3436.

Lusk G (1976): "The Elements of the Science of Nutrition." 4th ed. New York: Johnson Reprint Corporation.

Miller AT, Blyth CS (1954): Estimation of lean body mass and body fat from basal oxygen consumption and creatinine excretion. J Appl Physiol 5:73–78.

Miller D, Levine S, Bistrian B, D'Elia J (1983): Diagnosis of protein calorie malnutrition in diabetic patients on hemodialysis and peritoneal dialysis. Nephron 33:127–132.

Moghissi K, Hornshaw J, Teasdale PR, Dawes EA (1977): Parenteral nutrition in carcinoma of the esophagus treated by surgery: Nitrogen balance and clinical studies. Br J Surg 64:125–128.

Montgomery RD (1962): Muscle morphology in infantile protein malnutrition. J Clin Pathol 15:511–519.

Moran WH, Miltenberger FW, Shuayb WA, Zimmerman B (1964): Relationship of antidiuretic hormone secretion to surgical stress. Surgery 56:99–108.

Mullen JL, Buzby GP, Matthews DC, Smale BF, Rosato EF (1980): Reduction of operative morbidity and mortality by combined preoperative and postoperative support. Ann Surg 142:604–613.

Mullen JL, Gertner MH, Buzby GP, Goodheart GL, Rosato EF (1979): Implication of malnutrition in the surgical patient. Arch Surg 114:121–125.

Muller J, Dienst C, Brenner V, Pichlmaier H (1982): Preoperative feeding in patients with gastrointestinal carcinoma. Lancet 1:68–71.

Nixon DW, Heymsfield SB, Cohen AE, Kutner MH, Ansley J, Lawson DH, Rudman D (1980): Protein-calorie undernutrition in hospitalized cancer patients. Am J Med 68:683–690.

O'Keefe SJ, Carraker TE, El-Zayadi AR, Davis M, Williams R (1980): Malnutrition and immuno-competence in patients with liver disease. Lancet 2:613–617.

Padberg FT, Ruggiero J, Blackburn GL, Bistrian BR (1981): Central venous catheterization for parenteral nutrition. Ann Surg 193:264–270.

Peret J, Jacquot R (1972): Nitrogen excretion on complete fasting and on a nitrogen-free diet-endogenous protein. In Bigwood EJ (ed): "Protein and Amino Acid Functions." Oxford: Pergamon Press, pp 73–118.

Pomposelli JJ, Flores EA, Bistrian BR (1987): Dose response of recombinant mediators in the acute phase response. Clin Res 35(3):514A.

Pomposelli JJ, Flores EA, Bistrian BR (1988): The role of biochemical mediators in clinical nutrition and surigical metabolism. J Parenter Enteral Nutr 12:212–218.

Portnay GI, O'Brien JT, Bush J, Vagenakis AG, Azizi F, Arky RA, Ingbar SH, Braverman LE (1974): The effect of starvation on the concentration and binding of thyroxine and triiodothyronine in serum and on the response to TRH. J Clin Endocrinol Metab 39:191–194.

Rothschild MA, Oratz M, Schreiber SS (1971): Albumin synthesis. N Engl J Med 286:816–821.

Roza A, Shizgal HM (1984): The Harris-Benedict equation reevaluated: Resting energy requirements and the body cell mass. Am J Clin Nutr 40:168–182.

Runcie J, Hilditch TE (1974): Energy provision, tissue utilization, and weight loss in prolonged starvation. Br Med J 2:352–356.

Ryan RJ, Williams JD, Ansell BM, Bernstein LM (1957): The relationship of body composition to oxygen consumption and creatinine excretion in healthy and wasted men. Metabolism 6:365–377.

Schade DJ, Santiago JV, Skyler JS, Rizza RA (1983): Substrate and hormonal alterations in diabetes mellitus. In Schade DJ, Santiago JV, Skyler JS, Rizza RA (eds): "Intensive Insulin Therapy." Amsterdam: Excerpta Medica Offices, pp 36–68.

Schoenfeld P, Henry R, Laird N, Roxe D (1983): Assessment of nutritional status of the national cooperative dialysis study population. Kidney Int 23:580–588.

Scrimshaw NS, Taylor CE, Gordon JE (1968): Interactions of nutrition and infection. Geneva: WHO Scientific Monograph.

Shafrir E, Bergman M, Felig P (1987): The endocrine pancreas: Diabetes mellitus. In Felig P, Baxter J, Broadus A, Frohman L (eds): "Endocrinology and Metabolism." New York: McGraw-Hill Book Company, pp 1043–1178.

Shanbhogue RL, Bistrian BR, Jenkins RL, Jones C, Benotti P, Blackburn GL (1987): Resting energy expenditure in patients with end-stage liver disease and in normal population. J Parenter Enternal Nutr 11:305–308.

Stein T (1978): Cachexia, gluconeogenesis and progressive weight loss in cancer patients. J Theor Biol 73:51–52.

Studley HO (1936): Percentage of weight loss: A basic indicator of surgical risk in patients with chronic peptic ulcer. JAMA 106:458–460.

Talbot NB (1938): Measurement of obesity by the creatinine coefficient. Am J Dis Child 55:42–50.

Tocco-Bradley R, Georgieff M, Jones CT, Moldawer LL, Dinarello CA, Blackburn GL,

Bistrian BR (1988): Changes in energy expenditure and fat metabolism in rats infused with interleukin-1. Eur J Clin Invest 17:504–510.
Tomlinson B, Walton J, Rebeiz J (1969): The effects of aging and cachexia upon skeletal muscle—a histopathologic study. J Neurol Sci 9:321–346.
Tracey KJ, Beutler B, Lowry SF, Merryweather J, Wolpe S, Milsark IW, Hariri RJ, Fahey TJ, Zentella A, Albert JD, Shires GT, Cerami A (1986): Shock and tissue injury induced by recombinant human cachetin. Science 234:470–474.
Tracey KJ, Lowry SF, Fahey TJ, Albert JD, Foing Y, Hesse D, Beutler B, Manogue KR, Calvano S, Wei H, Cerami A, Shires GT (1987): Cachectin/tumor necrosis factor induces lethal shock and stres hormone responses in the dog. Surg Gynecol Obstet 164:415–422.
Vagenakis AG, Portnay GI, O'Brien JT (1977): Effect of starvation on the production and metabolism of thyroxine and triiodothyronine in euthyroid obese patients. J Clin Endocrinol Metab 45:1305–1309.
Viteri FE, Alvarado J (1970): The creatinine-height index: Its use in the estimation of the degree of protein depletion and repletion in protein-calorie malnourished children. Pediatrics 46:696–706.
Warren S (1932): The immediate causes of death in cancer. Am J Med Sci 184:610–615.
Waterlow JC, Neale RJ, Rowe L, Palin I (1972): Effect of diet and infection on creatine turnover in the rat. Am J Clin Nutr 25:371–375.
Williams RHP, Heatley RR, Lewis MH (1976): A randomized controlled trial of preoperative intravenous nutrition in patients with stomach cancer. Br J Surg 63:667–670.
Young GA, Hill GL (1979): Assessment of protein calorie malnutrition in surgical patients from plasma proteins and anthropometric measurements. Am J Clin Nutr 31:429–435.

Anthropometric Assessment
of Nutritional Status, pages 383–398

23
Anthropometric Assessment in an Adult Obesity Clinic

DAVID S. GRAY AND GEORGE A. BRAY
Department of Medicine, University of Southern California, Los Angeles, California 90033

INTRODUCTION

In addition of quantifying body dimensions, anthropometric measurements can be used to estimate body composition and fat distribution. The measurements in common use possess several advantages which make them especially suitable for use in the obesity clinic. Each of these, including weight and height, skinfolds, and body circumferences, will be discussed in detail below. In general they are inexpensive and require only simple and widely available equipment. They are portable and thus can be used in a variety of locations. Patients find most of the measurements quite acceptable, and they usually require very little time or technical expertise.

As estimates of body composition, anthropometric measures possess the disadvantage that they are indirect. Several alternative methods are available which are generally felt to give more accurate estimates of body composition. Table 1 lists a variety of body composition methods with estimates of their cost and ease of use as well as a global assessment of accuracy which takes into account both reliability and validity. The laboratory methods include underwater weighing, total body water determination, and ^{40}K counting (Lukaski, 1987). While these are in common use in research settings, they have not found general use in outpatient settings because of several disadvantages. They all require special equipment which is available only at a limited number of laboratories. They also tend to be expensive and time-consuming, and require technical expertise. Furthermore, there has been no demonstration that information gained from these measurements can significantly improve the management of obese patients in the outpatient setting. Thus, anthropometric measurements are more suitable for use in the obesity clinic.

Several considerations make the measurement or estimation of body composition important in the outpatient treatment of obesity. First, obesity is defined as an abnormal accumulation of body fat (Bray, 1976). Thus determination of body composition is implicit in the definition of obesity. Second, body

TABLE 1. Comparison of Methods of Estimating Body Fat and Its Distribution

	Cost[a]	Ease of use	Accuracy	Regional fat
Height and weight	$	Easy	High	No
Skinfolds	$	Easy	Low	Yes
Circumferences	$	Easy	Moderate	Yes
Density—immersion	$$	Moderate	High	No
—plethysmograph	$$$	Difficult	High	No
Water (^3H_2O, D_2O, $H_2{}^{18}O$)	$$	Moderate	High	No
Potassium (^{40}K)	$$$	Difficult	High	No
Conductivity (TOBEC)	$$$	Moderate	High	No
Bioelectric impedance	$$	Easy	High	No
Fat soluble gas	$$	Difficult	High	No
Computed tomography	$$$$	Difficult	High	Yes
Ultrasound	$$$	Moderate	Moderate	Yes
Neutron activation	$$$$	Difficult	High	No
Magnetic resonance	$$$$	Difficult	High	Yes

[a]$ = low cost; $$ = moderate cost; $$$ = high cost; $$$$ = very high cost.

composition has been shown repeatedly to relate to the health risks of obesity. As we will discuss in more detail below, both the amount of body fat and the anatomical distribution of that fat determine the amount of risk faced by an individual. Patients in higher risk categories should probably be treated more aggressively than those for whom obesity poses little or no problem. Therefore, if body composition determination can aid in risk assessment, it is of great importance in the obesity clinic. A third consideration is the determination of prognosis for successful treatment. This is a different and often overlooked area. Bjorntorp (1980) has suggested that fat cell morphology (particularly fat cell size and fat cell number) may predict the outcome of treatment for obesity. If some component of body composition relating to fat cell morphology can be measured anthropometrically, it is conceivable that a determination of prognosis could be made. A fourth point is the estimation of energy requirements. Resting energy expenditure is dependent to a large extent on body composition, and anthropometric measures have been used frequently to estimate or predict energy requirements (Owen et al., 1987). Such a determination can be of utility in the prescription of a caloric intake required for weight loss. The final consideration is the monitoring of progress during weight loss therapy. Since obesity is defined as increased body fat, and body fat relates to health risks, loss of body fat is a natural indicator of treatment success. It is also possible that measurement of changes in body fat distribution will be of benefit in determining the results of treatment. Anthropometric measurements also offer the potential advantage of separating fat from lean body mass. The amount of lean tissue lost along with body fat during weight loss therapy is often considered to relate to potential hazards of caloric restriction (Van Itallie and Yang, 1984). Thus, estimates of the quantity of both lean body mass and fat mass during weight loss would appear to be of great importance in the obesity clinic. In the sections to follow, each of the common anthropometric measurements will be discussed in light of these considerations.

WEIGHT AND HEIGHT

The most commonly used anthropometric measures in obesity clinics and medical practice in general are weight and height. They have the advantages of wide availability of equipment, ease and accuracy of use, and general acceptability to patients. In fact, most patients define obesity on the basis of body weight. The basic problem with these measures is that body weight is strongly correlated with body height, and for this reason is not a good measure of body fat. Two basic approaches have been used to overcome these difficulties.

The first is *relative weight.* This approach, which has been popularized by the insurance industry, involves dividing the patient's weight by a standard weight which is based on the patient's height. Relative weight has been used for many years and is generally accepted by the medical community and the population at large. It is a concept that is easy to understand, and it has been usefull to the insurance industry and in many epidemiologic studies, including the Framingham Study (Hubert et al., 1983). Nevertheless, the relative weight concept does have disadvantages. First, some sort of standard weight is required. The standard weights used most frequently are those published by the Metropolitan Life Insurance Company (1959, 1983), which are based on the weight associated with the lowest mortality at any given height. The appropriateness of their use has been debated (Russell et al., 1984). One problem is that it is not known exactly how closely an obese patient must approach the standard or acceptable weight for a satisfactory reduction in risk. A second problem is that tables of standard weights are required in order to determine relative weights, so there is no single standard for all patients.

This latter problem is addressed in part by the second basic approach to the use of weight and height, which is the *weight–height index.* This is defined as the weight divided by some power of height (W/H^p) (Benn, 1971). The power function (p) is selected for a population to give the maximum correlation with body fat and the minimum correlation with body height. When p is 2, the result is the body mass, or Quetelet index (kg/m^2), which is the most commonly used weight–height index. In fact, studies have shown that the body mass index (BMI) relates closely to body fat while being quite independent of height (Keys et al., 1972; Roche et al., 1981). Recently, Garrow and Webster (1985) have suggested that the BMI is actually a measure of body fat related to height rather than percent of body fat, and that this is a better measure of obesity than percentage body fat. While a value of 2 for p is a close approximation to the optimal, some authors have suggested that it is not the best to use, especially in children and possibly in women. In fact, analysis of the data from the NHANES I study conducted by the National Center for Health Statistics suggested that while a value for p of 2 was adequate for men, a value of 1.5 was preferable for women (Abraham et al., 1983). For the purpose of an obesity clinic, a standard value of 2 for p is more practical, and studies suggest that correlations with body fat are adequate (Garrow and Webster, 1985; Leonhardt et al., 1987). Because the calculation of body mass index is required each time a weight is determined, nomograms have been devised for this purpose which can easily be displayed near the scale (Fig. 1).

While the calculation of body mass index is more complex than that of relative weight, its interpretation is possibly more simple. As will be seen below, identical standard values can be used for all adult patients, both men women. Thus, once a body mass index is calculated, it can be related to a single set of easily memorized standards. For this reason, as well as its strong correlation with body fatness and increasing use in epidemiologic studies, we recommend the routine use of the body mass index in the obesity clinic.

Both relative weight and body mass index suffer from the fact that they are still measures of overweight and only estimates of body fat. A heavily muscled athlete will have a high value of either of these indices while he may have a very low fat content and none of the usual concomitants of obesity (Segal et al., 1987). If judgment is used, they both can give good approximations of the degree of obesity, and they both have been used in numerous epidemiologic studies to assess the degree of risk associated with obesity (Manson et al., 1987). It is interesting that the curves relating BMI to mortality for men and women are virtually superimposable (Fig. 2). This means that minimum mortality is associated with a body mass index of about 22 kg/m^2 in both sexes. We have divided this curve into BMI intervals of increasing risk which can be very easily remembered. Interestingly, for any given BMI, women will be fatter than men even though the risk of mortality is the same.

One of the strongest predictors of rate and amount of weight loss during caloric restriction is degree of overweight (Garrow et al., 1978). Thus weight–height of expected weight loss on a given caloric restricted regimen.

Estimation of energy requirements can be an important part of prescribing calorie-restricted diets. An attempt is often made to prescribe a fixed energy deficit (e.g., 500 kcal or more per day), and this requires knowledge of the patient's energy expenditure. Furthermore, the deficit actually incurred on an energy-restricted diet will determine the rate of weight loss (Garrow et al., 1978), so information about a patient's energy expenditure should give an indication of expected progress during weight reduction therapy. Body composition has repeatedly been shown to be a strong correlate of resting energy expenditure from which total daily energy expenditure can be estimated (Jequier and Schutz, 1983). Though many regression equations are available for this purpose, those recently published by Owen et al. (1987) offer the advantage of including only body weight and appear to be as accurate as any

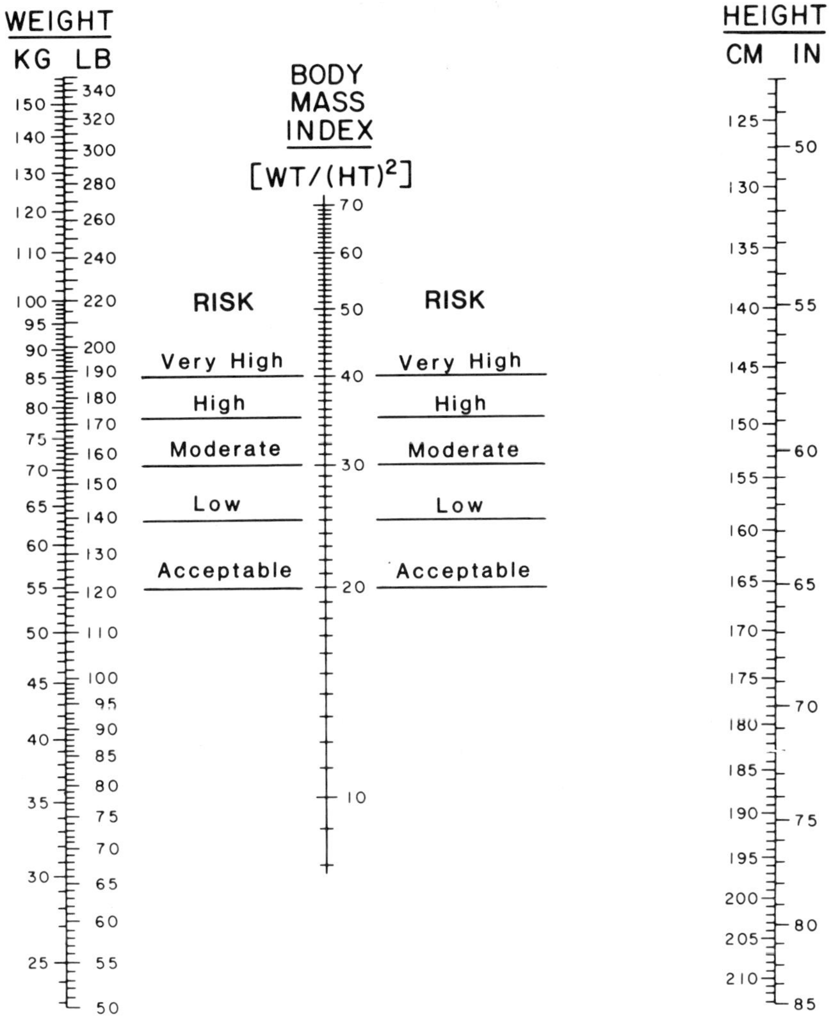

Fig. 1. Nomogram for determining body mass index (BMI). Place a straight edge between the column for weight and the column for height and read the BMI from the point where this straight edge crosses the body mass index line. (Copyright 1987, George A. Bray. Reproduced with permission.)

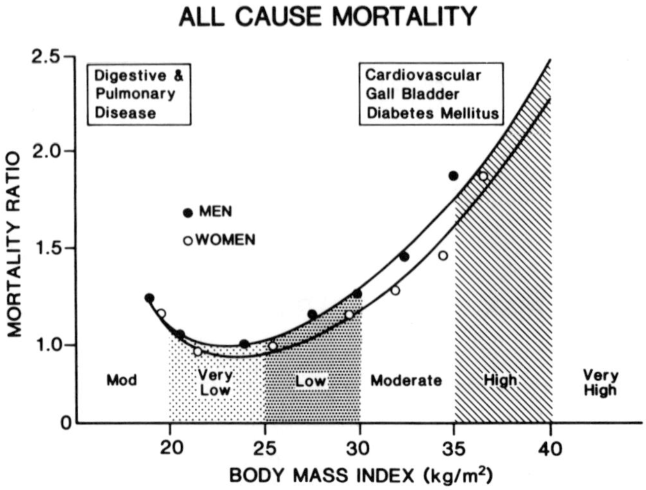

Fig. 2. Mortality ratio and body mass index. Data from the American Cancer Society study have been plotted for men and women to show the relationship of body mass index to overall mortality. At a body mass index below 20 kg/m^2 and above 25 kg/m^2 there is an increase in relative mortality. The major causes for this increased mortality are listed along with a division of body mass index groupings into various levels of risk. (Adapted from Lew and Garfinkel, 1979.)

others currently available. Table 2 presents a modification of these equations using rounded coefficients to simplify calculations and instructions for estimating total daily energy expenditure. Estimates of energy expenditure based on body composition are subject to considerable error and should be thought of only as rough guides.

TABLE 2. Estimation of Daily Energy Requirement (kcal/day)[a]

1. Calculation of resting metabolic rate (RMR)

$$\text{RMR (Men)} = 900 + 10 \times \text{(Weight in kg)}$$

$$\text{RMR (Women)} = 800 + 7 \times \text{(Weight in kg)}$$

2. Daily energy requirement = RMR × Activity factor

Activity level	Activity factor
Low (sedentary)	1.2
Moderate	1.4
High (regular exercise or manual labor)	1.6

[a]Adapted from Owen et al. (1987).

SKINFOLDS

Skinfold thickness measurement possesses many of the same advantages as weight and height measurement. The calipers are inexpensive and portable. The measurements are relatively simple to perform and quite acceptable to patients. Thus if use of skinfolds adds useful clinical information, they would appear to be ideal for the outpatient obesity clinic.

Many studies comparing the results of skinfold measurements to underwater weighing in the same subjects have been reviewed recently by Lohman (1981). These studies have yielded regression equations which use one or more skinfolds or the sum of several skinfolds to predict percent body fat. Thus, if one measures the appropriate skinfolds, an equation can be used to estimate a patient's body fat. Durnin and Womersley (1974) have provided their frequently used equations in the form of a table which gives the percent body fat value associated with different values for the sum of four skinfolds (biceps, triceps, subscapular, and suprailiac). Allen et al. (1956) pointed out the nonlinearity of the relationship between internal and external (subcutaneous) adiposity. This suggests that a simple linear regression may not be adequate, and the so-called generalized equations of Jackson et al. (1978, 1980) have included quadratic terms which may be more valid. Whichever equations are used, it is possible to obtain an estimate of body fatness from the use of skinfold measurements.

Skinfolds have been used in several epidemiologic studies relating body composition to disease risk, including those performed by the National Center for Health Stastistics (NHANES I) (NCHS, 1973). For example, Garn et al. (1983) used skinfolds among other indices of fatness in a prospective study in West Scotland. They demonstrated that lean individuals had excess deaths from cancer and obese individuals showed excess cardiovascular mortality. Studies such as this have demonstrated that fatness as distinguished from overweight can be related to mortality risk.

Skinfolds have also been used to measure body fat distribution. Mueller and Stallones (1981) used principal components analysis to evaluate skinfold data. This method looks for correlations between combinations of different skinfolds and groups together those which correlate well with each other. These investigators found that the skinfolds could be seperated into two groups, the first of which consisted of sums of skinfolds and related closely to body fatness. The second "component" of skinfold data consisted of differences between trunk and extremity skinfolds and was termed the *fat-patterning index.* The fat-patterning index showed no correlation with the total body fatness component.

The principal components method was used to analyze skinfold thickness data from the Paris Prospective Study, and it was found that both the total adiposity component and the fat-patterning component, which demonstrated trunk adiposity (compared to thigh), were greater in those subjects who developed coronary disease (Ducimetiere et al., 1986). In a study of Mexican-Americans, it was found that both the waist-to-hips circumference ratio (discussed later) and the subscapular-to-triceps skinfold ratio (an indicator of truncal versus peripheral fat distribution) were associated with high rates of diabetes mellitus, low HDL cholesterol levels, and high triglyceride levels (Haffner et al., 1987). Interestingly, data from the Honolulu Heart Program reveal that the risk of development of coronary disease is greater for those with a higher subscapular skinfold thickness at any level of body mass index (Donahue et al., 1987). Furthermore, when corrected for subscapular skinfold thickness, body mass index had no independent effect on coronary risk. These studies suggest that central body or truncal distribution of body fat may be a more important risk factor than total body fat. The waist-to-hips circumference ratio to be discussed in more detail below has received more attention as an indicator of fat distribution, but the use of trunk-to-limb skinfold ratios may be equally valid. In fact, the study by Haffner et al. (1987) suggested that the subscapular-to-triceps skinfold ratio and the waist-to-hips ratio were independent predictors of diabetes mellitus.

In addition to the use of skinfolds to estimate body fat and its distribution in the initial risk assessment of obese patients, their ease and rapidity of use make them ideal for monitoring progress during therapy. In light of the above discussion, it would be anticipated that the risks attendant to obesity would decrease in proportion to decreases in body fat and particularly centrally located body fat. Serial measurements during weight loss treatment can document and quantify these changes, although at this time there is inadequate data available to establish norms or goals for treatment. Furthermore, since skinfold measurements can provide an indirect estimate of lean body mass (body weight − fat mass), they could be used in principle to measure losses in the body protein compartment during weight loss. As mentioned earlier, many authors feel that losses of body protein or lean body mass should be limited as much as possible during therapeutic weight loss (Van Itallie and Yang, 1984).

There are several problems which must be considered when using skinfold thickness measurements. The first of these relates to measurement errors. In his review of the literature, Lohman (1981) stressed the importance of interobserver errors. While an experienced anthropometrist can obtain consistent measurements, there is commonly wide variation between values obtained by different observers. These may be due to differences in measurement technique as well as site selection. Measurement errors may be compounded by obesity. Bray et al. (1978) found greater interobserver differences between skinfold measurements taken on obese subjects than those taken on lean subjects. Repeated measurements on obese subjects showed differences ranging from 11% to 21.6%. In addition, it was impossible to obtain abdominal, subscapular, and suprailiac skinfolds on a significant number of obese patients because the calipers were not large enough to accommodate them.

The second problem with the use of skinfolds comes in the estimation of percent body fat. Regression equations which relate skinfold measurements to underwater weighing work very well on the population from which they were derived, but correlations tend to decrease when they are applied to other populations (Lohman, 1981). This may explain the wealth of equations available today. A review of this literature reveals that very few obese people have been included in the samples from which these equations were derived (Bray and Gray, 1988a). Thus considerable caution must be exercised in the use of existing equations for the prediction of body fatness from skinfold thicknesses in obese patients.

Martin et al. (1985) have recently published an autopsy study which evaluated the assumptions involved in the use of skinfolds for body composition determination. First, it is assumed that skinfolds are equally compressible at different sites and in different individuals. These authors found that compressibility determined by measuring adipose tissue depth at autopsy and comparing it to caliper-determined values varied from 34% to 64% at different sites and by similar amounts from one person to another. Caliper use also assumes a constant skin thickness from one site to another, but this study showed that skin thickness varied from 8.2% of the caliper reading (medial thigh) to 28.1% (subscapular). A third assumption of a constant thickness of the adipose tissue layer throughout the body is clearly not correct, pointing to the need to sample a variety of areas in order to make conclusions about whole body fatness. A fourth assumption is that internal fat, which is not measured by skinfold thicknesses, either makes up a constant proportion of total body fat or is very small compared to the subcutaneous fat mass. The data of Martin et al. (1985) suggest that there is a linear correlation between subcutaneous fat and internal fat and that the latter is about 15% of the former. However, their sample only included subjects with up to 35kg of subcutaneous fat. As mentioned above, Allen et al. (1956) using indirect methods concluded that internal fat makes up about 10% of total body fat in the lean, but could account for up to 65% of total body fat in the morbidly obese.

The final problem with the use of skinfolds for the measurement of total body composition comes from the effects of weight loss. Scherf et al. (1986) recently published a study in which body fat was estimated by skinfold measurements and compared to underwater weighing in patients who had lost more than 40 kg by caloric restriction. They concluded that the current equations significantly overestimated body fatness in these patients. This appears to be one more example of the lack of applicability of regression equations that were not derived specifically for the population to be measured.

These problems have led some authors to conclude that it would be better to use skinfold measurements by themselves and compare them to their own norms rather than to attempt to use them to make estimates of total body composition (Johnston, 1982; Martin et al., 1985). It is clear that numerous obstacles stand in the way of accurate prediction of body fatness from skinfold thicknesses. However, data cited above suggest that they may be valuable indicators of fat distribution patterns and their associated medical risks. Furthermore, if performed by one experienced observer, they may yield valuable data about trends in fatness over time within individuals.

CIRCUMFERENCES

The measurement of body circumferences with a tape measure poses the same advantages of portability, ease, and acceptability as skinfold thicknesses. In addition, circumference measurement appears to be more precise and less subject to interobserver errors than does skinfold determination, even in obese subjects (Bray et al., 1978). Thus if they yield valuable information, circumferences should be ideally suited for use in the obesity clinic.

Though some authors have suggested the use of circumferences at several locations for the determination of total body fatness (Weltman and Katch, 1975), they have found their biggest use in the estimation of body fat distribution. Prospective studies in Gothenburg, Sweden, have shown that both men and women who have a high ratio of waist to hip circumferences have increased risk of death, stroke, and ischemic heart disease (Larsson et al., 1984; Lapidus et al., 1984). Studies have shown that a greater waist-to-hips ratio is associated with higher blood pressure, glucose intolerance, and higher serum lipid levels (kissebah et al., 1982; Krotkiewski et al., 1983).

It is thus possible to characterize obese patients on the basis of the ratio of the circumferences of the abdomen or waist to the gluteal region or hips. These may be called the abdominal–gluteal ratio (AGR, also android–gynoid ratio) or the waist-to-hips ratio (WHR). A nomogram for calculating AGR is shown in Figure 3.

Patients with an elevated AGR (e.g., AGR $>$ 0.95 for men, and AGR $>$ 0.85 for women) are said to have abdominal, android, or male pattern of obesity, while patients with low AGR are said to have gluteal, gynoid, or female pattern of obesity (Gray and Bray, 1988). It appears from the literature cited above that the fat distribution pattern is more important than total adiposity in determining a patient's risk from obesity. Figure 4 depicts risk levels associated with different AGR according to age. Individuals with abdominal obesity are at greater risk of cardiovascular complications than those with gluteal obesity.

The explanation for the increased risks associated with abdominal obesity is unknown, but one theory is that abdominal fat calls are more metabolically active and thus tend to release more free fatty acids. These fatty acids could contribute to increased insulin resistance at the liver and elsewhere, and could possibly explain many of the metabolic phenomenon of increased AGR obesity (Larsson et al., 1984). In this context, it is interesting that Fujioka et al. (1987) have demonstrated that subjects with a greater ratio of intra-abdominal to subcutaneous fat as determined by abdominal CT scan have higher serum lipids and decreased glucose tolerance compared to those with relatively greater subcutaneous fat.

Since body fat distribution appears to be useful in the determination of health risks associated with obesity, it would be logical to postulate that a decrease in AGR with obesity treatment would be beneficial. Thus, the AGR should be a useful index for monitoring therapy. Unfortunately, data are not yet available to evaluate the effects of weight loss therapy on AGR and its associated risks.

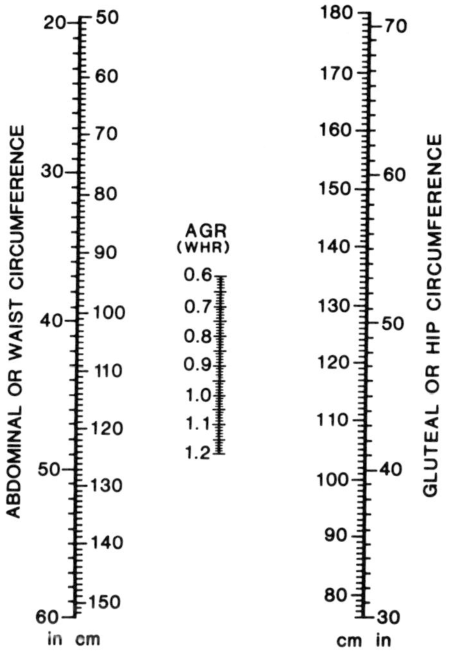

Fig. 3. Nomogram for determining abdominal (waist) to gluteal (hips) ratio. Place a straight edge between the column for waist circumference and the column for hip circumference and read the ratio from the point where this straight edge crosses the AGR (WHR) line. The waist or abdominal circumference is the smallest circumference below the rib cage and above the umbilicus, and the hips or gluteal circumference is taken as the largest circumference at the posterior extension of the buttocks. (Copyright 1987, George A. Bray. Reproduced with permission.)

SUMMARY AND RECOMMENDATIONS

Compared with laboratory methods for body composition determination, anthropometric measurements have distinct advantages for the obesity clinic. They are in general rapid, inexpensive, simple to perform, and quite acceptable to patients. Within the limitations discussed above, estimations can be obtained for body fat, lean body mass, and fat distribution. These in turn can be useful for determination of risk in individual patients and in some settings may be useful in determining prognosis of therapy and in monitoring progress over time.

The following measurements are recommended for general use in the obesity clinic. We use the methods outlined by Lohman et al. (1988). Body height and weight with calculation of body mass index are the most important measures. Circumferences are to be preferred over skinfold thicknesses, and the

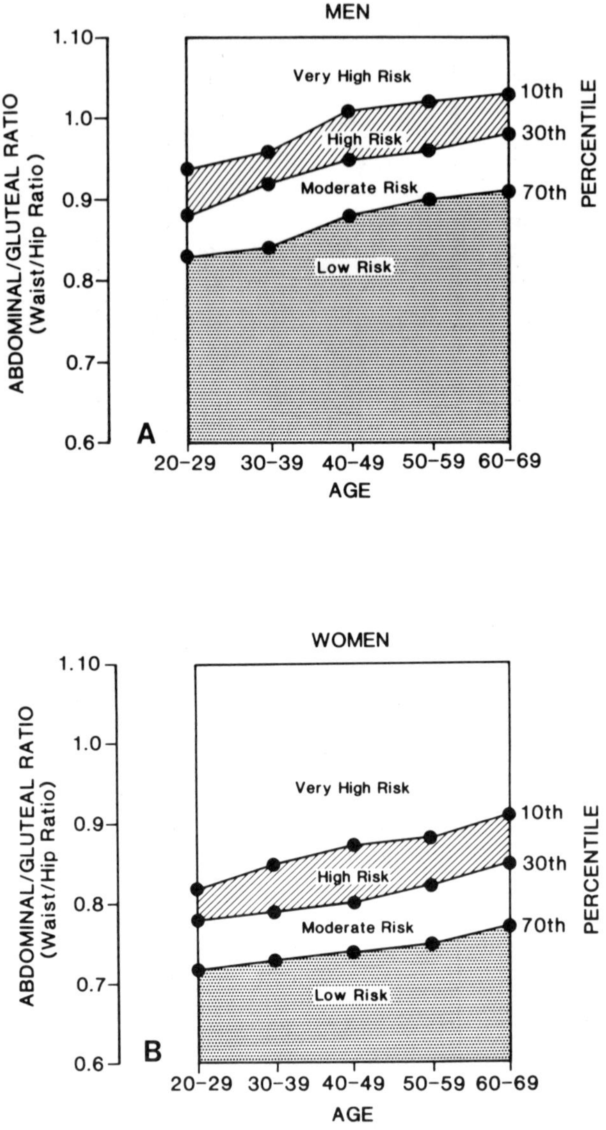

Fig. 4. Percentiles for fat distribution. The percentiles for the ratio of abdominal circumference to gluteal circumference (ratio of waist to hips) are depicted for men **(A)** and women **(B)** by age groups. The relative risk for these percentiles is indicated based on the available information. (Plotted from tabular data in the Canadian Standardized Test of Fitness, 3rd ed, 1986. Copyright 1987, George A. Bray. Reproduced with permission.)

abdomen and gluteus (hips) should be measured with calculation of abdominal–gluteal ratio. The issue of skinfold thicknesses is more complex because of the problems delineated above and the lack of adequate data to decide on their most appropriate use. If they are to be used to determine body fat, a minimum of four sites is probably necessary, with two trunk sites (e.g., subscapular and suprailiac or abdomen) and two limb sites (e.g., triceps and thigh or calf). For determination of skinfold distribution, the subscapular–triceps ratio may be the best, although a trunk and lower limb comparison might be just as good.

In order to use these measurements most efficiently to determine initial risk from obesity, we have developed an algorithm (Fig. 5). The patient is first classified on the basis of body mass index. Then the degree of risk is modified

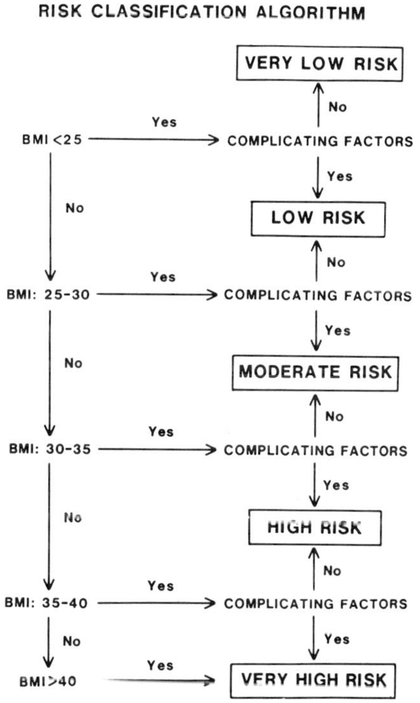

Fig. 5. Risk classification algorithm. The patient is first classified by body mass index (BMI) by moving down the left hand column. Then the risk is determined by the presence or absence of complicating factors. Complicating factors include an elevated abdominal–gluteal circumference ratio (AGR $>$ 0.95 in males, AGR $>$ 0.85 in females), hypertension, hyperlipidemia, glucose intolerance, cardiac disease, or other medical conditions. (Copyright 1987, George A. Bray. Reproduced with permission.)

by the presence or absence of complicating factors. The first of these is an elevated abdominal–gluteal circumference ratio (AGR > 0.95 in males, AGR > 0.85 in females), and others include hypertension, hyperlipidemia, glucose intolerance, cardiac disease, or other medical condition. The risks thus determined can serve as a guide to selection of appropriate therapy (Bray and Gray, 1988b).

REFERENCES

Abraham S, Carroll MD, Najjar MF, Fulwood R (1983): Overweight and obese adults in the United States. Vital and Health Statistics, DHHS Publication No. (PHS) 83-1680, National Health Survey Ser. 11, No. 230, pp 1–28.

Allen TH, Peng MT, Chen KP, Huang TF, Chang C, Fang HS (1956): Prediction of total adiposity from skinfolds and the curvilinear relationship between external and internal adiposity. Metabolism 5:346–352.

Benn RT (1971): Some mathematical properties of weight-for-height indices used as measures of adiposity. Br J Prev Soc Med 25:42–50.

Bjorntorp P (1980): Results of conservative therapy of obesity: Correlation with adipose tissue morphology. Am J Clin Nutr 33:370–375.

Bray GA (1976): "The Obese Patient." Philadelphia: WB Saunders.

Bray GA, Gray DS(1988a): Anthropometric measurements in the obese. In Lohman TG, Roche A, Martorell R (eds): "Anthropometric Standardization Manual". Champaign, Il: Human Kinetics, pp 131–136.

Bray GA, Gray DS (1988b): Obesity, II: Treatment. West J Med 149:555–571.

Bray GA, Greenway FL, Molitch ME, Dahms WT, Atkinson RL, Hamilton K (1978): Use of anthropometric measures to assess weight loss. Am J Clin Nutr 31:769–773.

Donahue RP, Bloom E, Abbott RD, Reed DM, Yano K (1987): Central obesity and coronary heart disease in men. Lancet 1:821–824.

Ducimetiere P, Richard J, Cambien F (1986): The pattern of subcutaneous fat distribution in middle-aged men and the risk of coronary heart disease: The Paris Prospective Study. Int J Obes 10:229–240.

Durnin JVGA, Womersley J (1974): Body fat assessed from total body density and its estimation from skinfold thickness: Measurements on 481 men and women aged from 16 to 72 years. Br J Nutr 32:77–97.

Fujioka S, Matsuzawa Y, Tokunaga K, Tarui S (1987): Contribution of intra-abdominal fat accumulation to the impairment of glucose and lipid metabolism in human obesity. Metabolism 36:54–59.

Garn SM, Hawthorne VM, Pilkington JJ, Pesick SD (1983): Fatness and mortality in the West of Scotland. Am J Clin Nutr 38:313–319.

Garrow JS, Durrant ML, Mann S, Stalley SF, Warwick PM (1978): Factors determining weight loss in obese patients in a metabolic ward. Int J Obes 2:441–447.

Garrow JS, Webster J (1985): Quetelet's index (W/H^2) as a measure of fatness. Int J Obes 9:147–153.

Gray DS, Bray GA (1988). Evaluation of the obese patient. In Burrows GD, Beaumont PJV, Casper R (eds): "Handbook of Eating Disorders, Part 2." Amsterdam, the Netherlands: Elsevier, pp 47–59.

Haffner SM, Stern MP, Hazuda HP, Pugh J, Patterson JK (1987): Do upper-body and centralized adiposity measure different aspects of regional body-fat distribution? Diabetes 36:43–51.

Hubert HB, Feinleib M, McNamara PM, Castelli WP (1983): Obesity as an independent risk factor for cardiovascular disease: A 26-year follow up of participants in the Framingham Heart Study. Circulation 67:968–977.

Jackson AS, Pollock ML (1978): Generalized equations for predicting body density of men. Br J Nutr 40:497–504.

Jackson AS, Pollock ML, Ward A (1980): Generalized equations for predicting body density of women. Med Sci Sports Excerc 12:175–182.

Jequier E, Schutz Y (1983): Long-term measurements of energy expenditure in humans using a respiration chamber. Am J Clin Nutr 38:989–998.

Johnston FE (1982): Relationships between body composition and anthropometry. Hum Biol 54:221–245.

Keys A, Fidanza F, Karvonen MJ, Kimura N, Taylor HL (1972): Indices of relative weight and obesity. J Chronic Dis 25:329–343.

Kissebah AH, Vydelingum N, Murray R, Evans DJ, Hartz AJ, Kalkhoff RK, Adams PW (1982): Relation of body fat distribution to metabolic complications of obesity. J Clin Endocrinol Metab 54:254–260.

Krotkiewski M, Bjorntorp P, Sjostrom L, Smith U (1983): Impact of obesity on metabolism in men and women: Importance of regional adipose tissue distribution. J Clin Invest 72:1150–1162.

Lapidus L, Bengtsson C, Larsson B, Pennert K, Rybo E, Sjostrom L (1984): Distribution of adipose tissue and risk of cardiovascular disease and death: A 12 year follow up of participants in the population study of women in Gothenburg, Sweden. Br Med J 289:1257–1261.

Larsson B, Svardsudd K, Welin L, Wilhelmsen L, Bjorntorp P, Tibblin (1984): Abdominal adipose tissue distribution, obesity, and risk of cardiovascular disease and death: 13 year follow up of participants in the study of men born in 1913. Br Med J 288:1401–1404.

Leonhardt W, Hanefeld M, Julius U, Schulze J, Fischer S, Weck M, Haller H (1987): Predictive value of the index of desirable body weight for total body fat mass as measured by dilution of tritiated water-problems and limitations. Int J Obes 11:221–228.

Lew EA, Garfinkel L (1979): Variations in mortality by weight among 750,000 men and women. J Chronic Dis 32:563–576.

Lohman TG (1981): Skinfolds and body density and their relation to body fatness: A review. Hum Biol 53:181–225.

Lohman TG, Roche A, Martorell R (1988): "Anthropometric Standardization Manual." Champaign, Ill: Human Kinetics.

Lukaski HC (1987): Methods for the assessment of human body composition: Traditional and new. Am J Clin Nutr 46:537–556.

Manson JE, Stampfer MJ, Hennekens CH, Willett WC (1987): Body weight and longevity: A reassessment. JAMA 257:353–358.

Martin AD, Ross WD, Drinkwater DT, Clarys JP (1985): Prediction of body fat by skin fold caliper: Assumptions and cadaver evidence. Int J Obes 9:31–39.

Metropolitan Life Insurance Company (1959): New weight standards for men and women. Stat Bull NY Metropolitan Life Insurance Co 40:1–4.

Metropolitan Life Insurance Company (1983): Metropolitan height and weight tables. Stat Bull NY Metropolitan Life Insurance Co 64:2–9.

Mueller WH, Stallones L (1981): Anatomical distribution of subcutaneous fat: Skinfold site choice and construction of indices. Hum Biol 53:321–335.

National Center for Health Statistics (1973): Plan and operation of the Health and Nutrition Examinatin Survey, United States, 1971–1973. Washington, DC: Health Services and Mental Health Administration. Vital and Health Statistics, Ser. 1. Nos. 10a, 10b. DHEW Publ. No. (HSM)73-1310.

Owen OE, Holup JL, D'Alessio DA, Craig ES, Polansky M, Smalley KJ, Kavle EC, Bushman MC, Owens LR, Mozzoli MA, Kendrick ZV, Boden GH (1987): A reappraisal of the caloric requirements of men. Am J Clin Nutr 46:875–885.

Roche AF, Siervogel RM, Chumlea WC, Webb P (1981): Grading body fatness from limited anthropometric data. Am J Clin Nutr 34:2831–2828.

Russell M, McGandy RB, Jelliffe D (1984): Reference weights: Practical considerations. Am J Med 76:767–769.

Scherf J, Franklin BA, Lucas CP, Stevenson D, Rubenfire M (1986): Validity of skinfold thickness measures of formerly obese adults. Am J Clin Nutr 43:128–135.

Segal K, Dunaif A, Gutin B, Albu J, Nyman A, Pi-Sunyer FX (1987): Body composition, not body weight, is related to cardiovascular disease risk factors and sex hormone levels in men. J Clin Invest 80:1050–1055.

Van Itallie TB, Yang M (1984): Cardiac dysfunction in obese dieters: A potentially lethal complication of rapid, massive weight loss. Am J Clin Nutr 39:695–702.

Weltman A, Katch V (1975): Preferential use of casing (girth) measures for estimating body volume and density. J Appl Physiol 38:560–563.

Anthropometric Assessment
of Nutritional Status, pages 399–418

24
Anthropometric Assessment of Nutritional Status in the Elderly

WM. CAMERON CHUMLEA
Division of Human Biology, Department of Pediatrics, Wright State University School of Medicine, Dayton, Ohio 45435

INTRODUCTION

Anthropometry is a very significant component in the assessment of an elderly person's nutritional status. The anthropometry in such an assessment provides noninvasive, indirect information about the amounts of subcutaneous adipose tissue and muscle mass in the body and the changes in body size that occur with old age (Clark et al., 1988). In the elderly, rapid changes in the amounts of adipose or muscle tissues or the extreme conditions of obesity or emaciation are significant health concerns (Kemm and Allcock, 1984; Fanelli 1987). Decreases in stature can indicate the possible development of osteoporosis, especially in women (Rossman, 1977). Obesity can occur among some elderly individuals as mobility decreases with old age (Patrick et al., 1982). Obesity places a burden on the locomotive and cardiovascular systems and also affects pulmonary function (Borkan et al., 1986). Emaciation in the elderly is also associated with reduced physical activity, but it increases the risk of morbidity and mortality, due in part to an association with depressed immune function (Mitchell and Lipschitz, 1982b; Fanelli, 1987; Clark et al., 1988). Furthermore, an anthropometric nutritional assessment of an elderly person is important because it can be used to help monitor the effects of nutritional intervention.

To use anthropometry to detect trends in nutritional status indicating the possible development of risk or to monitor the effectiveness of a nutritional intervention requires knowledge of the normal values for body measurements and the normal mean rates of change in those measurements with old age. There are only limited national reference data with which to compare an elderly person's anthropometric nutritional assessment, and only a few studies of nutritional status in the elderly have included anthropometry, direct measures of body composition, or a longitudinal design (Young et al., 1963; Durnin and Womersley, 1974; Friedlander et al., 1977; Steen et al., 1977, 1979; Abraham et al., 1978; Bastow, 1982; Garry et al., 1982; Chumlea et al., 1984b; Fanelli,

1987; Clark et al, 1988; Chumlea et al., 1988). Most such studies are also hampered by the problem of selecting an adequate number of "healthy" elderly persons who have aged "successfully" because of the increased prevalence of degenerative diseases with old age (Exton-Smith, 1982; Rowe and Kahn, 1987). Consequently, many study samples of the elderly are inherently biased and small.

To date, there is limited knowledge of the associations among measures of body size and composition in the elderly and especially for those over 85 years of age. In general, reported associations are not as significant or meaningful in the elderly as those reported for younger adults (Chumlea et al., 1984b). Correlations of triceps, subscapular, or suprailiac skinfolds with total or percent body fat in the elderly are less than corresponding values reported for younger adults (Wessel et al., 1963; Stoudt et al., 1965; Ward et al., 1975; Noppa et al., 1979; Roche et al., 1981), but correlations of waist or abdominal circumference with total body fat are larger than corresponding values in younger adults (Ward et al., 1975; Chumlea et al., 1984b). These differences between young adults and the elderly in corresponding associations among measures of body size and composition reflect the normal physiological effects of aging such as a reduction is stature (Rossman, 1977), or changes with age in the amount and distribution of lean tissue or internal and subcutaneous adipose tissue (Norris et al., 1963; Wessel et al., 1963; Young et al., 1963; Novak, 1972; Durnin and Womersley, 1974; Forbes, 1976; Borkan and Norris, 1977; Fisher et al., 1978). In addition, alterations in tissue elasticity (Grahame, 1970) and compressibility can effect measurement values (Himes et al., 1979).

In an anthropometric nutritional assessment of an elderly person, close attention needs to be given to techniques of collecting body measurements that minimize measurement errors. Improper anthropometric techniques can produce poor estimates of nutritional status or overestimates or underestimates of the effects of nutritional intervention in the elderly. This is because measurement errors for all body measurements are greater in the elderly and more so for circumferences and skinfolds of the trunk than in younger adults (Chumlea et al., 1984a). Greater compressibility and /or poor tissue separation in the elderly can significantly affect the reliability of skinfold measurements (Bowman and Rosenberg, 1982). Common anthropometric techniques can be effective in nutritional assessments of many elderly persons. However, these same measurements become increasingly difficult to collect and are prone to error in older or nonambulatory elderly persons. Common techniques may not be satisfactory at all for those who are nonambulatory or disabled.

A single observer taking replicate body measurements is effective, but two observers, measuring independently, are preferable (Cameron, 1978). It is also important to specify a limit on the acceptable range of intraobserver or interobserver differences and to repeat measurements if these limits are exceeded (Chumlea et al., 1984a). Interobserver differences are reported to exceed preset limits for the first pair of body measurements in 27% of a sample of elderly persons compared to only 19% of a sample of younger adults. In this study, the mean absolute interobserver errors for almost all the anthropometric variables were greater than those for the younger adults. Remeasurement of those for whom the interobserver errors exceeded preset limits reduced the prevalence of large interobserver errors to about 8% in each group (Chumlea et al., 1984a).

For the very old who are chair bound or bedfast due to arthritis, accidents, disease, or surgery, or for those who are unable to stand with the positioning needed to collect standard anthropometry, taking accurate and reliable anthropometric data using standard techniques is difficult. Some measurements, like stature or weight, are clearly inapplicable, or suitable equipment may not be available (Vir and Love, 1980; Bastow, 1982). The nutritional assessment of a nonambulatory elderly person, or of those ambulatory elderly persons who are too frail to stand for an examination, can be improved by the use of recumbent measurements. Recumbent anthropometry collected from nonambulatory elderly persons is as reliable as standing anthropometry. There are no significant systematic differences between paired values for corresponding recumbent and standing measures taken at the exact same body sites and with the recommended methodology (Chumlea et al., 1985c). Recumbent anthropometry can provide reliable nutritional assessments of elderly persons regardless of their levels of mobility (Chumlea et al., 1985b). It may appear easier to measure a nonambulatory elderly person who is confined to a wheelchair while seated. Except for midarm circumference, however, measurements are more reliably collected if the elderly person is removed from the wheelchair and placed in a recumbent position (Chumlea et al., 1985b).

RECOMMENDED ANTHROPOMETRIC ASSESSMENTS FOR THE AMBULATORY ELDERLY

The measurements recommended for an anthropometric nutritional assessment of an ambulatory elderly person are stature, weight, midarm circumference, triceps and subscapular skinfold thicknesses, and calf circumference. Midarm circumference and triceps and subscapular skinfold thicknesses provide measures of subcutaneous adipose tissue thickness on the arm and trunk. Midarm circumference together with triceps skinfold can also be used to compute the cross-sectional area of muscle in the upper arm. Calf circumference is an important measure of the general loss of muscle in response to a reduction in physical activity (Fentem et al., 1976; MacLenman et al., 1980; Patrick et al., 1982). Detailed descriptions of the standard techniques for each of these body measurements are found in the *Anthropometric Standardization Reference Manual* (Lohman et al., 1988). However, there are some particular points applicable to measuring stature and weight in the elderly that are not covered in the manual.

Stature

To measure stature properly, an elderly person should be able to stand upright without assistance with bare heels close together, legs straight, arms at the sides, shoulders relaxed, and wearing minimal clothing so that posture can be seen clearly. Large amounts of adipose tissue on the buttocks in many elderly persons will allow only the heels and buttocks to touch the measuring wall. It is more important that the elderly person stand erect than that all body parts make contact with the wall.

In some elderly persons, particularly women, the spinal column may be so curved that the headboard of the measuring device cannot be positioned on the crown of the head. When stature cannot be measured, knee height, a recumbent measurement, can be used to estimate stature.

Weight

Weight is the most commonly recorded body measurement, and is critical in assessing nutritional status (Butterworth and Blackburn, 1975; Heber, 1986). Weight is a gross measure of the mass of body tissues and fluids, and serial measures of weight can record changes in these body constituents. An increase in weight may indicate developing obesity or edema, while decreases in weight can signify the presence, severity, or progress of disease or a nutritional disorder. Despite the nutritional importance of measuring body weight, it is reported that body weight was not recorded in about 22% of cases of adults receiving nutritional support because the patients were nonambulatory, too ill, or equipment was not available or unreliable (Guenter et al., 1982). Ambulatory elderly persons can be weighed on an upright balance beam scale, but if an elderly person can only sit, a movable wheelchair balance beam scale can be used. Bed scales are available for measuring the weight of bedfast elderly persons.

RECUMBENT ANTHROPOMETRY FOR THE NONAMBULATORY ELDERLY

Five recumbent measurements are recommended for an anthropometric nutritional assessment of a nonambulatory elderly person: knee height, calf circumference, midarm circumference, and triceps and subscapular skinfold thicknesses. This sequence of measurements is also recommended because it reduces the time needed to collect the measurements and limits any discomfort or inconvenience to the subject.

Recumbent measures should be taken from the left side of an elderly person lying on a bed or an examination table with adequate support for the arms and legs. The left side of the body is recommended because this is the side from which the reference data were collected, but measurers should have access to both sides of the body. Measurements can be collected from the right side of the body and compared to reference data because of the absence of significant differences between corresponding measurements taken from opposite sides of the body (Martorell et al., 1988). One should select a side of the body and not change unless necessary because of a broken limb, paralysis, a cast, etc.

Knee Height

Knee height is used to help estimate the stature of an elderly person who cannot stand or who has such spinal curvature that a measurement of stature would be misleading or is not possible. Knee height does not change with age

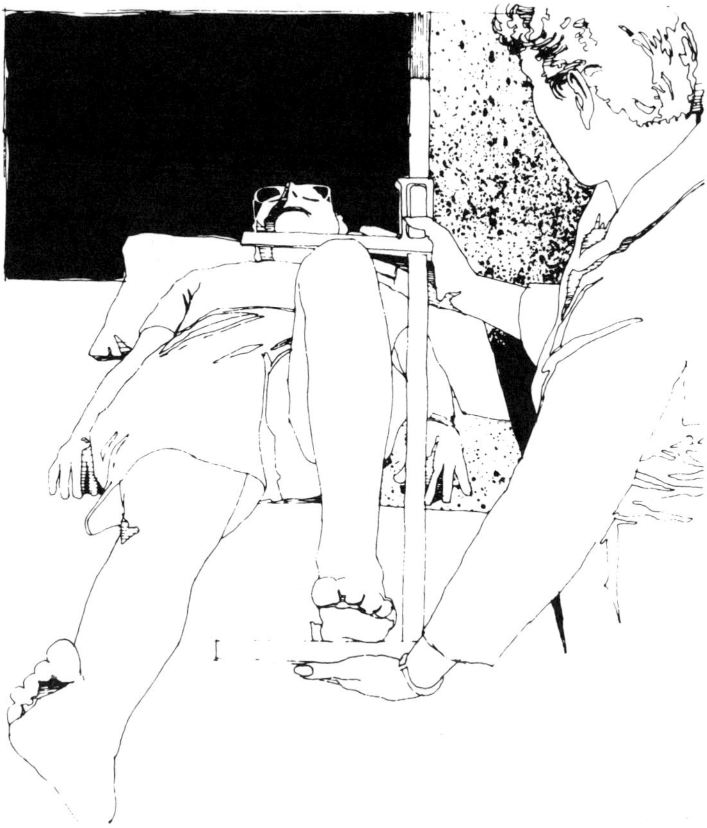

Fig. 1. Position of the Mediform sliding caliper for the measurement of knee height. (Reproduced with permission of Ross Laboratories, Columbus, Ohio 43216, © Ross Laboratories.)

in adults and is highly correlated with stature. Knee height can also be used to compute an estimate of body weight. Equations to estimate stature and body weight from knee height are discussed later.

Knee height is measured accurately and reliably with a specific sliding broad-blade caliper[1] (Chumlea, 1985). The elderly person is positioned supine with the left knee and left ankle each bent to a 90° angle. The shaft of the caliper needs to be placed so that it passes over the lateral malleolus and just posterior to the head of the fibula. It is important that the shaft of the caliper be held parallel to the shaft of the tibia and pressure applied to compress the tissues (Fig. 1).

[1]Caliper available from Medical Express, 5150 S.W. Griffith Dr., Beaverton, OR 97005, 800-633-3676.

Calf Circumference

Calf circumference is measured with the body in the same position as for measuring knee height. The loop of an inelastic tape is used to locate the largest circumference of the calf (Fig. 2). It is important, however, that the tape not be tight around the calf, because that compresses the tissues.

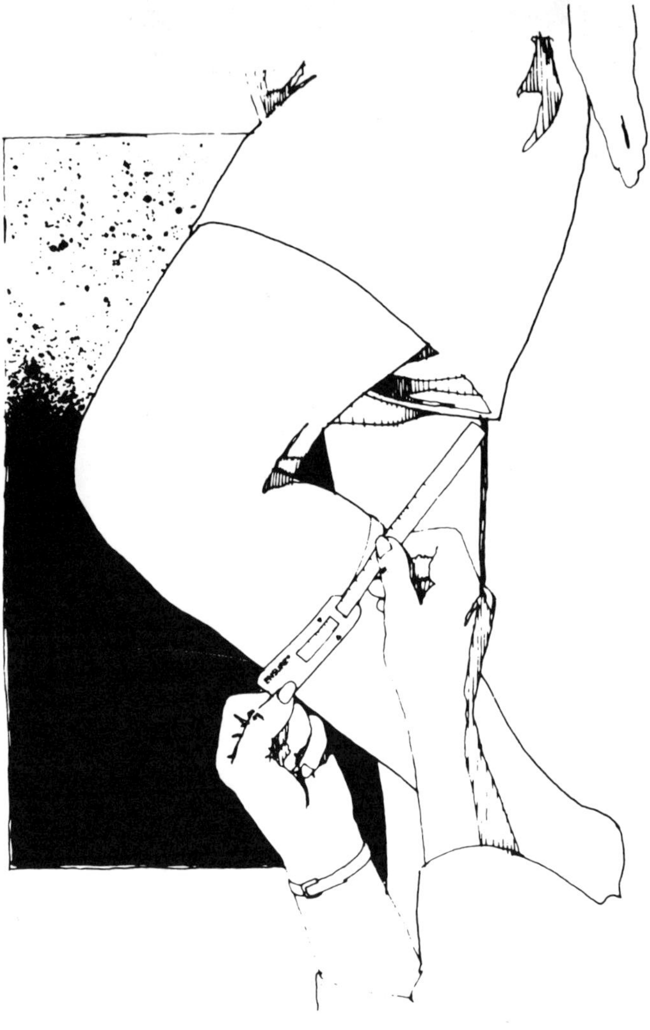

Fig. 2. Measurement of calf circumference. (Reproduced with permission of Ross Laboratories, Columbus, Ohio 43216, © Ross Laboratories.)

Midarm Circumference

The circumference of the upper arm is measured at its midpoint. With the subject supine, the left arm is bent to a 90° angle at the elbow, and the forearm placed palm down across the trunk. The upper arm should be approximately parallel to the trunk. Using an insertion tape[2], the measurer locates and marks the midpoint of the upper arm (Fig. 3).

It is important that the left arm then be extended alongside the supine body, with the palm facing up, and the arm raised slightly off the surface of the bed or examination table by placing a sandbag or towel under the elbow (Fig. 4). Again, the tape is pulled just snug around the arm, but *not* so tight that the tissues are compressed.

Triceps Skinfold Thickness

This measurement and subscapular skinfold thickness are taken with the elderly person lying on the right side, with the right arm extending from the front of the body. The trunk should be in a straight line, and the legs bent and tucked up slightly. The left arm rests along the trunk, palm down (Fig. 5). An imaginary line through the acromion processes should be perpendicular to the bed. There are a variety of skinfold calipers available for measuring subcutaneous adipose tissue thickness, and a listing of these can be found in the *Anthropometric Standardization Reference Manual* (Lohman et al., 1988). For spring-loaded skinfold calipers, readings should be taken at about three seconds, but in some elderly persons the skinfold caliper may take longer to stabilize, particularly if the tissue is edematous.

The triceps skinfold thickness measurement is taken on the back of the left arm over the triceps muscle, at the level marked as the midpoint for the circumference measurement. Values of repeated triceps skinfold thickness measurements can vary markedly if they are made at different sites.

It is important that the measurer gently grasps a double fold of skin and subcutaneous adipose tissue between the fingers and thumb and that the fold of skin be on the back of the arm, in the midline and parallel to the long axis of the upper arm (Fig. 6). In order to avoid errors due to parallax, the measurer should bend down to read the caliper.

Subscapular Skinfold Thickness

This measurement is also taken with the elderly person in the same body position as for measuring the triceps skinfold. The subscapular skinfold thickness is measured just posterior to the inferior angle of the left scapula. Again, the measurer gently grasps a double fold of skin and subcutaneous adipose tissue between the fingers and thumb, on a line from the inferior angle of the left scapula to the left elbow (Fig. 7).

[2]Insertion tapes available from Ross Laboratories, 625 Cleveland Avenue, Columbus, OH 43215, 614-227-3333.

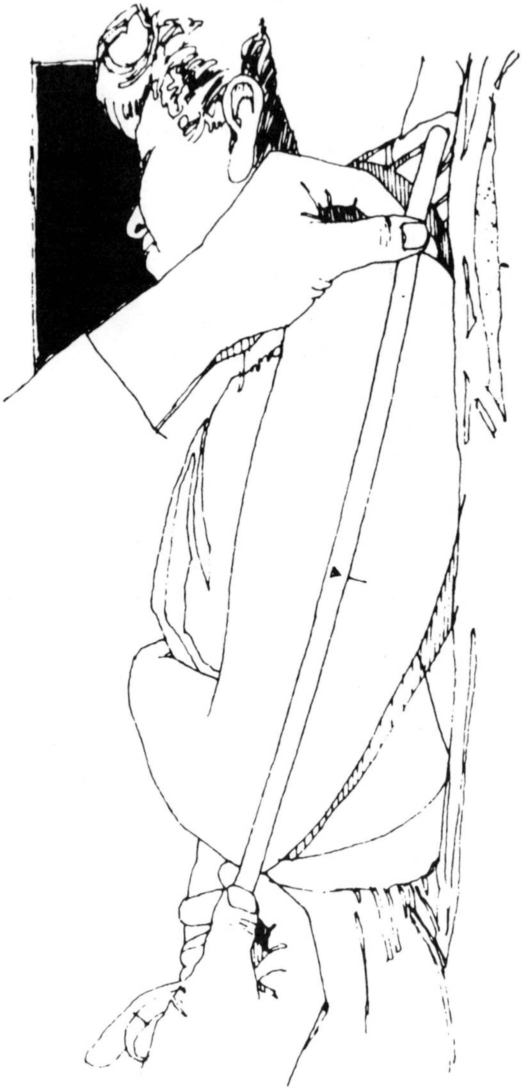

Fig. 3. Locating the midpoint of the upper arm with an insertion tape. (Reproduced with permission of Ross Laboratories, Columbus, Ohio 43216, © Ross Laboratories.)

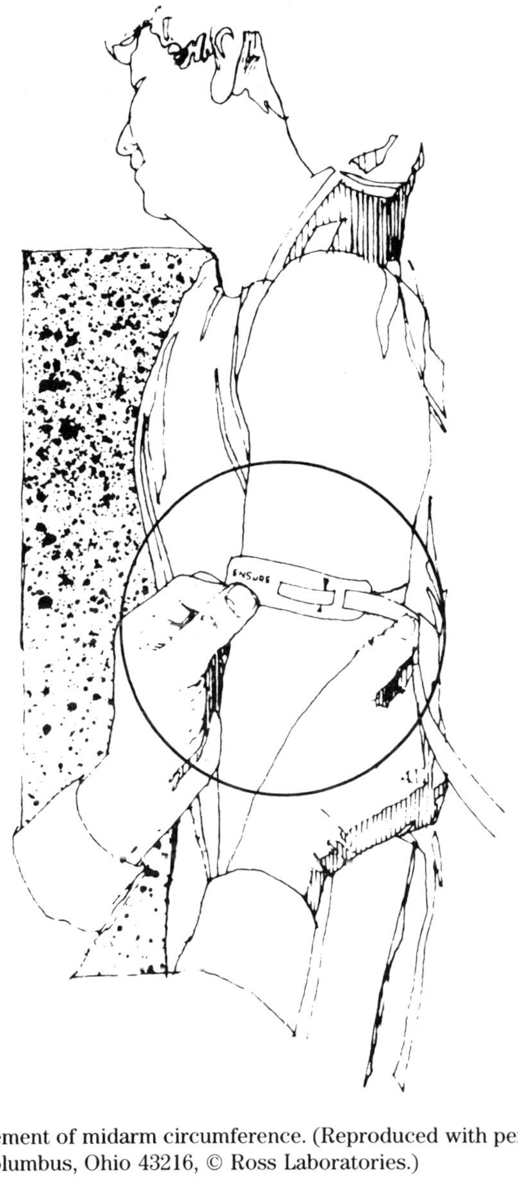

Fig. 4. Measurement of midarm circumference. (Reproduced with permission of Ross Laboratories, Columbus, Ohio 43216, © Ross Laboratories.)

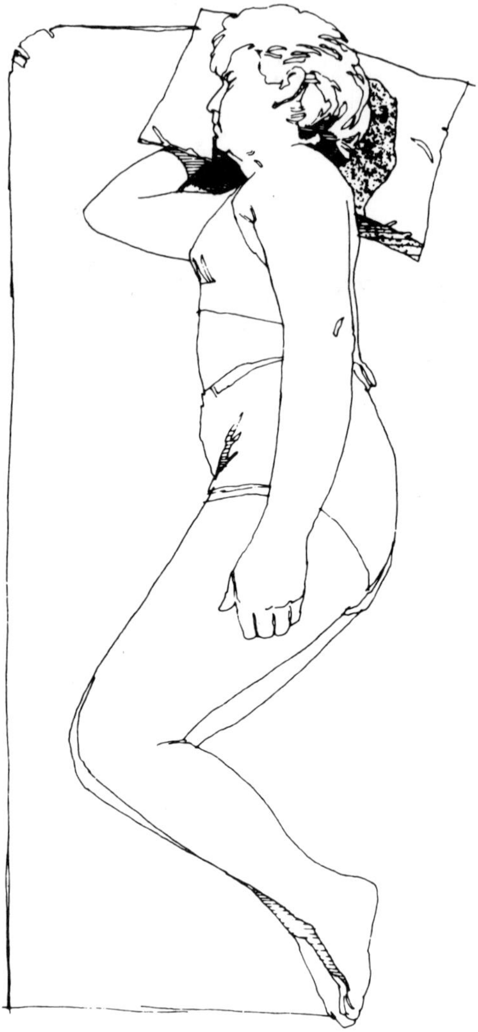

Fig. 5. Position of the body for triceps and subscapular skinfold measurements. (Reproduced with permission of Ross Laboratories, Columbus, Ohio 43216, © Ross Laboratories.)

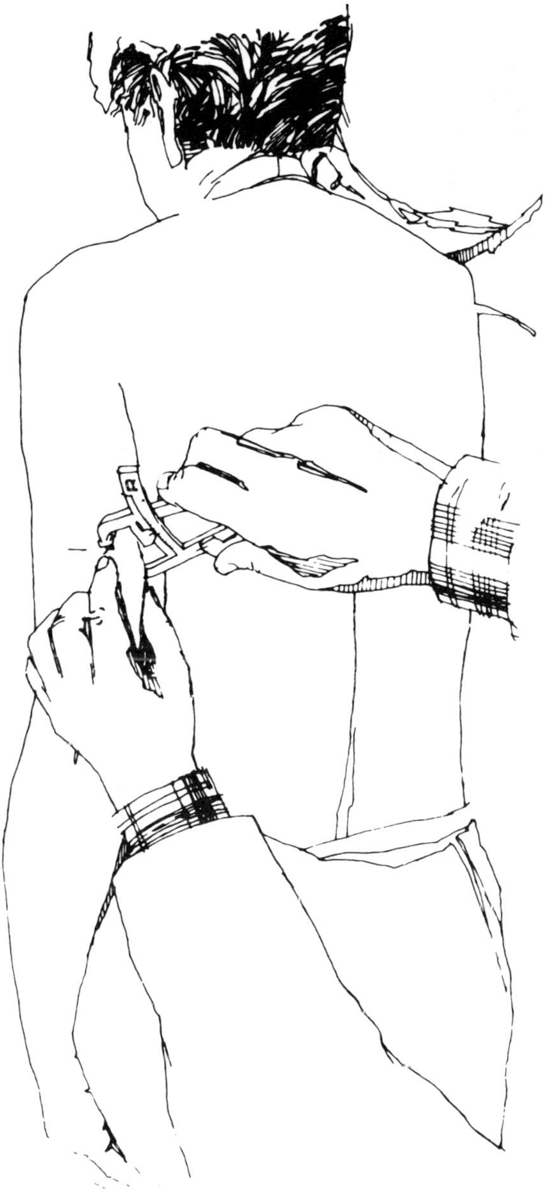

Fig. 6. Measuring the triceps skinfold. (Reproduced with permission of Ross Laboratories, Columbus, Ohio 43216, © Ross Laboratories.)

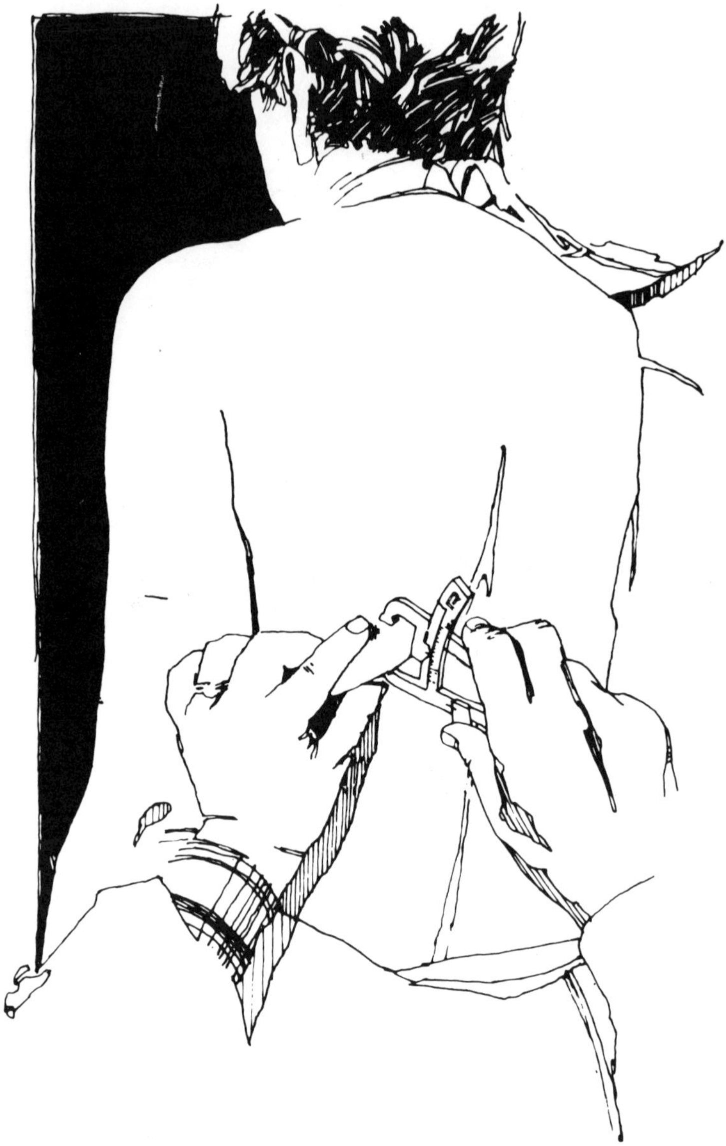

Fig. 7. Measuring the subscapular skinfold. (Reproduced with permission of Ross Laboratories, Columbus, Ohio 43216, © Ross Laboratories.)

ANTHROPOMETRIC INDICES OF NUTRITIONAL STATUS IN THE ELDERLY

The recommended body measurements can be used to derive additional quantitative values or indices that are useful in assessing the nutritional status of an elderly person. Estimates of stature and body weight can be computed if they cannot be measured. An index of obesity can be derived by dividing weight by stature squared (W/S^2), and midarm muscle area can be calculated also.

Stature From Knee Height

The knee height measurement is used to estimate the stature of an elderly person who is bedfast or chair bound or one who has such spinal curvature that an accurate stature measurement cannot be obtained. The estimated stature can then be used in indexes such as W/S^2 or in estimates of basal energy expenditure (Harris and Benedict, 1919; Benedict, 1928; Boothby et al., 1936; Dubois, 1936; Blackburn et al., 1977; Long et al., 1979).

Arm span has been proposed as a substitute for a measure of stature because it is highly correlated with stature and changes little with age (Brown and Wigzell, 1963; Dequeker et al., 1969). However, arm span is not recommended because it is too difficult to measure reliably in nonambulatory elderly persons or in those with significant chest of spinal deformities (Mitchell and Lipschitz, 1982b). Total arm length has also been proposed as a substitute for stature (Mitchell and Lipschitz, 1982a), but knee height is the preferred measurement. Knee height is a component of stature, and it is more highly correlated with stature than total arm length or other arm length measurements (Zoreb et al., 1963). Also, the interobserver reliability for knee height is better than that for arm length measurements (Chumlea et al., 1985a).

To estimate stature requires the elderly person's knee height, age, and sex. The knee height measurement is in centimeters, age is rounded to the nearest whole year, and the computed value of stature is in centimeters.

$$\text{Stature for men} = (2.02 \times \text{knee height}) - (0.04 \times \text{age}) + 64.19$$
$$\text{Stature for women} = (1.83 \times \text{knee height}) - (0.24 \times \text{age}) + 84.88$$

The 90% error bounds for estimates of stature are about 6.0 cm for both men and women. These estimation equations were developed from a sample not nationally representative of elderly persons in the Unites States, so caution is indicated if they are applied to other groups of elderly persons (Chumlea et al., 1985a).

Weight From Anthropometry

When the weight of an elderly person cannot be measured because of infirmity or fractures requiring traction or a cast, it can be estimated from anthropometric data. The necessary measurements are calf circumference (Calf C), knee height (knee H), midarm circumference (MAC), and subscapular skinfold thickness (Subsc SF). Most of these body measurements are in common clinical use, are indices of the actual constituents of body composition, and are important in assessing anthropometric nutritional status in the elderly (Blackburn et al., 1977; Chumlea et al., 1985a, 1985c, 1986; Lohman et al., 1988). Estimates of weight for an elderly person can also be used in indexes such as W/S^2 or in calculations of energy expenditure using the Harris-Benedict equation (1919). There are separate equations for men and women.

$$\text{Body weight for men} = (.098 \times \text{Calf C}) + (1.16 \times \text{Knee H}) + (1.72 \times \text{MAC}) + (0.37 \times \text{Subsc SF}) - 81.69$$

$$\text{Body weight for women} = (1.27 \times \text{Calf C}) + (0.87 \times \text{Knee H}) + (0.98 \times \text{MAC}) + (0.4 \times \text{Subsc SF}) - 62.35$$

These equations have a 95% probability of estimating the weight of an elderly man or woman to within plus or minus 8.96 kg or 7.60 kg, respectively (Chumlea et al., 1988). Besides the equations presented here, there are two equations for estimating the weight of elderly persons that use only two or three body measurements. This allows the selection of an equation to estimate weight based upon those measurements that actually can be collected from an elderly person. However, the errors of prediction are larger with the use of less than four predictor variables or if insufficient attention is given to measurement technique (Chumlea et al., 1988).

Weight Divided by Stature Squared

Weight divided by stature squared (W/S^2), an index of obesity, is the best simple indicator of total body fat and an excellent indicator of the amount of body fat expressed as a percentage of body weight (Roche et al., 1981). A person with a high W/S^2 value has a greater probability of having more body fat than a person with a relatively low W/S^2 value. For some elderly persons, W/S^2 may not be completely useful because of decreases in stature with age (Dequeker et al., 1969), and because associations between weight and present stature are problematic depending upon the degree of spinal curvature. Stature can be a measure of questionable value in some elderly persons or impossible to measure in others, but since stature can be estimated reliably from knee height and age (Chumlea et al., 1985a), W/S^2 should be considered an index of obesity in the elderly. The complete interpretation of the importance of W/S^2 in the elderly is uncertain until associations between W/S^2 and body fatness from densitometry have been determined in large representative samples.

Midarm Muscle Area

Midarm muscle area (MAMA) is an index of the amount of muscle or lean tissue in the body. Midarm muscle area is computed using measurements of midarm circumference and triceps skinfold in the following formula:

$$\text{Midarm muscle area (cm}^2) = \frac{\text{Midarm circumference (cm)} - \Pi \times \dfrac{\text{Triceps}^2 \text{ Skinfold (mm)}}{10}}{4\,\Pi}$$

This formula can be used with recumbent measurements of midarm circumference and triceps skinfold because of the absence of significant systematic differences between corresponding standing and recumbent measurements (Chumlea et al., 1985b). This formula does produce an overestimated MAMA when compared to actual values from computerized tomographic cross-sections at the midpoint of the upper arm in young adults, and Heymsfield and associates (1979, 1982) recommend the use of corrected formulae for estimating MAMA. However, these corrected formulae have not been validated in the elderly (Heymsfield, et al., 1982).

REFERENCE DATA FOR THE ELDERLY

Anthropometric nutritional assessment data and indices of W/S^2 and MAMA can help to identify those elderly persons who may be at nutritional risk for obesity or who have inadequate protein reserves. Such data are more informative and understandable if they are plotted on reference charts for the elderly. A complete anthropometric nutritional assessment record for an elderly person consists of a combination of tabulated and plotted measurements. Assessment data should be recorded on the appropriate chart, along with any information relevant to measurement problems or the techniques used (Chumlea et al., 1987; Fig. 8). The charts simplify the comparison of current data with previous data.

Anthropometric nutritional assessment reference charts are used to plot an elderly person's anthropometric values by year between ages 65 and 90 years. Plotting the data facilitates communication with the elderly individual about nutritional status, possible intervention, and follow-up. Plotting serial nutritional anthropometric assessment values can also reveal an abnormal change that warrants further evaluation (Chumlea et al., 1987). If values appear unusual compared to earlier ones or compared to the reference data, the elderly person should be remeasured to verify the current results. An actual change in an anthropometric value can signal a potential shift in nutritional status. Such a change would have been missed if earlier measurements had not been plotted for comparison. Unusual values and/or patterns of change in nutritional anthropometry are useful in identifying, as early as possible, those elderly persons who need diagnostic tests and nutritional intervention. Serial assessment can also help monitor the effectiveness of nutritional intervention.

The anthropometric nutritional assessment of an elderly person ought to be compared with an appropriate reference sample similar to the population to which the person belongs. Such comparisons may be misleading if the indi-

Weight

Table 2. Percentiles for Weight in kg (and lb)

Men				Women			
Age (years)	95%	50%	5%	Age (years)	95%	50%	5%
65	102.0 (224.9)	79.5 (175.0)	62.6 (138.0)	**65**	87.1 (192.0)	66.8 (147.3)	51.2 (112.9)
70	99.1 (218.5)	76.5 (168.7)	59.7 (131.6)	**70**	84.9 (187.2)	64.6 (142.4)	49.0 (108.0)
75	96.3 (212.3)	73.6 (162.3)	56.8 (125.2)	**75**	82.8 (182.5)	62.4 (137.6)	46.8 (103.2)
80	93.4 (205.9)	70.7 (155.9)	53.9 (118.8)	**80**	80.6 (177.7)	60.2 (132.7)	44.7 (98.5)
85	90.5 (199.5)	67.8 (149.5)	51.0 (112.4)	**85**	78.4 (172.8)	58.0 (127.9)	42.5 (93.7)
90	87.6 (193.1)	64.9 (142.8)	48.1 (106.0)	**90**	76.2 (168.0)	55.9 (123.2)	40.3 (88.8)

Fig 16. Percentiles for weight of elderly men.

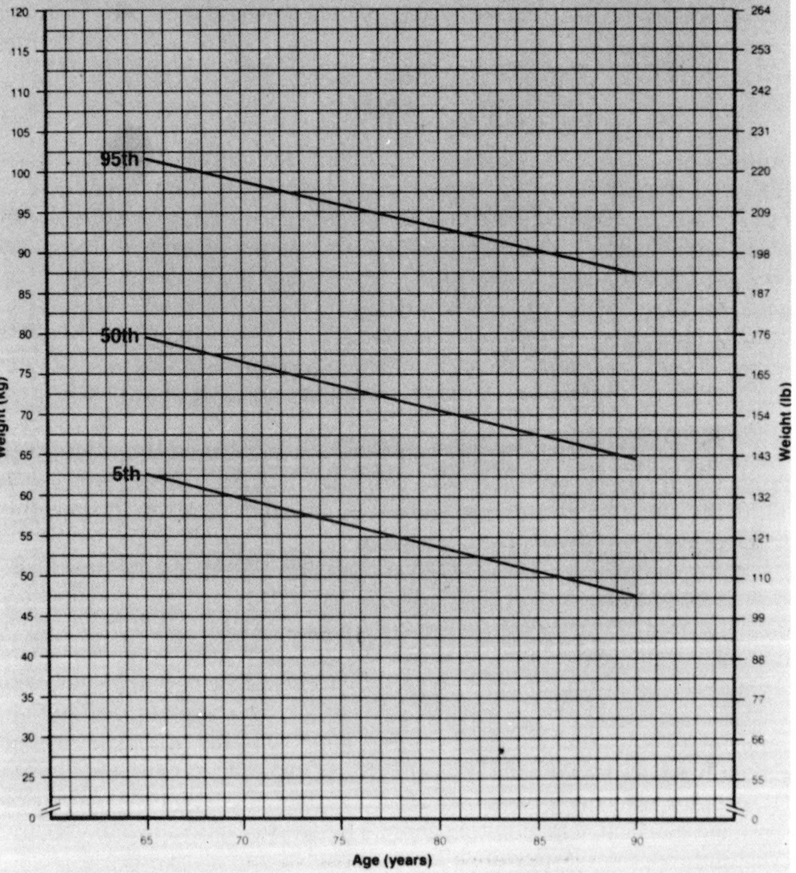

Fig. 8. Charts for plotting anthropometric data for elderly man. (Reproduced with permission of Ross Laboratories, Columbus, Ohio 43216 © Ross Laboratories.)

vidual belongs to a group different from the reference sample. The limited reference data in the recommended charts were derived from a sample of 269 elderly white persons who were not unusual in body size. At corresponding ages, the anthropometric data for these elderly persons do not differ significantly from those reported by the National Center for Health Statistics (Abraham et al., 1978; Chumlea et al., 1985c). Similar national reference data for a representative sample of persons aged 75 years and older are lacking, and the only reference data for recumbent anthropometry are the examples reported here (Chumlea et al., 1985c, 1987). It is not known whether this set of nutritional anthropometric assessment charts can be used for elderly blacks or Hispanics in the United States (Chumlea et al., 1987). This is because differences exist among younger black, white, and Hispanic American adults in distributions of triceps and subscapular skinfolds and in the W/S^2 index (Cronk and Roche, 1982; Malina et al., 1983). The anthropometric assessment techniques, indices, and limited reference data presented here, when combined with the other components of a nutritional assessment, can provide a very good picture of the nutritional status or change in nutritional status for an elderly person regardless of his of her level of mobility. Although these reference data are not completely applicable to black and Hispanic elderly persons, they can be used effectively to monitor changes in the nutritional status of elderly persons, regardless of race.

ACKNOWLEDGEMENTS

This research was supported by Grant HD-12252 from the National Institutes of Health, Bethesda, Maryland, and by Ross Laboratories, Columbus, Ohio.

REFERENCES

Abraham S, Johnson CL, Najjar MF (1978): Weight and height of adults 18–74 years of age. Vital and Health Statistics Ser. 11 No. 211. Rockville, Md: DHEW Publication No. (PHS) 79-165.

Bastow MD (1982): Anthropometrics revisited. Proc Nutr Soc 41:381–388.

Benedict FG (1928): Basal metabolism data on normal men and women (Series II) with some considerations of the use of prediction standards. AM J Physiol 85:607–613.

Blackburn GL, Bristrian BR, Maini BS, Schlamm HT, Smith MF (1977): Nutritional and metabolic assessment of the hospitalized patient. J Parenter Enteral Nutr 1:11–22.

Boothby WM, Berkson SR, Dunn HL (1936): Studies of the energy metabolism of normal individuals: A standard for basal metabolism with nomogram for clinical application. Am J Physiol 116:468–473.

Borkan GA, Norris AH (1977): Fat distributions and the changing body dimensions of the adult male. Hum Biol 49:495–514.

Borkan GA, Sparrow D, Wisniewski C, Vokonos PS (1986): Body weight and coronary disease risk: Patterns of risk factor change associated with long-term weight change. Am J Epidemiol 124:410–419.

Bowman BB, Rosenberg IH (1982): Assessment of the nutritional status of the elderly. Am J Clin Nutr 35:1142–1151.

Brown OT, Wigzell FW (1963): The significance of span as a clinical measurement. "Current Achievements in Gariatrics." Conference on Medical and Surgical Aspects of Aging. London: Cassell, pp 246–251.

Butterworth CE, Blackburn GL (1975): Hospital malnutrition. Nutr Today 10:8–18.

Cameron N (1978): The methods of auxological anthropometry. In Falkner F, Tanner JM (eds): "Human Growth. Vol 2, Postnatal Growth." New York: Plenum Press, pp 35–90.

Chumlea WC (1985): Accuracy and reliability of a new sliding caliper. Am J Phys Anthropol 68:425–427.

Chumlea WC, Garry PJ, Hunt WC, Rhyne RL (1988): Distribution of serial changes in stature and weight in a healthy elderly population. Hum Biol 60:917–925.

Chumlea WC, Guo S, Roche AF, Steinbaugh ML (1988): Prediction of body weight for the nonambulatory elderly. J Am Diet Assoc 88:564–588.

Chumlea WC, Roche AF, Mukherjee D (1986): Some anthropometric indices of body composition for elderly adults. J Gerontol 41:36–39.

Chumlea WC, Roche AF, Mukherjee D (1987): "Nutritional Assessment in the Elderly Through Anthropometry." Columbus, Ohio: Ross Laboratories.

Chumlea WC, Roche AF, Rogers E (1984a): Replicability for anthropometry in the elderly. Hum Biol 56:329–337.

Chumlea WC, Roche AF, Steinbaugh ML (1985a): Estimating stature from knee height for persons 60 to 90 years of age. J Am Geriatr Soc 33:116–120.

Chumlea WC, Roche AF, Steinbaugh ML, Mukherjee D (1985b): Errors of measurement for methods of recumbent nutritional anthropometry in the elderly. J Nutr Elderly 5:3–11.

Chumlea WC, Roche AF, Webb P (1984b): Body size, subcutaneous fatness and total body fat in older adults. Int J Obes 8:313–317.

Chumlea WC, Steinbaugh ML, Roche AF, Mukherjee D, Gopalaswamy N (1985c): Nutritional anthropometric assessment in elderly persons 65 to 90 years of age. J Nutr Elderly 4:39–51.

Clark GC, Rappaport JI, DiScala C, Lamothe DA, Blackburn GL (1988): Nutritional support of the chronically ill elderly female at risk for elective or urgent surgery. J Am Coll Nutr 7:17–26.

Cronk CE, Roche AF (1982): Race- and sex-specific reference data for triceps and subscapular skinfolds and weight/stature^2. Am J Clin Nutr 35:347–354.

Dequeker JV, Baeyers JB, Claessens J (1969): The significance of stature as a clinical measurement of aging. J Am Geriatr Soc 17:169–179.

Dubois EF (1936): "Basal Metabolism in Health and Disease." 3rd ed. Philadelphia: Lea & Febiger.

Durnin JVGA, Womersley J (1974): Body fat assessed from total body density and its estimation from skinfold thickness: Measurements on 481 men and women aged from 16 to 72 years. Br J Nutr 32:77–97.

Exton-Smith AN (1982): Epidemiological studies in the elderly: Methodological considerations. Am J Clin Nutr 35:1273–1279.

Fanelli MT (1987): The ABC's of nutritional assessment in older adults. J Nutr Elderly 6:33–40.

Fentem PH, Jones PRM, MacDonald IC, Scriven PM (1976): Changes in the body composition of elderly men following retirement from the steel industry. J Physiol 258:29P–30P.

Fisher S, Hendricks DG, Mahoney AW (1978): Nutritional assessments of senior rural Utahans by biochemical and physical measurements. Am J Cliin Nutr 31:667–672.

Forbes GB (1976): The adult decline in lean body mass. Hum Biol 48:161–173.

Friedlander JS, Costa PT, Bosse R, Ellis E, Rhoado JG, Stoudt HW (1977): Longitudinal physique changes among healthy white veterans at Boston. Hum Biol 48:541–558.

Garry PJ, Goodwin JS, Hunt WC, Hooper EM, Leonard AG (1982): Nutritional status in a healthy elderly population: Dietary and supplemental intakes. Am J Clin Nutr 36:319–331.

Grahame R (1970): A method for measuring human skin elasticity in vivo with observations on the effects of age, sex and pregnancy. Clin Sci 39:223–238.

Guenter PA, Moore K, Crosby LO, Buzby GP, Mullen JL (1982): Body weight measurement of patients receiving nutritional support. J Parenter Enteral Nutr 6:441–443.

Harris JA, Benedict FG (1919): "A Biometric Study of Basal Metabolism in Man." Washington, DC: Carnegie Institute of Washington.

Heber D (1986): Assessing nutritional status of the elderly. Diagnosis 8:41–62.

Heymsfield SB, McManus C, Smith J, Stevens V, Nixon DW (1982): Athropometric measurement of muscle mass: Revised equations for calculating bone-free arm muscle area. Am J Clin Nutr 36:680–690.

Heymsfield SB, Olalson RP, Kutner MH, Nixon DW (1979): A radiographic method of quantifying protein-caloric malnutrition. Am J Clin Nutr 32:693–702.

Himes JH, Roche AF, Siervogel RM (1979): Compressibility of skinfolds and the measurement of subcutaneous fatness. Am J Clin Nutr 32:1734–1740.

Kemm JR, Allcock J (1984): The distribution of supposed indicators of nutritional status in elderly patients. Age Aging 13:21–28.

Lohman T, Martorell R, Roche AF (1988): "Anthropometric Standardization Reference Manual." Champaign, Ill Human Kinetics.

Long CL, Schaffel N, Gieger JW (1979): Metabolic response to injury and illness: Estimation of energy and protein needs from indirect calorimetry and nitrogen balance. J Parenter Enteral Nutr 3:452–456.

MacLenman WJ, Hall MRP, Timothy JI, Robinson M (1980): Is weakness in old age due to muscle wasting? Age Aging 9:188–192.

Malina RM, Little BB, Stern MP, Gaskill SP, Hazuda HP (1983): Ethnic and social class differences in selected anthropometric characteristics of Mexican American and Anglo adults: The San Antonio heart study. Hum Biol 55:867–883.

Martorell R, Mendoza F, Mueller WH, Pauson IG (1988): Which side to measure: Right or left. In Lohman TG, Roche AF, Martorell R (eds): "Anthropometric Standarization Reference Manual." Champaign, Ill: Human Kinetics, pp 87–92.

Mitchell CO, Lipschitz DA (1982a): Arm length measurement as an alternative to height in nutritional assessments of the elderly. J Parenter Enteral Nutr 6:226–229.

Mitchell CO, Lipschitz DA (1982b): Detection of protein caloric malnutrition in the elderly. Am J Clin Nutr 35:398–406.

Noppa H, Anderson M, Bengtsson C, Bruce A, Isaksson B (1979): Body composition in middle-aged women with special reference in the correlation between body fat mass and anthropometric data. Am J Clin Nutr 32:1388–1395.

Norris AH, Lundy T, Shock NW (1963): Trends in selected indices of body composition in men between the ages 30 and 90 years. Ann NY Acad Sci 110:623–639.

Novak LP (1972): Aging, total body potassium, fat-free mass and cell mass in males and females between ages 18 and 85 years. J Gerontol 27:438–443.

Patrick JM, Baasey EJ, Fentem PH (1982): Changes in body fat and muscle in manual workers at the retirement. Eur J Appl Physiol 49:187–196.

Roche AF, Siervogel RM, Chumlea WC, Webb P (1981): Grading body fatness from limited anthropometric data. Am J Clin Nutr 34:2831–2838.

Rossman I (1977): Anatomic and body composition changes with aging. In Finch CE, Hayflick L (eds): "Handbook of the Biology of Aging." New York: Van Nostrand, pp 189–221.

Rowe JW, Kahn RL (1987): Human Aging: Usual and successful. Science 237:143–149.

Steen B, Bruce A, Isaksson B, Levin T, Ivanborg A (1977): Body composition in 70-year-old males and females in Gothenburg, Sweden—a population study. Acta Med Scand 611 (suppl):87–112.

Steen GB, Isaksson B, Svanberg A (1979): Body composition at 70 and 75 years of age. A longitudinal population study. J Clin Exp Gerontol 1:185–200.

Stoudt HW, Damon A, McFarland RA, Roberts J (1965): Weight, height and selected body dimesions of adults. "Vital and Health Statistics series II, No.8." Rockville, Md: DHEW Publication No. (PHS) 1000.

Vir SC, Love AHG (1980): Anthropometric measurements in the elderly. Gerontology 26:1–8.

Ward GM, Krzywicki HJ, Rahman DP, Quaas RL, Nelson RA, Consolazio CF (1975): Relationship of anthropometric measurements to body fat as determined by densitometry, potassium-40, and body water. Am J Clin Nutr 28:162–169.

Wessel JA, Ufer A, Van Huss WD, Cederquist D (1963): Age trends of various components of body composition and functional characteristics in women 29–69year. Ann NY Acad Sci 110:608–622.

Young CM, Blondin J, Tensuan R, Fryer JH (1963): Body composition studies of "older" women thirty to seventy years of age. Ann NY Acad Sci 110:589–607.

Zoreb PA, Prime FJ, Harrison A (1963): Estimation of height from tibial length. Lancet 1:195–196.

Index